Recent Results in Cancer Research

96

Adjuvant Chemotherapy of Breast Cancer

Edited by H.-J. Senn

With 98 Figures and 91 Tables

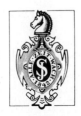

Springer-Verlag
Berlin Heidelberg New York Tokyo 1984

Papers presented at the 2nd International Conference
on Adjuvant Chemotherapy of Breast Cancer,
Kantonsspital St. Gallen, Switzerland, March 1−3, 1984.

Professor Dr. Hans-Jörg Senn
Kantonsspital St. Gallen
Medizinische Klinik C
CH-9007 St. Gallen, Switzerland

Sponsored by the Swiss League against Cancer

ISBN 3-540-13738-6 Springer-Verlag Berlin Heidelberg New York Tokyo
ISBN 0-387-13738-6 Springer-Verlag New York Heidelberg Berlin Tokyo

Library of Congress Cataloging in Puplication Data. Main entry under title: International
Conference on Adjuvant Chemotherapy of Breast Cancer (2nd: 1984: Saint Gall, Switzer-
land) Adjuvant chemotherapy of breast cancer. (Recent results in cancer research; 96)
"Papers presented at the 2nd International Conference on Adjuvant Chemotherapy of Breast
Cancer, Kantonsspital St. Gallen, Switzerland, March 1−3, 1984, sponsored by the Swiss
League against Cancer" − T.p. verso. Includes bibliographies and index. 1. Breast-Can-
cer-Adjuvant treatment-Congresses. 2. Breast-Cancer-Chemotherapy-Congresses. I. Senn,
Hansjörg. II. Schweizerische Nationalliga für Krebsbekämpfung und Krebsforschung.
III. Title. IV. Series: Recent results in cancer research; v. 96. [DNLM: 1. Adjuvants,
Immunologic-therapeutic use-congresses. 2. Adjuvants, Pharmaceutic-therapeutic use-con-
gresses. 3. Breast Neoplasms-drug therapy-congresses. W1 RE106P v. 96 / WZ 267 I45
1984a] RC261.R35 vol. 96 616.99′4s [616.99′449061] 84-20206 [RC280.B8]

Typesetting and printing: v. Starck'sche Druckereigesellschaft m.b.H., Wiesbaden
Binding: J. Schäffer OHG, Grünstadt
2125/3140−5 4 3 2 1 0

Contents

List of Contributors*

Alberto, P.   175[1]
Amgwerd, R.   90
Amman, J.   90
Andersen, K. W.   117
Baral, E.   197
Barrelet, L.   175
Beling, U.   197
Bigler, R.   90
Blumenschein, G. R.
   129, 141
Bonadonna, G.
   34, 66, 178, 188
Brambilla, C.   178
Brincker, H.   117
Brooks, R. J.   133
Brunner, K. W.   175, 224
Bulbrook, R. D.   74
Bush, H.   74
Buzdar, A. U.   129, 141
Carbone, P. P.   218
Carstensen, J.   197
Cavalli, F.   175
Chaudary, M.   74
Creux, G.   90
Crowther, D.   74
Dykes, D. J.   1
Enderlin, F.   90
Engelhart, G.   90
Fentiman, I. S.   74
Fischerman, K.   117

Fisher, B.   8, 55
Fisher, E. R.   55
Foulkes, M.   166
Friberg, S.   197
Garewal, H. S.   133
Gelber, R. D.   102
George, W. D.   74
Giordano, G. F.   133
Glas, U.   197
Glucksberg, H.   166
Goldhirsch, A.   204
Gray, R.   110
Griswold, D. P.   1, 46
Hartmann, W. H.   30
Hayward, J. L.   74
Heinz, C.   90
Heusinkveld, R. S.   133
Hochuli, E.   90
Holdener, E. E.   188
Hortobagyi, G. N.   129, 141
Høst, H.   48
Howat, J. M. T.   74
Howell, A.   74, 188
Huh, N.   18
Jackson, R.   133
Jones, S. E.   133, 148, 188
Jungi, W. F.   90, 175
Kaigas, M.   197
Kemmer, S. R.   133
Ketchel, S. J.   133

---

* The address of the principal author is given on the first page of each
   contribution
1 Page on which contribution begins

Introduction

H.-J. Senn

Adjuvant Chemotherapy (ACT) of breast cancer has now emerged as one of the controversial subjects in clinical and also experimental oncology.

Driven by growing frustration about stagnating cure rates in breast cancer [1, 4] and stimulated by elegant demonstration of highly curative effects of adjuvant systemic therapy in animal models [6, 11] and in several childhood neoplasias [15], researchers introduced ACT to the primary treatment of breast cancer with great hope some 15 years ago. After a first wave of isolated "historic" trials with generally limited but in one case remarkable success [5, 9], a second generation of ACT studies was initiated by NSABP investigators and oncology centers in Europe [2, 6, 13]. These trials were well conducted statistically and diagnostically, and all in the early 1970s included a surgical control arm.

Early and intermediate beneficial effects on relapse-free survival (RFS) after 2–3 years median observation time then prompted a whole series of ACT studies in breast cancer. These "third-gener-ation" studies usually regarded some positive influence of ACT as a given fact, dropping surgical control regimens and comparing different ACT regimens, hopefully in a prospective, randomized way

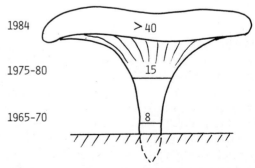

Fig. 1. The mushrooming of adjuvant studies in breast cancer

[reviews in 3, 14]. The "mushrooming" of ACT studies in breast cancer during the last 10 and especially 5 years is demonstrated in Fig. 1, and it gets really cumbersome even for the insider to keep on top of the multitude of sometimes conflicting data.

Since early optimistic therapeutic expectations [8] were met only in part [2, 6, 14], more or less scientifically qualified critique arose against the present concept of ACT in breast cancer, sometimes even questioning the experimental basis of this therapeutic approach in man [7, 10, 12]. Benefical effects of ACT in human breast cancer could − with a few exeptions − be seen only in certain patient subpopulations, which, moreover, varied from study to study with different ACT regimens. The interpretation of results became increasingly difficult and their long-expected translation into clinical practice nearly impossible [3, 14]. As a consequence of this unforeseen complication of the clinical research in ACT of breast cancer, there is growing confusion among investigators, physicians, and surgeons and also among the public. It is interesting to see (at least in the German-speaking world) that the same public media which 6−8 years ago critized the medical research community heavily for "unethically withholding new curative treatment from women after mastectomy for breast cancer" now condemn cancer researchers for their "unethical and unnecessary exposing of patients to unsuccessful and harmful drugs".

It seemed therefore most appropriate to again bring leading specialists and spokesmen from major study groups and centers together for an international working conference, which we called the "Second International Conference on Adjuvant Chemotherapy in Breast Cancer". We are fully aware of the fact that there are many such meetings going on all over the world, and we have many times participated in them as moderators and speakers. However, although some outstanding experts are usually involved, we felt the definite need to gather them *all* together and to organize a complete and critical discussion of the present merits and limitations of ACT in operable breast cancer in the light of nearly 20 years experience. We have done so in the place where 10 years ago the first Swiss adjuvant breast cancer trial (the OSAKO trial 06/74) was initiated. In addition, 6 years have passed since in March 1978 we gathered around 60 oncologists from eight leading groups and centers at the skiing resort of Wildhaus near St. Gallen to discuss evolving problems of ACT in breast cancer. Important years have now gone by, and over 20 groups are engaged worldwide in currently more than 40 trials. For this reason we welcomed for this second working conference more than 250 medical oncologists, surgeons, gynecologists, pathologists, and basic researchers to present and discuss their most recent data. It is our hope that the proceedings of this unique conference on a critical topic in present-day oncology will constitute a helpful basis in the search for more appropriate curative treatment in breast cancer, the most prevalent type of cancer in the female population.

References

1. Baum M (1976) The curability of breast cancer. Br Med J i: 439
2. Bonadonna G, Valagussa P, Rossi A, et al. (1978) Are surgical adjuvant trials going to alter the course of breast cancer? Semin Oncol 5: 450
3. Bonadonna G, Valagussa P (1982) Adjuvant therapy in primary breast cancer. In: Carter SK, Glatstein E, Livingstone RB (eds) Principles of cancer treatment. McGraw-Hill, New York, p 315
4. Cutter SJ, Myers H, Green SB (1975) Trends in survival rates in patients with cancer. N Engl J Med 293: 122
5. Fisher B, Slack NH, Ravdin RG, et al. (1968) Surgical adjuvant chemotherapy in cancer of the breast. Results of a decade of cooperative investigation. Ann Surg 168: 337
6. Fisher B (1977) Biological and clinical considerations regarding the use of surgery and chemotherapy in the treatment of primary breast cancer. Cancer 40: 574
7. Haybittle JL (1983) Is breast cancer ever cured? Rev Endocrine Related Cancer 14: 13
8. Holland JF (1976) Major advance in breast cancer therapy. N Engl J Med 294: 440
9. Nissen-Meyer R, Kjellgren K, Månsson B, et al. (1982) Adjuvant chemotherapy in breast cancer. Recent Results Cancer Res 80: 142
10. Rubens RD, Hayward JL, Knight RK, et al. (1983) Controlled trial of adjuvant chemotherapy with melphalan for breast cancer. Lancet i: 839
11. Schabel FM (1975) Concepts for systemic treatment of micrometastases. Cancer 35: 15
12. Sauter C (1983) Hat die heutige adjuvante zytostatische Chemotherapie bei radikal operierten Mammakarzinompatientinnen versagt? Schweiz Med Wochenschr 113: 414
13. Senn HJ, Mayr AC (1979) Adjuvant chemotherapy in breast cancer – Swiss cooperative studies. Cancer Treat Rev (Suppl) 6: 79
14. Senn HJ (1982) Current status and indications for adjuvant chemotherapy in breast cancer. Cancer Chemother Pharmacol 8: 139
15. Sutow WW, Sullivan MP (1976) Childhood cancer – the improving prognosis. Postgrad Med 59: 131

The Preclinical Scientific Basis for Adjuvant Chemotherapy in Breast Cancer

D. P. Griswold Jr., W. R. Laster Jr., M. W. Trader, and D. J. Dykes

Southern Research Institute, 2000 Ninth Avenue, South, P.O. Box 55305, Birmingham, AL 35255-5305, USA

The relatively slow and limited regression of solid tumor masses following and during chemotherapy initially led many to believe, because of the long duration of treatment implied to be necessary by these slow regressions, that chemotherapeutic cure of a solid tumor was impractical if not impossible. However, with the later realization that solid tumor mass reduction grossly underestimates the fraction of a tumor cell population killed by chemotherapy [6], it became evident that chemotherapy may be more effective than had been anticipated. Furthermore, it has been well documented that curability is inversely proportional to the size of the tumor cell population [4]. Thus, it was anticipated that tumor debulking followed by chemotherapy, aimed at destruction of surviving tumor stem cells, would lead to cure for a significant fraction of appropriately staged breast cancer patients. The first clinical trials, however, were disappointing [3].

A few years later, some again believed that carcinoma of the breast would be the first curable solid tumor of major importance. That optimism was based on knowledge that the primary tumor is in a surgically accessible site, that improving diagnostic procedures offered the possibility of early detection, that a significant portion of the tumors is responsive to relatively nontoxic hormonal therapy or ablation, and that, importantly, from the chemotherapists' viewpoint, at least a half-dozen first-line chemotherapeutic agents had been shown to be effective against these cancers. This optimism was also supported by increasing successes that resulted from (a) chemotherapy of other malignancies, e.g., Hodgkin's disease and acute lymphatic leukemia in children, (b) experimental adjuvant chemotherapy studies in solid tumor model systems in animals [4, 10, 13], and (c) adjuvant chemotherapy trials in other human neoplasms [2, 7]. Certainly, some success has been realized in the adjuvant therapy of breast cancer, both in relapse-free survival (RFS) time and overall survival [1]. Nevertheless, progress has not been as rapid or as great as was anticipated several years ago. In spite of improved RFS, recurrence of metastatic and local lesions remains a critical problem, and cure has become an elusive goal.

Cure may require reduction of the total body burden of tumor cells to less than one since it has been shown that fatal cancer of several histological types and in several animal species can be established from a single cancer cell [12]. By implication, metastasis and recurrences may also result from the survival or translocation of a single cell. If that is true, how can therapy be planned to destroy all viable tumor stem cells? What are the obstacles that stand in that path?

Recent Results in Cancer Research. Vol. 96
© Springer-Verlag Berlin · Heidelberg 1984

Several obstacles to improved therapeutic results have been identified. Two of the most critical are diagnostic limitations that preclude the identification and follow-up of micrometatases and the relatively poor basis for selection of the chemotherapeutic agent(s) for initial treatment − thus the continuing interest in the development and application of assays for the determination of the drug sensitivity of individual patients' tumors. Other identifiable obstacles may be broadly classified into three areas: (a) difficulties in disease staging, (b) inability to adequately quantitate viable, clonogenic tumor cell population size before or after treatment, and (c) pharmacologic limitations that encompass a variety of problems.

Staging

Levitt [8] recently noted that "a large number of clinically unsuspected metastases may account for our inability to adequately stage disease . . ." Similarly, the possible inclusion of patients with no metastases in groups to be treated may further cloud the interpretation of the results of that adjuvant treatment. It has been well documented with a number of metastasizing animal tumors that there is a direct relationship between time from primary tumor implant and the existence and extent of metastatic disease [4]. Unfortunately, as the percentage of those animals with metastasis approaches 100%, the fraction of animals with metastatic tumor burden that is beyond the curative potential of currently available adjuvant therapy has also increased [5]. On the other hand, when staging is adjusted to include animals at lower risk for metastasis, the variance of existence of metastatic disease increases. Thus, "cure" as measure of the success of treatment becomes less meaningful. In the latter circumstance, cure would be a function of the percentage of low-risk animals (or patients) included in the adjuvant therapy group.

Quantitation

There has been recent criticism, partly for ethical reasons, of use of the measurement RFS in adjuvant therapy trials [15]. Perhaps that criticism is partly justified (but for a different reason) in that this parameter, as well as others that are used clinically and preclinically, does not provide an accurate measure of clonogenic tumor cell populations that survive adjuvant treatment. In fact, quantitative problems begin with patient selection and disease staging for adjuvant therapy. The success of adjuvant therapy of micrometastatic disease may also be misjudged on the basis of such commonly used parameters. In a typical experimental surgical adjuvant chemotherapy trial in which metastatic disease was staged to include some animals with minimal disease, one would typically expect to see an increased cure rate, above that provided by surgery alone, in those instances where the adjuvant treatment provided a marked increase in median survival time or RFS. Often there is a direct correlation between increased median survival time and cure rate, and this has been well documented (see [9] for a review of this subject). There are also instances where increased median survival time is not accompanied by any change in cure rate (Fig. 1). A number of factors may account for this, some of which are well recognized.

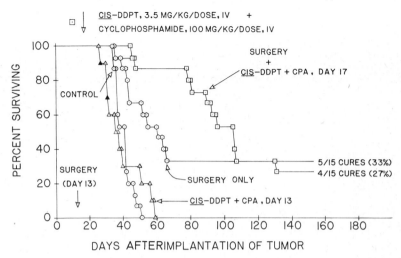

Fig. 1. Response of SC implanted colon tumor 26 to surgery with and without *cis*-DDPt + cyclophosphamide treatment. Tumors were 400–1,000 Mg at the time of surgical removal. (Reproduced with permission of Raven Press)

Some Reasons for Increased RFS with Little or No Overall Benefit

The existence of a metastatic tumor burden of sufficient size that it is beyond the reach of therapeutic curability is one factor accounting for increased RFS with little or no overall benefit; this is demonstrated in Fig. 2. The B16 melanoma is a very refractory tumor, and tumors of 10^7 cells or greater are rarely eradicated regardless of drug or treatment schedule. Both tumor growth delay and increased survival time may occur without cure. Also in Fig. 2 may be seen the difficulty of attempting to directly estimate the net tumor cell kill from commonly used endpoints, such as increased survival time or tumor growth delay. In this example, those parameters are similar for each of the three treatment schedules used, yet the net fraction of each of the tumor cell populations that was killed is markedly different.

Relatively limited antitumor activity of most drugs is not unusual [11]. The therapeutic indices (TI) and LD_{90}/LD_{10} ratios at the optimal treatment schedule for each of 12 agents that were used to treat intraperitoneally (ip) implanted L1210 leukemia are listed in Table 1. The median TI value is 3.2 and the median LD_{90}/LD_{10} ratio is 2.0. Using these median values, a plot (Fig. 3) was made showing the composite dosage-mortality curve in relationship to the minimal effective dose and the nonlethal dosage range in which a minimal (40% increase life span) antitumor effect can be seen. The narrow range of drug dosage over which an antitumor effect can be achieved without unacceptable host toxicity is readily apparent.

The mutation of tumor cells leading to the overgrowth of a drug-resistant subpopulation is another factor that will limit the applicability of an otherwise effective drug treatment regimen [5]. This obstacle, however, can be overcome by the proper choice and mix of drugs to which the tumor cells are not likely to be cross-resistant. Table 2 shows the drug-sensitivity profiles for drug-sensitive and -resistant lines of P388 leukemia and three commonly used anticancer drugs. These data clearly show that each tumor line selected for resistance to one of the three drugs retains its sensitivity to the other two. A combination

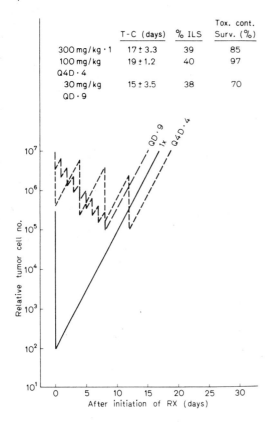

	T-C (days)	% ILS	Tox. cont. Surv. (%)
300 mg/kg · 1	17 ± 3.3	39	85
100 mg/kg Q4D · 4	19 ± 1.2	40	97
30 mg/kg QD · 9	15 ± 3.5	38	70

Fig. 2. Idealized response of SC implanted B16 melanoma to cyclophosphamide when used in three different treatment regimens; based on three or more experiments per treatment schedule

Table 1. Therapeutic indices (TI)[a] from optimal drug treatment of mice with 10^5 L1210 cells, IP and LD_{90}/LD_{10} ratios from dosage-mortality studies in non-tumor-bearing BDF1 (C57BL/6 × DBA/2) mice (reproduced with permission of Raven Press)

	TI	LD_{90}/LD_{10} ratios
5-Fluorouracil	5.6	1.1
Methotrexate	3.5	6.8
Ara-C	> 2.8	2.0
Cyclophosphamide	3.0	2.1
MeCCNU	10.5	2.4
BCNU	8.0	2.0
CCNU	3.2	2.1
Mitomycin-C	2.0	1.7
Melphalan	5.8	2.0
DTIC	3.1	2.4
Hexamethylmelamine	< 1.0	1.7
Adriamycin	1.0	1.7
Median	3.2	2.0

$$^a TI = \frac{LD_{10} \ (mg/kg)}{Minimum \ effective \ dose \ (ILS_{40} - mg/kg)}$$

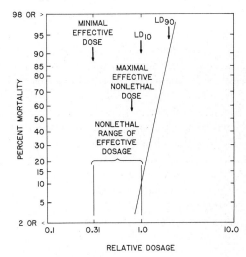

Fig. 3. Dosage-mortality curve from data in Table 1. (Reproduced with permission of Raven Press)

Table 2. Log$_{10}$ change in the body burden of drug-sensitive and drug-resistant leukemia P388 stem cell populations by drug treatment at ≤ LD$_{10}$ doses

	Cyclophosphamide	BCNU	L-PAM
P388/0	−7	−7	−7
P388/Cyclophosphamide	−1	−7	−7
P388/BCNU	−6	−1	−6
P388/L-PAM	−7	−7	−1

Table 3. Response of advanced IP-implanted P388 leukemia to simultaneous combination treatment with cyclophosphamide, BCNU, and melphalan (L-PAM)

Drug (IP)	Optimal dosage (mg/kg)	Tumor-free survivors
Cyclophosphamide	250	0/10
BCNU	25	0/10
L-PAM	20	0/10
Cyclophosphamide	138	
BCNU	15	18/20
L-PAM	8	
Cyclophosphamide	110	
BCNU	12	19/20
L-PAM	6.4	
Cyclophosphamide	91	
BCNU	10	15/20
L-PAM	5.3	

A single dose of each agent was given singly or in combination on day 5 after tumor implant when the tumor cell population was estimated to be about 2.8×10^8 cells

chemotherapy trial was undertaken to determine the effect of this three-drug combination on the potential curability of a large body burden (2.8×10^8 cells at start of treatment) of P388 leukemia. Partial results are shown in Table 3. When given singly, cyclophosphamide reduced the tumor cell population by about 8 $\log_{10}$ units but was not curative. Similarly, BCNU reduced the cell population by about 7 $\log_{10}$ units but was not curative. Treatment with L-PAM (melphalan) only held this large tumor cell population static. Previous data have shown that large populations of P388 leukemia contain some cells resistant to BCNU and some resistant to cyclophosphamide, but that those cells retain their sensitivity to L-PAM. It is probable that the therapeutic synergism observed in this trial resulted from use of drugs to which these cells are not cross-resistant.

Other factors that appear to be obstacles to curability include anatomic and pharmacologic barriers that preclude the attainment of minimal effective drug concentrations for a sufficient time to effect cell kill. Alternatively, resting cells (G_0 or long residence times in G_1), which characteristically may be found in solid tumors, may not be killed by certain antimetabolites or may have sufficient time to repair after exposure to highly reactive agents [14]. These possibilities are less well understood and documented than is specific biochemical resistance.

In conclusion, some pertinent observations may be summarized as follows:

1. Cure is inversely proportional to tumor burden, but the relationship is not always linear.
2. The random nature of metastasis assures that staging will tend to include patients without metastatic disease in low-risk groups or patients in high-risk groups with a metastatic burden beyond the curative potential of the drugs used.
3. Parameters commonly used for the measurement of the effects of treatment may not accurately determine the net tumor cell reduction achieved.
4. Good initial response to treatment, e.g., increased RFS, without overall benefit may result from:
   a) Tumor burden being too great or limited drug cytotoxicity
   b) Selection and overgrowth of drug-resistant tumor cells
   c) Pharmacologic- and/or population-kinetic barriers
5. Further improvement in adjuvant chemotherapy may require high-dose, combination drug therapy tailored for the individual (based on pharmacologic determinations), in addition to improved diagnostic and drug selection technology.

Acknowledgements. Previously unpublished results reported herein were carried out under contract N01-CM-97309, Drug Evaluation Branch, Division of Cancer Treatment, National Cancer Institute, National Institutes of Health, Bethesda, MD 20205.

References

1. Bonadonna G, Gasparini M, Rossi A (1980) Adjuvant therapies of postsurgical minimal residual disease. In: Mathe G, Muggia FM (eds) Cancer chemo- and immunopharmacology. 1. Chemopharmacology. Springer, Berlin Heidelberg New York, pp 8–25 (Recent results in cancer research, vol 74)
2. Cortes EP, Holland JF, Wang JJ, Sinks LF, Blom J, Senn H, Bank A, Glidewell O (1974) Amputation and adriamycin in primary osteosarcoma. N Engl J Med 291: 998–1000
3. Fisher B, Ravdin RG, Ausman AK, Slack NH, Moore GE, Noer RF (1968) Surgical adjuvant chemotherapy in cancer of the breast: Results of a decade of cooperative investigation. Ann Surg 168: 337–356

4. Griswold DP Jr (1975) The potential for murine tumor models in surgical adjuvant chemotherapy. Cancer Chemother Rep 5: 187–204
5. Griswold DP Jr, Schabel FM Jr, Corbett TH, Dykes DJ (1981) Concepts for controlling drug-resistant tumor cells. In: Fidler IJ, White RJ (eds) Design of models for testing cancer therapeutic agents. Van Nostrand Reinhold, New York, pp 215–224
6. Griswold DP Jr, Schabel FM Jr, Wilcox WS, Simpson-Herren L, Skipper HE (1968) Success and failure in the treatment of solid tumors. I. Effects of cyclophosphamide (NSC-26271) on primary and metastatic plasmacytoma in the hamster. Cancer Chemother Rep 52: 345–387
7. Jaffe N, Frei E III, Traggis D, Bishop Y (1974) Adjuvant methotrexate and citrovorum-factor treatment of osteogenic sarcoma. N Engl J Med 291: 994–997
8. Levitt SH (1983) Pattern of failure in breast cancer. Cancer Treat Symp 2: 123–129
9. Martin DS (1981) The scientific basis for adjuvant chemotherapy. Cancer Treat Rev 8: 169–189
10. Mayo JG, Laster WR Jr, Andrews CM, Schabel FM Jr (1972) Success and failure in the treatment of solid tumors. III. "Cure" of metastatic Lewis lung carcinoma with methyl-CCNU (NSC-95441) and surgery-chemotherapy. Cancer Chemother Rep 56: 183–195
11. Schabel FM Jr, Griswold DP Jr, Corbett TH, Laster WR Jr (1983) Increasing therapeutic response rates to anticancer drugs by applying the basic principles of pharmacology. Pharmacol Ther 20: 283–305
12. Schabel FM Jr, Simpson-Herren L (1978) Some variables in experimental tumor systems which complicate interpretation of data from in vivo kinetic and pharmacologic studies with anticancer drugs. In: Schabel FM Jr (ed) Fundamentals in cancer chemotherapy. Karger, Basel, Antibiotics and chemotherapy, vol 23, pp 113–129
13. Shapiro DM, Fugmann RA (1957) A role for chemotherapy as an adjuvant to surgery. Cancer Res 17: 1098–1101
14. Skipper HE, Schabel FM Jr (1984) Tumor cell heterogeneity: Implications with respect to classification of cancers by chemotherapeutic effect. Cancer Treat Rep 68: 43–61
15. Smith IE (1983) Adjuvant chemotherapy for early breast cancer. Br Med J 287: 379–380

The Clinical Scientific Basis of Adjuvant Chemotherapy in Breast Cancer

B. Fisher*

NSABP National Surgical Adjuvant Project for Breast and Bowel Cancers,
Biostatistical Center, Suite 730, 3515 Fifth Avenue, Pittsburgh, PA 15213, USA

Introduction

It is possible to trace over the course of this century two main developmental pathways associated with the therapy of women with operable breast cancer. One charts the results from laboratory and clinical investigations which have permitted formulation, testing, and acceptance of an alternative biological hypothesis to replace the Halsted theory which is based on anatomical principles. That paradigmatic change accounts for the revolution in the local-regional management of the disease. The second developmental pathway associated with the therapy of breast cancer is that related to the use of systemic chemotherapy. It orginated from an awareness that only by distant disease control could there be an improvement in outcome for breast cancer patients. Acceptance of this concept has resulted in a major change in breast cancer research and treatment. It has led to the implementation of clinical trials to evaluate the efficacy of different systemic treatment regimens employed as adjuncts to operation. The first clinical trial of adjuvant therapy for breast cancer was begun in 1958 and within the past decade such controlled studies have proliferated at a furious pace. It seems appropriate to pause and reflect upon what has provided the basis for past and present efforts and to comment upon these considerations which might be employed for future efforts.

The Basis for the First Generation of Adjuvant Therapy Trials

The historical background that provided the basis for the first generation of clinical trials of adjuvant therapy is worthy of more than casual consideration. The earliest study of tumor cells in the blood was performed in 1869 by Ashworth [1], who found the cells in a patient with malignant skin tumors. Excluding a few sporadic case reports of abnormal cells in the blood of patients with tumors, little interest in tumor cells in the blood was entertained. In 1955 Fisher and Turnbull [2] reported the presence of tumor cells in the blood of cancer patients, and a surge of interest took place.

---

* Refer to papers in References for listing of NSABP investigators and institutions contributing to these studies

Recent Results in Cancer Research. Vol. 96
© Springer-Verlag Berlin · Heidelberg 1984

In the few years following these studies, many investigators found tumor cells in the peripheral blood of patients with operable and advanced lesions, in hepatic vein blood, in the blood of patients with all types of neoplasms, and in the blood of children with cancer. Of special interest are the studies that demonstrated the presence of cancer cells in the blood during pelvic and rectal examinations, uterine curettage, transurethral resection, while cleaning the skin over a tumor prior to operation, and during the operation itself [3].

It was believed that tumor cells dislodged during operation were a prime factor in the failure to cure, despite meticulous surgical skill, and that if such hematogenous circulating tumor cells were destroyed, improved results would follow. With reports of favorable effects of chemotherapeutic agents on the destruction of disseminated tumor cells in experimental animals [4], a rationale for embarking upon clinical trials of adjuvant therapy was established. At that time it was considered that chemotherapy cell kill was related to zero order kinetics.

Further support for the use of systemic therapy was obtained from the early investigations of Shapiro and Fugmann [5] who worked with a mammary adenocarcinoma. They noted that although surgical removal of tumors or the use of 6-mercaptopurine failed to "cure" animals with tumors, the combination of the two resulted in a 57% "cure" rate.

Armed with this information there was reason for hypothesizing that the use of adjuvant chemotherapy would lower recurrence and improve the survival of breast cancer patients. Consequently, in 1957, representatives of 23 institutions in the United States, under the auspices of the National Institutes of Health, Cancer Chemotherapy National Service Center, adopted a common protocol to determine the efficacy of administering chemotherapy in conjunction with curative cancer surgery to decrease recurrence and extend survival of patients with breast cancer. It was anticipated that such a therapeutic regimen could destroy the tumor cells dislodged into the blood and lymph during surgical manipulation. The effort became known as the National Surgical Adjuvant Breast Project (NSABP). This title has since been used to identify the cooperative group in the United States that for 25 years has carried out clinical trials to evaluate a variety of treatment modalities in the management of patients with primary breast cancer.

The results of that first effort demonstrated both a decrease in recurrence and an improvement in survival in one subgroup of patients [6]. The observation in retrospect is of historic importance in that it was the first demonstration that the natural history of breast cancer could be perturbed by the use of adjuvant chemotherapy. It also indicated that there was a difference in patient subset response to a therapy, a prediction of future findings. Disappointment with the overall results, however, led to the conclusion that the hypothesis had not been confirmed. Subsequent events revealed that the hypothesis was still valid, but that the premise upon which the first testing was based was inappropriate. It became appreciated that the killing of surgically disseminated tumor cells was probably less important than was the response of existing micrometastases to cytotoxic agents.

In general, the 1960s were nonproductive. They produced virtually no substantive clinical information which demonstrated that adjuvant chemotherapy was or was not of benefit for adult solid tumors. Advanced disease was the arena for the use of chemotherapy. It was in that forum that evidence accumulated which indicated that the use of multiple agents produced a greater remission rate than did single drugs. From that information a rationale was evolving which was to influence future trials of adjuvant chemotherapy. At the same time there was considerable research activity going on which was able to have significant consequences.

The Basis for a Second Generation of Adjuvant Therapy Trials

It became apparent that the original hypotheses upon which adjuvant chemotherapy was based were inadequate. Cells disseminated at the time of surgery are less important than the micrometastases already established. In the 1960s new concepts were formulated, which led to a second generation of chemotherapy trials. Following is an overview of those principles, which are primarily related to tumor cell kinetics, and which for the most part, still provide the biological basis for the use of adjuvant chemotherapy.

Mendelsohn [7], then Skipper and Schabel [8, 9] defined the concept of a growth fraction in tumor cell populations. They hypothesized that tumors are made up of three cell compartments.

1. *Compartment A* consists of proliferating clonogenic cells undergoing active anabolism. Cells in compartment A help to increase total cell number in a tumor population. Tumor growth occurs when proliferating cells in the compartment exceed cell loss. Cell cycle-specific chemotherapeutic agents destroy cells in this compartment.
2. *Compartment B* is composed of a population of nonproliferative cells not engaged in active anabolism. These cells do not contribute to population growth but are in equilibrium with cells in compartment A, and they retain their potential for proliferation. Although sensitive to cell cycle-nonspecific agents to some extent, they are more resistant to cytostatic manipulation. For cell cycle-specific agents to effectively control tumor growth, cells in compartment A must be depleted. Transformation of noncycling cells in compartment B to proliferating cells in compartment A results. These cells then become vulnerable to chemotherapeutic agents.
3. *Compartment C* is composed of permanently nonproliferating, nonclonogenic cells, which do not contribute to tumor growth, only to tumor volume, and consequently seem to be less clinically significant.

The growth fraction of a tumor has been defined as the ratio of proliferating to nonproliferating cells: $A/(B + C)$. The greater the growth fraction, the more sensitive a cell population is to chemotherapy. The growth fraction of a given population of cells in a growing solid tumor is neither constant nor related to total tumor volume. The changing growth rate of tumor cells fits the Gompertz equation, which described exponential tumor growth that is exponentially inhibited. With increasing tumor volume, tumor growth fraction progressively decreases, and the tumor doubling time increases, resulting in a loss of sensitivity to chemotherapy. Micrometastases, with a population of $\leq 10^6$ cells, have been shown to approach exponential log-phase (non-Gompertzian) growth. Micrometastasis cells are more sensitive to chemotherapy than are those of their more crowded counterparts in large primary tumors.

The killing of cells by chemotherapeutic agents follows first-order kinetics: regardless of size, a constant proportion of the total tumor cell population remaining is killed following each administration of a constant quantity of drug. First-order kinetics apply only to those populations that grow exponentially with constant growth fractions and tumor doubling times (i.e., micrometastases as opposed to large-volume primary tumors).

Another factor that determines the responsiveness of a tumor population to chemotherapy is the variation of cell-cycle time or the degree of synchronization of cell cycles. Cells that cycle at similar velocities (synchronized) have the greatest sensitivity to chemotherapy. Conversely, the more heterogeneously synchronized the population, the less likely it is to respond effectively to chemotherapy. The reduction of the tumor cell population by surgical removal or radiation of a primary tumor may affect the growth fraction and synchronization of cells in micrometastases so profoundly that they become more sensitive to chemotherapy.

Endpoints utilized in clinical trials to test the effectiveness of chemotherapy against either late or early disease may fail to reflect important events occurring at the cellular level. A 50% regression of a measurable tumor mass resulting from administration of a chemotherapeutic agent may be associated with a 99.99% reduction in clonogenic cells. In early disease, administration of drugs as adjuvants may be associated with overall results (a disease-free interval or survival). Although not as dramatic, the results may be of greater biological importance.

Skipper [9] estimated that about 75% of women with stage II breast cancers, who harbor between 10^6 and 10^7 residual cells following primary tumor removal, could benefit from single-agent therapy. Thus, based on kinetic studies and data derived from animal tumor models, the logical starting point for evaluating the worth of adjuvant chemotherapy in breast cancer is implementation of clinical trials utilizing single agents. After determining the effectiveness of single agents, multiple agents can then be evaluated.

Following is a summary of information regarding tumor-cell kinetics, which provided a rational basis in the early 1970s for planning meaningful protocols of adjuvant chemotherapy and led us to adopt our clinical-trial strategy.

1. Growth fractions and doubling times of primary tumors may differ from those in micrometastases. Consequently, responsiveness to chemotherapy may differ.
2. The magnitude of response of a primary tumor in the plateau of Gompertzian growth need not reflect the response of micrometastases in exponential growth.
3. First-order kinetics relative to the cell kill by cytocidal agents apply to those cells with constant growth fractions in exponential growth (i.e., micrometastases of $\leq 10^6$ cells).
4. The degree of synchronization of cell-cycle times of a primary tumor and those of its micrometastases may differ. On this basis, primary tumor and its micrometastases may respond to cyclical chemotherapy differently.
5. Ablation of a primary tumor with resultant decrease in total tumor cell population may alter the growth characteristics of residual micrometastases. A decrease in tumor-doubling time may result. Such changes may enhance the sensitivity of micrometasases to chemotherapy.
6. Micrometastases approaching exponential-growth kinetics could be sensitive to single-agent chemotherapy. Consequently, there exists the rationale for first evaluating the effect of single agents as adjuvants.

We were in accord with Skipper that "it would be foolhardy to expect to hit upon the best drug(s) and best regimens in the first, second or third clinical trials designed and carried out. Hopefully, such trials could be planned in a manner so that we learn and improve design and end-results in a stepwise fashion" [10]. While the prevailing concept at the time was that increasing numbers of chemotherapeutic agents would directly increase therapeutic response, our premise was that since the residual tumor burden would be variable, and it had been suggested by Skipper that tumor cell populations between 10^6 and 10^7 cells could be amenable to single-agent chemotherapy, it was possible that subsets of patients could be as responsive to single agents as to combinations of drugs. An awakening awareness of the phenomenon of tumor "heterogeneity" also suggested to us the possibility that there might be a variable response to a therapeutic regimen by different patient subsets. There then arose new premises for the use of adjuvant chemotherapy.

Testing During the 1970s

The next decade saw the vigorous testing of the adjuvant chemotherapy hypothesis by means of numerous clinical trials [review, 11]. The results of those studies have been under constant scrutiny and review and have been the subject of continuous comparison. Even prior to the establishment of its worth, adjuvant chemotherapy became the paradigm for the treatment of micrometastatic disease. It is now appropriate to decide whether evidence has accumulated which lends support to the hypothesis that adjuvant chemotherapy is of value and whether new data have arisen which would modify the prevailing hypothesis or establish new premises for future testing. It is also appropriate to consider whether there is evidence that a new paradigm for the treatment of systemic disease is in the making.

Information from all of the major trials indicates that the natural history of breast cancer has been altered. There is justification to conclude that the original hypothesis has been confirmed − *but only partially so*. The results from a clinical point of view may be disappointing since no "penicillin effect" has been observed. When one considers the empiricism employed in those trials, however, any positive result at all seems remarkable. In none was there a preliminary determination of optimal drug dose. The scheduling, length of administration, decisions concerning drug-dose reduction and escalation were arbitrary. Consequently, the results obtained may reflect the application of less than optimal methodology.

Some of the findings in the plethora of data appear to have a particular biological importance. It is clearly apparent that there is a heterogeneous response to a particular chemotherapeutic regimen. Some subsets of patients are benefited to a greater or lesser degree than others or not at all. This disparate therapeutic response is concordant with evidence characterizing the biological heterogeneity between and within tumors [12].

A major premise upon which the trials of the 1970s were based was that increasing the number of agents in combination would increase the effectiveness of the therapy. It is our opinion that this thesis has not been entirely borne out by the findings. In some subsets of patients one or two drugs have been as effective as three or five. In others two, three, or five agents have produced similar results, while in others any number used in combination have failed to demonstrate an effect.

Recent Considerations for a New Generation of Adjuvant Therapy Trials

Trials carried out in the last decade are almost passé. While they were being conducted, new laboratory and clinical research provided information which modifies old premises and gives rise to new ones.

Concerning Tumor Receptors

Findings relative to the estrogen receptor (ER) and progesterone receptor (PR) content of tumors have added a new dimension to breast-cancer biology. Receptor values are of prognostic importance not only in untreated patients but in adjuvant therapy-treated patients as well. Our own studies indicate that the heterogeneity of response to adjuvant therapy is not *only* related to the number of positive nodes, age, and tumor characteristics but is also influenced by tumor ER and PR [13].

It is our opinion that for the more effective use of receptor information in a next generation of trials it is necessary to determine whether disparate levels of ER in tumors are due to changes in the proportion of cells expressing the receptor or to variation in the amount of receptor in the cell population with ER. To answer that question and others relative to ER it is necessary to determine the receptor in single, intact viable cells. For several years we have been incubating suspensions of mouse or human mammary tumor cells with a ligand consisting of a fluorescein moiety coupled to position 17 of estrone (17-FE) [14]. Cells binding ligand demonstrate fluorescence. The proportion of cells in human breast cancers varied in our series from 3% to 58%. Moreover, the location of the fluorescence was not the same in all ER-positive tumor cells, further indicating the heterogeneity of the cell population. This methodology makes it possible to evaluate host influences on tumor-cell ER as well as to relate ER to other cellular activities such as DNA synthesis. It should be a goal of laboratory research to develop methodology capable of determining individual cellular production of, for example, markers, enzymes, CEA, etc., in human tumors rather than estimating those values in the tumor as a whole.

Hypothesis for the Use of Perioperative Therapy

Perioperative therapy provides another example of how laboratory and clinical research interacts. Several different biological premises provide justification for considering the use of perioperative chemotherapy. One relates to the effect which removal of a primary tumor has on the growth kinetics of metastases. Our studies have demonstrated that within 24 hours following removal of a primary C3H mammary tumor there is an increase in the labelling index (LI) of a distant tumor focus which persists for between 7 and 10 days [15]. There is also a decrease in tumor doubling time and a measurable increase in tumor size which becomes apparent about a week following tumor removal. The tumor growth is probably a result of the conversion of noncycling cells in G_0 phase into proliferating cells; cells which should be more vulnerable to cytostatic agents. The rapidity of the onset of the kinetic changes and their relatively short duration provides a suitable rationale for the use of chemotherapy as soon as possible following tumor removal. Investigations carried out by us in an animal model have, indeed, indicated that chemotherapy had a more favorable effect when given on the day of tumor removal than 3 days later when the LI of metastases were at a peak and it was least effective when given at a time when the LI had returned to the preoperative level [16]. The greatest benefit occurred when the chemotherapy was given prior to operation. Use at that time completely prevented the increase in LI, more effectively suppressed tumor growth, and prolonged survival to a greater extent than was noted under any other circumstance. This suggests that for more effective control of metastases chemotherapy had best be employed before or at the time of primary tumor removal. Aside from the therapeutic ramifications of the findings, their biological import requires assessment. Elucidation of the mechanism whereby removal of a primary tumor exerts its effect on metastases is worthy of investigation. What mediates such a phenomenon and what characterizes the cells that respond to the stimulus? It hardly needs pointing out that the kinetic changes observed by us and by others [17, 18] in animal models provide no assurance that a similar phenomenon takes place following removal in the human or even that the temporal pattern of the kinetic changes in the animal and in the patient (should they occur) are similar.

Of interest are our laboratory investigations which show that a change in the porportion of cells containing a certain marker may be associated with a change in the proportion of cells demonstrating other markers. We have noted that the increase in ^{3}HTdR-labeled cells is accompanied by a decrease in those demonstrating ER.

Another justification for perioperative therapy is based upon the contention of Goldie and Coldman, that as a tumor-cell population increases there is an ever-expanding number of drug-resistant phenotypic variants which become more difficult to eradicate [19]. In that concept "every minute counts." Consequently, combinations of non-cross-resistant drugs should be administered when a tumor population contains as few cells as possible. The Goldie somatic mutation theory seems to provide an alternative and independent explanation to that evoking cell kinetic principles as the basis for drug resistance. The two are not, however, mutually exclusive. With the growth of a tumor not only are the absolute numbers of resistant cells increased but so is the percentage of resistant cells in the total cell population. The latter is presumed to occur because resistant phenotypes not only multiply as a result of their own intrinsic growth rates but as a consequence of the addition of new mutations from the pool of nonresistant (sensitive) cells [20]. Following tumor removal, as a consequence of the enhanced proliferation of cells, it becomes more likely that the number of resistant phenotypes will increase in the metastatic population. Thus, appropriate perioperative therapy should not only destroy cells made more sensitive by their kinetic alteration but at the same time, by preventing cell proliferation, prevent an increase of resistant cells.

A third justification for the use of perioperative therapy relates to repeated observations that surgical manipulations result in "showers" of circulating tumor cells. It has been reported that the presence of such cells is *not* related to patient outcome [21−23]. Examination of the studies providing evidence for such a conclusion, however, reveals that they were "no contests" and could not have determined what the consequences of finding circulating cells might be. Insufficient patients with too short a follow-up time were inappropriately analyzed. Most important, outcome was related to the presence or absence of circulating tumor cells without regard for other variables which could have influenced prognosis.

Findings from two clinical trials employing perioperative chemotherapy have provided evidence to indicate that there may be a benefit from such therapy. Our own [6], employing thiotepa on the day of surgery and for 2 successive days thereafter, demonstrated an improvement in both disease-free survival and survival in some patients − the first evidence indicating the worth of adjuvant chemotherapy. A Scandinavian trial [24] in which cyclophosphamide was administered for 6 consecutive days starting on the day of operation also indicated an advantage. It cannot be too emphatically stated, however, that neither of those trials provide evidence that perioperative therapy is any better than the same therapy given at a later time. Neither trial had the proper control group to answer that question, i.e., a group of similar patients treated precisely the same way but at an interval following operation.

Since such therapy is apt to neutralize only events which are transient, i.e., cells disseminated and kinetic alterations occurring during the perioperative period, it may be conjectured as to how much more beneficial such treatment will be than that which is conventionally given a few weeks to a month following operation. Is that "lead time" apt to significantly alter an outcome which is more likely determined by events prior to operation? In that regard, one may contemplate many of the suppositions of the Goldie hypothesis which does not, to my knowledge, have its basis in findings from in vivo experimental systems but, rather, has been derived from computer modeling. How can that concept relate to breast cancer metastases if they possess a relatively small growth fraction or do not grow at a constant rate? If gene amplification is a mechanism leading to resistance, earlier use of drugs may result in the more rapid emergence of resistant cells. Despite these speculations, a trial of perioperative therapy is likely to provide more definitive biological information relative to human neoplasms than will additional in vitro and in vivo models. If it is revealed from a study that has truly been a contest (a proper evaluation) that there is no benefit to the use of perioperative therapy, then it may be concluded that the biological consequences of primary tumor removal or of circulating tumor cells released at the time of operation are not likely to be of clinical significance and that further research in that aspect of metastasis should be diminished or redirected.

Concerning New Kinetic Considerations

As was recently noted, the rationale which governed the design of adjuvant chemotherapy protocols to date assumes that micrometastases grow according to Gompertzian kinetics. A further assumption presumes that micrometastatic foci are more sensitive to chemotherapy by the virtue of their more-rapid growth rates. Moreover, it was hypothesized that small tumors which approximate exponential growth are more likely to undergo mutations than larger tumors which are growing more slowly. A further principle upon which the first generation of adjuvant clinical trials was based assumed that chemotherapeutic agents act by killing a constant proportion of cells rather than a constant number. As a consequence of this "log kill hypothesis," the use of repetitive prolonged therapy was instituted. It was conjectured that optimal kill requires maximum dosage of the agents employed and that combinations of therapeutically non-cross-resistant agents would be superior to drugs used alone. It would seem that many of those kinetic considerations have been inadequate to predict the clinical behavior of breast cancer and to supply guidelines for using currently available chemotherapeutic agents with greater effectiveness.

Recently, Speer, Retsky, and associates (personal communication) reevaluated the Gompertz equation as a valid representation of human breast cancer growth by employing computer-simulated models. They observed that if the popularly accepted parameters for log kill are introduced into the Gompertz equation, the time required for a tumor to grow from one cell to a volume large enough for clinical detection would be far too short (approximately 4 months) in one such model. Even if a range of parametric values were substituted into the Gompertzian equation, none of the curves generated would result in the growth of a tumor from one cell to clinical detection in a time in excess of 1 year. It seems that the Gompertz equation does not describe the growth pattern of clinical breast cancer. Thus, the Goldie and Coldman hypothesis which assumes that tumor growth simulates bacteria in their exponential growth phase may not be substantiated by this model. Based on these observations, Speer et al. have devised a stochastic numerical model which simulates breast-cancer growth as observed in the clinical setting. The model proposes that Gompertzian kinetics are relevant but that from time to time and in a random fashion there occurs a spontaneous change in the growth rate so that the overall growth pattern of a tumor occurs in a stepwise fashion. According to this model the average time for the tumor burden to increase from one cell to clinical detection is in the range of 8 years. The model proposed that resistance to chemotherapy in patients with resected breast cancer may be due to cells in G_0 rather than to other mechanisms of resistance including the development of mutations. The consideration that tumors might grow in "spurts" instead of in a steady progression has resulted in an alternative hypothesis which simulates natural history data in breast cancer. The model has enabled the simulation of a population of individuals with breast cancer possessing behavioral characteristics that encompass a broad spectrum of the disease with all its heterogenous aspects.

Whether one employs a stochastic or deterministic kinetic model to simulate breast cancer growth, it appears evident that there is a longer lag period between the origin and clinical appearance of a tumor than could be explained by the simplistic application of Gompertzian kinetics. Thus, some of the more modern kinetic models of breast cancer suggest that there are periods in the life history of a tumor in which no growth is evident.

If a major cause of resistance to chemotherapy is indeed due to large numbers of cells in the G_0 state, there must exist a number of time periods when a metastasis is not changing in size. If this is the case, adjuvant chemotherapy regimens based on the simpler growth kinetic theories might be predictably inadequate. The use of a low-dose continuous regimen would be effective only during growth spurts and would result in nothing more than the induction of toxicity during plateau phases.

Whether the described model can or cannot survive the criticisms of other kinetic and mathematical "modelers" is not as important as the fact that it proposes a possible explanation for the inordinately long intervals observed between primary-tumor removal and the detection of metastases. That phenomenon may be related to the possibility that micrometastases do indeed grow in "spurts."

Comment

This overview has attempted to indicate that there has been and must continue to be a biological rationale for the conduct of clinical trials using adjuvant chemotherapy. The firmer the laboratory and clinical research findings, which provide the basis for the trial, the more likely that major gains will be made.

We continue to consider our clinical trials of adjuvant therapy to be research endeavors of the highest order. Chemotherapeutic agents or combinations of agents employed in such trials may be considered to be "probes" to identify subpopulations whose metastases have cells with common or differing biological properties. Such therapeutic probes cull from a population of heterogeneous tumors, responders and nonresponders, and provide direction for further investigation to determine why there is a difference in response between and within subgroups.

Acknowledgements. This work was supported by USPHS grants R-01-CA-12027, contract N01-CB-23876, and by American Cancer Society grant RC-13.

References

1. Ashworth TR (1869) A case of cancer in which cells similar to those in the tumors were seen in the blood after death. Aust Med J 14: 146
2. Fisher ER, Turnbull RB Jr (1955) Cytologic demonstration and significance of tumor cells in the mesenteric venous blood in patients with colorectal carcinoma. Surg Gynecol Obstet 100: 102–108
3. Delarue NC (1960) The free cancer cell. Cancer Med Assoc J 82: 1175–1182
4. Cruz EP, McDonald GO, Cole WH (1956) Prophylactic treatment of cancer: the use of chemotherapeutic agents to prevent tumor metastasis. Surgery 40: 291–296

5. Shapiro DM, Fugmann RA (1957) A role of chemotherapy as an adjunct to surgery. Cancer Res 17: 1098−1101
6. Fisher B, Ravdin RG, Ausman RK, Slack NH, Moore GE, Noer RJ (1968) Surgical adjuvant chemotherapy in cancer of the breast: results of a decade of cooperative investigation. Ann Surg 168: 337−356
7. Mendelsohn ML (1960) The growth fraction: a new concept applied to tumors. Science 132: 1496
8. Skipper HE, Schabel FM Jr (1973) Quantitative and cytokinetics studies in experimental tumor models. In: Holand JR, Frei E III (eds) Cancer medicine. Lea and Febiger, Philadelphia, pp 629−650
9. Skipper HE (1971) Kinetics of mammary tumor cell growth and implications for therapy. Cancer 28: 1479−1499
10. Skipper HE (1971) Some thoughts on surgery-chemotherapy trials against breast cancer. In: Monograph 1, Southern Research Institute, Birmingham, AL
11. Fisher B, Redmond C, Abramson N, Bowman D, Compbell T, Desser R, Dimitrov N, Frelick R, Geggie P, Glass A, Plotkin D, Prager D, Stolbach L, Wolter J and other NSABP investigators (1983) Topics in oncology: advances in adjuvant chemotherapy of breast cancer. In: Fairbanks VF (ed) Current hematology II. Wiley, New York, pp 415−446
12. Fisher B (1980) Laboratory and clinical research in breast cancer − a personal adventure: the David A. Karnofsky memorial lecture. Cancer Res 40: 3863−3874
13. Fisher B, Redmond C, Brown A, Wickerham DL, Wolmark N, Allegra J, Escher G, Lippman M, Savlov E, Wittliff J and Fisher ER, with the contributions of Plotikin D, Bowman D, Wolter J, Bornstein R, Desser R, Frelick R and other NSABP investigators (1983) Influence of tumor estrogen and progesterone receptor levels on the response to tamoxifen and chemotherapy in primary breast cancer: J Clin Onc 1: 227−241
14. Fisher B, Gunduz N, Zheng S, Saffer EA (1982) Fluoresceinated estrone binding by human and mouse breast cancer cells. Cancer Res 42: 540−549
15. Gunduz N, Fisher B, Saffer EA (1979) Effect of surgical removal on the growth and kinetics of residual tumor. Cancer Res 39: 3861−3865
16. Fisher B, Gunduz N, Saffer EA (1983) Influence of the interval between primary tumor removal and chemotherapy on kinetics and growth of metastases. Cancer Res 43: 1488−1492
17. Schiffer LM, Braunschweiger PG, Stragand JJ (1978) Tumor cell population kinetics following noncurative treatment. Antibiotics Chemother 23: 148−156
18. Simpson-Herren L, Sanford AH, Holmquist JP (1976) Effects of surgery on the cell kinetics of residual tumor. Cancer Treat Rep 60: 1749−1760
19. Goldie JH, Coldman AJ (1979) A mathematic model for relating the drug sensitivity of tumors to their spontaneous mutation rate. Cancer Treat Rep 63: 1727−1733
20. Goldie, JH (1982) Drug resistance and chemotherapeutic strategy. In: Owens AH Jr, Coffey DS, Baylin SB (eds) Tumor cell heterogeneity: origins and implications. Academic, New York, pp 115−125
21. Engell HC (1959) Cancer cells in the blood. A five to nine year follow-up study. Ann Surg 149: 457−461
22. Ritchie AC, Webster DR (1961) Tumor cells in the blood. In: Proceedings of the 4th Canadian Conference. Academic, New York
23. Salsbury AJ (1975) The significance of the circulating cancer cell. Cancer Treat Rev 2: 55−72
24. Nissen-Meyer R, Kjellgren K, Malmio K, Mansson B, Norin T (1978) Surgical adjuvant chemotherapy. Results with one short course with cyclophosphamide after mastectomy for breast cancer. Cancer 41: 2088−2098

Molecular and Cellular Mechanisms Underlying Ineffective Cancer Chemotherapy

M. F. Rajewsky and N. Huh

Institut für Zellbiologie (Tumorforschung), Universität Essen, Gesamthochschule, Hufelandstrasse 55, 4300 Essen 1, Federal Republic of Germany

The title of this contribution is not meant to imply that cancer chemotherapy is generally ineffective; rather, we intend to discuss some of the mechanisms, at the molecular and cellular level, that are obstacles to effective treatment of malignant tumors and leukemias with chemical agents. Basically we remain confronted with the fact that no form of cytocidal chemical treatment can at present be targeted exclusively to the malignant cells contained within the large number of normal cells in the organism ($\sim 10^9$ malignant cells in 1 g of tumor tissue vs $\sim 5 \times 10^{13}$ normal cells, in the adult). This limits the applicable dose of a cytotoxic agent to a level compatible with the survival of sufficient numbers of (stem) cells of the most critical normal-cell systems (hemopoietic and immune system, intestinal epithelia). A much more favorable situation would, of course, arise if agents were to become available that would interact specifically with proliferation-competent cells of a malignant tumor, but not with any of the critical normal cells. This is presently not the case, although cytotoxic monoclonal antibodies (Mab), or Mab coupled to cytocidal agents, which are directed against cell-surface components of particular types of tumor or leukemic cells are becoming available (see [48a, 103]). With appropriately chosen antitumor cell surface Mab, cytotoxic damage to normal cells may be restricted to cell subpopulations sharing the respective cell-surface antigens (usually cell type- and differentiation stage-specific determinants) with the malignant cells. Coelimination of such cross-reacting normal-cell subpopulations may be tolerable provided they do not represent irreplaceable stem cells of critical cell lineages. However, even if tumor cell-specific agents such as cell surface-directed Mab were generally available, there would remain the problem of reaching all of the malignant cells via systemic application, i.e., of achieving a sufficiently high concentration of the cytocidal agent in their microenvironment. In contrast to the cells in normal tissues, the accessibility of tumor cells via the capillary system and by diffusion is often poor, particularly in tumors of larger size. The differences in tumor vs normal tissue architecture and vascularization constitute one of the obstacles to effective cancer chemotherapy.

Tumor Heterogeneity

Cellular heterogeneity, both inter- and intratumoral, has become a catchword often referred to in relation to the limitations of cancer therapy [21, 39, 41−43, 62, 63, 67, 68].

Recent Results in Cancer Research. Vol. 96
© Springer-Verlag Berlin · Heidelberg 1984

However, this general term needs more precise definition. Although malignant tumors and leukemias in most cases derive from one single clone of cells [26, 69], there is clear evidence that by the time of detection and treatment of malignant disease the population of malignant cells is usually composed of multiple cell subpopulations differing with regard to many of the phenotypic properties that we have learned to recognize. This cellular diversity apparently results from a pronounced "plasticity" of malignant phenotypes as compared with the stable phenotypes of normal cells, i.e., a remarkable capacity for adaptation to changing microenvironmental conditions, reminiscent to a certain extent of the properties of cells at early stages of development and differentiation [46, 48, 99]. Malignant cells generally have an abnormal nuclear DNA content (see [4]), and a decreased genetic stability is thus widely assumed to be responsible for their phenotypic variability [62]. However, epigenetic changes and altered regulatory mechanisms may also play an important role. Before considering more precisely some of their properties in relation to cancer chemotherapy, we must acknowledge that, with few exceptions (see, e.g., [4, 29, 89]), our information on phenotypically differing cell subpopulations in tumors comes from analyses of cultured cell lines established from primary or metastatic tumors. However, given both the different microenvironmental conditions in cell culture and the frequent generation of phenotypic variants in malignant cell populations, such in vitro analyses hardly provide a faithful picture of the relative proportions and properties of cell subpopulations within individual tumors. Indeed, the biological behavior of malignant tumors (and their drug sensitivity) in vivo may be influenced to a significant extent by cell subpopulation interactions of different kinds (e.g., via short-range humoral factors or direct cell-cell contacts) which are unlikely to operate in the same way under cell culture conditions [43, 66, 67].

Besides the well-established inter- and intratumoral genotypic variability in terms of aneuploidy and karyotype abnormalities [79, 81, 113], heterogeneity of malignant cell populations has been observed with respect to a large variety of phenotypic properties. These include the morphological appearance of tumor cells (in cell culture and in tissues); their biochemical properties; their cell-surface receptors (e.g., for lectins) and hormone receptors; their immunogenicity and ability to escape the humoral and cellular immune reactions of the host; their tumorigenicity (in terms of the number of cells required to produce a tumor upon reimplantation into either isogeneic or immune-deficient or immune-suppressed hosts); their capacity to invade adjacent normal tissues and to metastasize; their capacity to communicate via intercellular communication channels (gap junctions); to synthesize specialized products (e.g., growth factors, pigment); and to respond to various differentiation stimuli (see, e.g., [11, 21, 45, 50, 84, 96]), the latter aspect being of particular interest as a basis for an alternative (or combined modality) approach to the use of cytocidal agents in cancer therapy. A very important obstacle to the successful clinical management of malignant disease is the large inter- and intratumor variability with respect to the relative sensitivity or resistance of malignant cell populations to cytocidal agents, including the development (selection for) drug-resistant cell subpopulations in the course of therapy (see, e.g., [42, 90]). From the recognition of this unfortunate situation stems the current trend towards the application of (more or less empirically designed) combinations chemotherapy as well as of combination of different treatment modalities [14, 31, 33, 34, 63, 68]. We shall briefly discuss three aspects of tumor cell heterogeneity that are of particular importance in relation to cancer chemotherapy, namely (a) the proliferative characteristics of malignant cell systems, (b) drug resistance on the basis of DNA (gene) amplification, and (c) the capacity of malignant cells for enzymatic repair of DNA structurally modified by chemotherapeutic agents.

Proliferative Parameters Relevant to Cancer Chemotherapy

The importance for chemotherapy of the proliferative characteristics of malignant tumors and leukemias, and of their variability, derives from the fact that most of the cytocidal agents presently used are more effective against proliferating cells (*P*-cells) than nonproliferating cells (*Q*-cells; see [5, 22, 23, 70−72, 93, 101]). Agents preferentially directed against *P*-cells usually interfere with molecular processes associated with particular phases of the cell cycle, i.e., G_1, S (DNA replication), G_2 or M (mitosis). These agents are, therefore, often termed cell cycle phase-specific, referring to the selective drug sensitivity exhibited by the target cells during a defined cell cycle-phase (not necessarily) identical with the cell cycle phase during which cell death subsequently occurs. A number of agents are antimetabolites, i.e., inhibitors of specific pathways of nucleic acid or protein synthesis (e.g., methotrexate (MTX), a potent inhibitor of dihydrofolate reductase (DHFR); [3, 8]) others (e.g., alkylating agents) bind to cellular DNA, thereby causing various types of structural DNA alterations (see, e.g., [16, 55, 74, 108]).

Several of the proliferative characteristics of malignant cell systems complicate successful chemotherapy [23, 70−72, 93, 101]. (a) Proliferating tumor cells proceed through the cell cycle asynchronously, i.e., cells in all phases of the cell cycle will be present when a cell cycle phase-specific drug is administered. (b) The distributions of intermitotic times of the *P*-cells in malignant tumors are generally broad, with large inter- and intratumor variations (including differences between primary tumors and individual metastases). (c) The size of the proliferative fraction (number of *P*-cells/total cell number) in malignant tumors is variable, but often surprisingly low (< 50%), while (d) the overall rate of cell loss (by cell death, exfolation, etc.) is usually surprisingly high (sometimes > 90% of the increase in cell number due to cell division is compensated by cell loss; note that in a normal, nonexpanding "steady state" cell system this value is 100%). No conclusive information is available regarding the relative rates of cell loss from the *P*-compartments vs the *Q*-compartments of malignant cell populations. (e) Although most of the *Q*-cells in tumors (but not necessarily in leukemias) are considered to have left the *P*-compartment due to nutrient deprivation (insufficient vascularization of the tumor tissue), other mechanisms (e.g., cell differentiation) may also be important determinants for the $P \rightarrow Q$ transition. Therefore, the reversibility of the *Q*-state (i.e., the probability of resuming a proliferative state), both in response to an improved nutritive situation and/or due to other as yet undefined control mechanisms, and the life expectancy of *Q*-tumor cells, remain important issues to be studied in more detail. It has been established, however, that *Q*-cells in tumors can be "recruited" into the cell cycle following chemotherapy [44, 52, 101]. Like the cells in the *P*-compartment, the *Q*-cell subpopulation thus recruited into cycle contains so-called clonogenic cells (i.e., cells capable of clonal proliferation; "tumor stem cells"), the fraction of which is again subjected to considerable intertumor variations. Tumor cells with a clonogenic potential (which are also responsible for the growth of metastases) must be the prime target of cancer therapy; yet these cells may be temporarily hidden in the *Q*-compartment and thus less accessible to cytocidal drugs.

Drug Resistance on the Basis of DNA (Gene) Amplification

The presence of drug-resistant cell subpopulations in malignant tumors, and their selective growth, or development, in the course of chemotherapy, are often responsible for ultimate therapeutic failure and thus represent one of the most serious problems associated with cancer therapy (see, e.g., [39, 42, 63, 68, 90]). For the most part in tumors of experimental animals and in cell culture systems, variant cells have been found whose increased drug resistance is due respectively, to (a) impaired drug uptake or increased outward drug transport (see, e.g., [17, 27, 38, 86, 92]); (b) increased intracellular enzymatic drug inactivation (see, e.g., [14, 94]); (c) reduced or lacking expression of drug-activating enzymes [12]; (d) structurally altered target enzymes with reduced affinity to the respective drugs [20, 25, 35, 36, 40, 49]; or (e) an elevated cellular concentration of target enzymes (increased rate of enzyme synthesis, e.g., due to amplification of the genes coding for the respective enzymes [2, 3, 7, 9, 15, 30, 37, 47, 53, 64, 82, 83, 95, 104]; and (f) an increased cellular capacity for DNA repair (see below).

Of the various molecular mechanisms that can render malignant cells drug resistant, the overproduction of target enzymes for specific inhibitors via amplification of the corresponding cellular genes deserves particular attention. Since the original work by Schimke and his group [3, 82, 83] who demonstrated that MTX-resistant cultured mouse cells contained an increased number of DHFR gene copies and exhibited a marked overproduction of DHFR, many studies — mainly on malignant human and rodent cell lines cultured in the presence of the respective enzyme inhibitors — have shown amplification of genes (with flanking DNA sequences of varying lengths) coding for different enzymes (e.g., DHFR; adenosine deaminase; glutamine synthetase; asparagine synthetase; and the multifunctional CAD protein, a polypeptide containing the enzymes carbamyl phosphate synthetase, aspartase transcarbamylase, and dihydroorotase [104]). The degree of enzyme overproduction can be very high (up to 10^4-fold); similarly copy numbers of the order of 10^2-10^3 have been observed for the corresponding amplified genes in extreme cases (see [30]). In many instances, amplified DNA sequences can be recognized microscopically in chromosome preparations, in the form of "double minute" chromosomes (DMs), extended homogeneously staining regions (HSRs), or abnormally banding regions [9, 10, 105]. However, neither the precise molecular mechanisms leading to the amplification of DNA sequences in eukaryotic cells are presently well-understood (although various models have been advanced [28, 78, 83, 97, 102, 111]), nor is there a definitive answer to the question of whether the selective pressure of a given agent (or a combination of agents) on the target cell population leads to a selective growth advantage for cells with previously amplified DNA sequences, or rather amplification is a direct consequence of drug interactions with the cells.

In spite of the strong suggestive evidence cited above, and although amplification obviously occurs in human malignant cells (see, e.g., [9, 30, 83]), it also remains undecided whether DNA amplification does indeed represent a major mechanism underlying the acquisition of drug resistance in human tumors. Barsoum and Varshavsky [6] have recently shown that the incidence of colony-forming, MTX-resistant, mouse 3T6 cells varies considerably depending on the conditions of selection, and can be greatly enhanced by certain physiological factors (e.g., insulin or epidermal growth factor), by a phorbol ester tumor promoter, and by transient cytotoxic treatment (which increases the probability of disproportionate DNA replication). On the basis of these data, which may be highly relevant to cancer chemotherapy, it appears possible that the development of drug resistance is also a function of the cellular microenvironment in the tumor tissue, and that the probability of the development of drug-resistant malignant cell subpopulations might be reduced by altering these conditions.

Capacity of Malignant Cells for Enzymatic Repair of DNA Structurally Modified by Chemotherapeutic Agents

By virtue of the interaction of their reactive metabolites with target-cell DNA, many DNA-reactive anticancer drugs cause DNA damage by specific alterations of DNA structure. These alterations may be toxic and lead to cell death.

Alternatively they may be mutagenic or, for example, interfere with the patterns of mRNA processing and DNA methylation, or cause inappropriate rearrangements at the level of genes and chromosomes, or disproportionate DNA replication leading to DNA amplification (see, e.g., [32, 55, 77, 88, 108]). The reaction products of a variety of chemical agents with DNA, notably of the alkylating N-nitroso compounds (see, e.g., [74, 88]), have been well characterized; however, in many other cases detailed structural analyses of the DNA adducts are still lacking. It may be predicted that all chemically induced structural alterations persisting in cellular DNA constitute potentially lethal damage, although the relative importance of different types of DNA lesions in terms of causing cell death is still a matter of discussion (see, e.g., [58, 85]). Error-free enzymatic repair of potentially lethal DNA damage caused both by DNA-reactive chemical agents (see, e.g., [32, 59]) or by ionizing radiation (see, e.g., [109]), is obviously an important cellular determinant in relation of the efficacy of cancer therapy. Malignant cells exhibiting low DNA repair capacity will accumulate more DNA damage, and be subjected to a higher mutation rate (in part lethal mutations, in part mutations leading to the establishment of phenotypically variant cell subpopulations, possibly including variants with increased repair capacity), while a high capability to repair potentially lethal DNA lesions will render malignant cells more resistant to the cytocidal effects of DNA-reactive agents. Not surprising in view of the large variety of structural alterations of DNA effected by different types of chemicals, the complex enzymology of DNA repair is still far from being fully understood. However, in the case of the repair of DNA damage caused by alkylating N-nitroso compounds, more precise information on the mechanisms and enzymes involved has become available during the past years (see, e.g., [59, 74]). These analyses are now being facilitated, and carried to the level of individual cells, by the development of high-affinity Mab specifically directed against defined DNA adducts [1, 76].

Is there evidence for inter- and intratumor variability with regard to the capacity of malignant cells to repair chemically modified DNA? As might be predicted, the available experimental data indicate that cellular DNA repair capacity is indeed part of the large spectrum of phenotypic properties that can vary in cancer cells. The repair of one of the best-studied DNA alkylation products, O^6-alkyldeoxyguanosine (O^6-alkyldGuo; see, e.g., [59, 74]), may serve as a case in point. Formation of this monoadduct appears, for example, to precede the appearance of DNA interstrand cross-links in cells exposed to chloroethylnitrosourea [24, 98, 114]. O^6-alkyldGuo is enzymatically removed from the DNA of normal rodent and human cells at different rates; most rapidly by hepatocytes, most slowly, if at all, by brain cells (see, e.g., [65, 74, 75]). We would expect this cell type-dependent capability to remove O^6-alkyldGuo to be reflected by similar intertumor variations, if the respective "O^6-alkyldGuo repair-phenotypes" of the normal cells of origin were retained in the cells through the multistep process of malignant transformation and remain stably expressed in the tumor cells. Note, however, that neither the range of variation of DNA repair capacity for different types of DNA adducts is well-established for the individual cells of normal tissues, nor has this range been sufficiently well defined with respect to interindividual variability within human populations [56, 61, 87, 100].

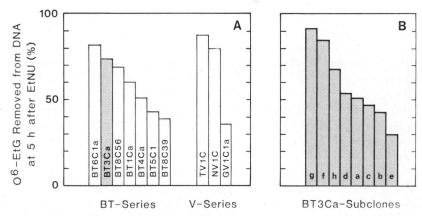

Fig. 1A, B. Cellular capacity for enzymatic removal from DNA of the alkylation product O^6-ethyldeoxyguanosine (O^6-EtdGuo), from malignant neuroectodermal cell lines induced by in vivo exposure of fetal BDIX-rat brain cells to N-ethyl-N-nitrosourea (EtNU). **A** *Abscissa:* Cloned cell lines *BT1Ca, Bt3Ca, BT4Ca, BT6C1a,* and *GV1C1a;* and cell lines *BT5C1, BT8C* (passage 39 and 56, respectively), *TV1C,* and *NV1C. Ordinate:* Percentage of O^6-EtdGuo removed from DNA at 5 h after a 20 min-incubation of near-confluent cells with EtNU (100 µg/ml), resulting in an "initial" O^6-EtdGuo/deoxyguanosine molar ratio in DNA of $\sim 8 \times 10^{-6}$ (= 100%). **B** *Abscissa:* Subclones *(a–h)* of cell line *BT3Ca* (see *A*). *Ordinate:* As in *A*

Furthermore, the stable expression of DNA repair enzymes in tumor cells appears unlikely in view of the general instability of malignant phenotypes.

Regarding the rate of enzymatic removal of O^6-alkyldGuo from cellular DNA, considerable differences have indeed been observed between a number of malignant cell lines in culture, including cell lines derived from human tumors [18, 19, 85, 91, 110, 112, 114], and in primary human tumor cells [110], ranging from the absence of measurable repair activity (Mer⁻ phenotype [18]) to various degrees of repair proficiency. Tumor cells are thus apparently capable of repairing chemically induced DNA lesions to varying degrees. Interestingly, we have recently found [47a] that a panel of malignant neuroectodermal rat cell lines (BT- and V-lines [57, 73]; see. Fig. 1A) remove the alkylation product O^6-ethyldeoxyguanosine (O^6-EtdGuo) from their DNA very efficiently, in fact in all cases more efficiently than rat liver (the normal rat tissue with the highest capacity for enzymatic removal of O^6-alkyldGuo from DNA). These malignant neuroectodermal cell lines originate from fetal (18th day of prenatal development) BDIX-rat brain cells and have either undergone tumorigenic conversion in cell culture after exposure to the alkylating N-nitroso carcinogen N-ethyl-N-nitrosourea (EtNU) in vivo (BT-lines) or are derived from neural tumors that developed in vivo after prenatal EtNU-exposure of BDIX-rats (V-lines). Both pre- and postnatal brain cells are, however, deficient with regard to the enzymatic removal of O^6-alkyldGuo from DNA [60, 73]. It appears, therefore, that in this cell system malignant transformation (or some as yet undefined stage of the process of malignant transformation preceding the ultimate development of tumorigenic phenotypes) is associated with the activation of O^6-alkyldGuo repair. Since these O^6-alkyldGuo repair-proficient neuroectodermal tumor cells were maintained and analyzed in cell culture, it should, however, also be investigated whether the expression of DNA repair enzymes may be modified by the continuous cultivation of (malignant) cells on plastic surfaces. The same studies on the capacity for O^6-EtdGuo repair of the malignant neuroectodermal BT- and V-rat cell lines have also provided information on the stability of the "O^6-EtdGuo repair-phenotype" of these cells [47a]. Subcloning in semisolid agar medium of one of the repair-proficient clonal BT-lines (BT3Ca) resulted in a panel of eight subclones which, upon reanalysis, again exhibited varying rates of O^6-EtdGuo removal from DNA (see Fig. 1B). This rapid diversification of cellular O^6-EtdGuo repair capacities in the course of the cell generations required for subcloning indicates instability of the O^6-alkyldGuo repair phenotype. This observation supports the assumption that malignant cell subpopulations varying with respect to DNA repair capacity may continuously develop in the course of tumor growth and progression.

E. coli (and other bacteria) respond to multiple exposures to low doses of alkylating agents with an increased expression of DNA repair enzymes ("adaptive response" [13]). This, in turn, leads to an increased resistance to subsequent high doses of these agents in terms of cell killing and mutagenesis. Could a similar "adaptive resistance" ensue after repeated application of chemotherapeutic drugs in cancer patients? In this respect it is of interest that the induction of an "adaptive response" has recently been reported for some transformed mammalian cell lines [51, 80], including rat hepatoma cells [59]. It remains to be seen whether this phenomenon is of general importance in relation to the chemotherapy of human cancer.

Conclusions

The phenotypic heterogeneity of cell subpopulations and individual cells in malignant cell systems, and the plasticity of malignant phenotypes (i.e., the extraordinary capability of cancer cells for adaptation to changing microenvironmental conditions), represent major problems for chemotherapy with cytotoxic drugs. Major obstacles to successful chemotherapy are the lack of drug specificity for malignant cells vs critical normal (stem) cells, the differential accessibility of tumor cells for drugs administered systemically, the variable proliferative characteristics of tumor cell populations, the selection for (or development of) drug-resistant tumor cell subpopulations in the course of chemotherapy, and the differential capacity of cancer cells for DNA repair. It appears difficult to overcome these problems completely with current chemotherapeutic approaches, although progress may be expected from further optimization of therapeutic procedures in certain areas.

Acknowledgements. Research in the authors' laboratory was supported by the Deutsche Forschungsgemeinschaft (SFB 102/A1 and A9).

References

1. Adamkiewicz J, Ahrens O, Huh N, Nehls P, Spiess E, Rajewsky MF (1984) High-affinity monoclonal antibodies for the specific recognition and quantitation of deoxynucleosides structurally modified by N-nitroso compounds. In: N-Nitroso compounds: Occurrence and biological effects. IARC Scientific Publ, Internat Agency for Res on Cancer, Lyon (in press)
2. Albrecht AM, Biedler JL, Hutchison DJ (1982) Two different species of dihydrofolate reductase in mammalian cells differentially resistant to amethopterin and methasquin. Cancer Res 32: 1539–1546

3. Alt FW, Kellems RE, Bertino JR, Schimke RT (1978) Selective multiplication of dihydrofolate reductase genes in methotrexate-resistant variants of cultured murine cells. J Biol Chem 253: 1357–1370
4. Barlogie B, Raber MN, Schumann J, Johnson TS, Drewinko B, Swartzendruber DE, Göhde W, Andreeff M, Freireich EJ (1983) Flow cytometry in clinical cancer research. Cancer Res 43: 3982–3997
5. Barranco SC, Novak JK (1974) Survival response of dividing and nondividing mammalian cells after treatment with hydroxyurea, arabinosylcytosine, or adriamycin. Cancer Res 34: 1616–1618
6. Barsoum J, Varshavsky A (1983) Mitogenic hormones and tumor promoters greatly increase the incidence of colony-forming cells bearing amplified dihydrofolate reductase genes. Proc Natl Acad Sci USA 80: 5330–5334
7. Beach LR, Palmiter RD (1981) Amplification of the metallothionein-I gene in cadmium-resistant mouse cells. Proc Natl Acad Sci USA 78: 2110–2114
8. Bertino JR (1963) The mechanism of action of the folate antagonists in man. Cancer Res 23: 1286–1306
9. Biedler JL, Spengler BA (1976) Metaphase chromosome anomaly: Association with drug resistance and cell-specific products. Science 191: 185–187
10. Biedler JL (1982) Evidence for transient or prolonged extrachromosomal existence of amplified DNA sequences in antifolate-resistant, vincristine-resistant, and human neuroblastoma cells. In: Schimke RT (ed) Gene amplification. Cold Spring Harbor Laboratory, Cold Spring Harbor, New York, pp 39–95
11. Breitman TR, Kenne BR, Hemmi H (1983) Retinoic acid-induced differentiation of fresh human leukemic cells and the human myelomonocytic leukemic cell lines, HL-60, U-937, and THP-1. Cancer Surveys 2: 263–291
12. Brockman RW (1974) Mechanisms of resistance. In: Sartorelli AC, Johns DG (eds) Antineoplastic and immunosuppressive agents. Springer, Berlin, pp 352–410
13. Carins J, Robins P, Sedgwick B, Talmud P (1981) Inducible repair of alkylated DNA. Progr Nucleic Acids Res Mol Biol 26: 237–243
14. Cheng Y-C, Brockman RW (1983) Mechanisms of drug resistance and collateral sensitivity: Bases for development of chemotherapeutic agents. In: Cheng Y-C et al. (eds) Development of target-oriented anticancer drugs. Raven Press, New York, pp 107–117
15. Cowan KH, Goldsmith ME, Levine RM, Aitken SC, Douglass E, Clendeninn N, Nienhuis AW, Lippman ME (1982) Dihydrofolate reductase gene amplification and possible rearrangement in estrogen-responsive methotrexate-resistant human breast cancer cells. J Biol Chem 257: 15079–15084
16. Crooke ST, Prestayko AW (eds) (1980) Cancer and chemotherapy, vol I. Academic, New York
17. Danø K (1973) Active outward transport of daunomycin in resistant Ehrlich ascites tumor cells. Biochim Biophys Acta 323: 466–483
18. Day RS III, Ziolkowski CHJ, Scudiero DA, Meyer SA, Lubiniecki AS, Girardi AG, Galloway SM, Bynum GD (1980) Defective repair of alkylated DNA by human tumor and SV40 transformed human cell strains. Nature 288: 724–727
19. Day RS III, Yarosh DB, Ziolkowski CHJ (1984) Relationship of methyl purines produced by MNNG in adenovirus 5 DNA to viral inactivation in repair-deficient (Mer⁻) human tumor cell strains. Mutat Res 131: 45–52
20. Derse D, Bastow KF, Cheng Y-C (1982) Characterization of the DNA polymerase induced by a group of herpes simplex virus type I variants selected for growth in the presence of phosphonoformic acid. J Biol Chem 257: 10251–10260
21. Dexter DL, Calabresi P (1982) Intraneoplastic diversity. Biochim Biophys Acta 695: 97–112
22. Drewinko B, Patchen M, Yang L-Y, Barlogie B (1981) Differential killing efficacy of twenty antitumor drugs on proliferating and nonproliferating human tumor cells. Cancer Res 41: 2328–2333

23. Epifanova OI, Smolenskaya IN, Polunovsky VA (1978) Responses of proliferating and nonproliferating Chinese hamster cells to cytotoxic agents. Br J Cancer 37: 377–385

24. Erickson LC, Laurent G, Sharkey NA, Kohn KW (1980) DNA crosslinking and monoadduct repair in nitrosourea-treated human tumour cells. Nature 288: 727–729

25. Eriksson S, Gudas LJ, Ullman B, Clift SM, Martin DW Jr (1981) Deoxy-ATP-resistant ribonucleotide reductase of mutant mouse lymphoma cells. J Biol Chem 256: 10184–10188

26. Fialkow PJ (1980) Clonal and stem cell origin of blood cell neoplasms. Contemp Hematol Oncol 1: 1–46

27. Flintoff WF, Davidson SV, Siminovitch L (1976) Isolation and partial characterization of three methotrexate-resistant phenotypes from Chinese hamster ovary cells. Somat Cell Genet 2: 245–261

28. Flintoff WF, Livingston E, Duff C, Worton RG (1984) Moderate-level gene amplification in methotrexate-resistant Chinese hamster ovary cells is accompanied by chromosomal translocations at or near the site of the amplified DHFR gene. Mol Cell Biol 4: 69–76

29. Foulds L (1956) The histologic analysis of mammary tumors of mice. II. The histologic of responsiveness and progression. J Natl Cancer Inst 17: 713–756

30. Fox M (1984) Gene amplification and drug resistance. Nature 307: 212–213

31. Frei E, III (1982) Models and the clinical dilemmas. In: Fidler J, White R (eds) Design of models for testing cancer therapeutic agents. Van Nostrand, New York, pp 248–259

32. Friedberg EC, Bridges BA (eds) (1983) Cellular responses to DNA damage. Liss, New York

33. Goldie JH, Coldman AJ, Gudauskas GA (1982) Rationale for the use of alternating non-crossresistant chemotherapy. Cancer Treatm Rep 66: 439–449

34. Goldin A (1980) Combined chemotherapy. Oncology (Suppl 1) 37: 3–8

35. Gupta RS, Flintoff WF, Siminovitch L (1977) Purification and properties of dihydrofolate reductase from methotrexate-sensitive and methotrexate-resistant Chinese hamster ovary cells. Can J Biochem 55: 445–452

36. Haber DA, Beverly SM, Kiely ML, Schimke RT (1981) Porperties of an altered dihydrofolate reductase encoded by amplified genes in cultured mouse fibroblasts. J Biol Chem 256: 9501–9510

37. Hänggi UJ, Littlefield JW (1976) Altered regulation of the rate of synthesis of dihydrofolate reductase in methotrexate-resistant hamster cells. J Biol Chem 251: 3075–3080

38. Harrap KR, Hill BT, Furness MES, Hart LI (1971) Sites of action of amethopterin: Intrinsic and acquired drug resistance. Ann NY Acad Sci 186: 312–324

39. Hart IR, Fidler IJ (1981) The implications of tumor heterogeneity for studies on the biology and therapy of cancer metastasis. Biochim Biophys Acta 651: 37–50

40. Heidelberger Ch, Kaldor G, Mukherjee KL, Danneberg PB (1960) Studies on fluorinated pyrimidines. XI. In vitro studies on tumor resistance. Cancer Res 20: 903–909

41. Heppner GH, Dexter BL, De Nucci T, Miller FR, Calabresi P (1978) Heterogeneity in drug sensitivity among tumor cell subpopulations of a single mammary tumor. Cancer Res 38: 3758–3763

42. Heppner GH (1979) The challenge of tumor heterogeneity. In: Bulbrook RD, Taylor DJ (eds) Commentaries on research in breast cancer. Liss, New York, pp 177–191

43. Heppner GH, Miller BE, Miller FR (1983) Tumor subpopulation interactions in neoplasmas. Biochim Biophys Acta 695: 215–226

44. Hermens AF, Barendsen GW (1978) The proliferative status and clonogenic capacity of tumour cells in a transplantable rhabdomyosarcoma in the rat before and after irradiation with 800 rad of x-rays. Cell Tissue Kinet 11: 83–100

45. Hoal E, Wilson L, Dowdie EB (1982) Variable effects of retinoids on two pigmenting human melanoma cell lines. Cancer Res 42: 5191–5195

46. Holtzer H, Rubinstein N, Fellini S, Yeoh G, Chi S, Birnbaum J, Okayama M (1975) Lineages, quantal cell cycles and the generation of cell diversity. Q Rev Biophys 8: 523–557

47. Hunt SW, Hoffee PA (1983) Amplification of adenosine deaminase gene sequences in deoxycoformycin-resistant rat hepatoma cells. J Biol Chem 258: 13185–13192

47a. Huh, Rajewsky MF (in preparation)
48. Ibsen KM, Fishman WH (1979) Developmental gene expression in cancer. Biochim Biophys Acta 560: 243−280
48a. Immunol Rev 62: 5−185, 1982
49. Jackson RC, Niethammer D (1977) Acquired methotrexate resistance in lymphoblasts resulting from altered kinetic properties of dihydrofolate reductase. Eur J Cancer 13: 567−575
50. Jetten AM, De Luca LM (1983) Induction of differentiation of embryonal carcinoma cells by retinol: Possible mechanisms. Biochim Biophys Res Comm 114: 593−599
51. Kaina B (1982) Enhanced survival and reduced mutation and aberration-frequencies induced in V79 Chinese hamster cells pre-exposed to low levels of methylating agents. Mutat Res 93: 195−211
52. Kallman RF, Combs CA, Franko AJ, Furlong BM, Kelley SD, Kemper HL, Miller RG, Rapacchietta D, Schoenfeld D, Takahashi M (1980) Evidence for the recruitment of noncycling clonogenic tumor cells. In: Meyn RE, Withers HR (eds) Radiation biology in cancer research. Raven, New York, pp 397−414
53. Kaufman RJ, Brown PC, Schimke RT (1979) Amplifid dihydrofolate reductase genes in unstably methotrexate-resistant cells are associated with double minute chromosomes. Proc Natl Acad Sci USA 76: 5669−5673
54. Klein C, Klein E (1984) Oncogene activation and tumor progression. Carcinogenesis 5: 429−435
55. Kohn KW (1979) DNA as a target in cancer chemotherapy: Measurement of macromolecular DNA damage produced in mammalian cells by anticancer agents and carcinogens. Meth in Cancer Res 16: 291−345
56. Krokan H, Haugen Å, Myrnes B, Guddal PH (1983) Repair of premutagenic DNA lesions in human fetal tissues: Evidence for low levels of O^6-methylguanine-DNA methyltransferase and uracil-DNA glycosylase activity in some tissues. Carcinogenesis 4: 1559−1564
57. Laerum OD, Rajewsky MF (1975) Neoplastic transformation of fetal rat brain cells in culture following exposure to ethylnitrosourea in vivo. J Natl Cancer Inst 55: 1177−1187
58. Laval F, Lavel J (1984) Adaptive response in mammalian cells: Cross-reactivity of different pretreatment and cytotoxicity as contrasted to mutagenicity. Proc Natl Acad Sci USA (in press)
59. Lehmann AR, Karran P (1981) DNA repair. Int Rev Cytol 72: 101−146
60. Müller R, Rajewsky MF (1983) Elimination of O^6-ethylguanine from the DNA of brain, liver, and other rat tissues exposed to ethylnitrosourea at different stages of prenatal development. Cancer Res 43: 2897−2904
61. Myrnes B, Giercksky KE, Krokan H (1983) Interindividual variation in the activity of O^6-methylguanine-DNA methyltransferase and uracil DNA-glycosylase in human organs. Carcinogenesis 4: 1565−1568
62. Nowell PC (1976) The clonal evolution of tumor cell populations Acquired genetic lability permits stepwise selection of variant sublines and underlies tumor progression. Science 194: 23−28
63. Owens AH Jr, Coffey DS, Baylin SB (eds) Tumor cell heterogeneity: Origins and implications. Bristol-Meyers Cancer Symposia. Academic, New York
64. Padgett RA, Wahl GM, Coleman PF, Stark GR (1979) N-(phosphonacetyl)-L-aspartate-resistant hamster cells overaccumulate a single mRNA coding for the multifunctional protein that catalyzes the first steps of UMP synthesis. J Biol Chem 254: 974−980
65. Pegg AE (1983) Alkylation and subsequent repair of DNA after exposure to dimethylnitrosamine and related carcinogens. Rev Biochem Toxicol 5: 83−133
66. Poste G, Doll J, Fidler IJ (1981) Interactions between clonal subpopulations affect the stability of the metastatic phenotype in polyclonal populations of B16 melanoma cells. Proc Natl Acad Sci USA 78: 6226−6230
67. Poste G, Tzeng J, Doll J, Greig R, Rieman D, Zeidman I (1982) Evolution of tumor cell heterogeneity during progressive growth of individual lung metastases. Proc Natl Acad Sci USA 79: 6574−6578

68. Poste G, Greig R (1983) The experimental and clinical implications of cellular heterogeneity in malignant tumors. J Cancer Res Clin Oncol 106: 159–170

69. Rabes HM, Bücher Th, Hartmann A, Linke I, Dünnwald M (1982) Clonal growth of carcinogen-induced enzyme deficient preneoplastic cell populations in mouse liver. Cancer Res 42: 3220–3227

70. Rajewsky MF (1972) Proliferative parameters of mammalian cell systems and their role in tumor growth and carcinogenesis. Z Krebsforsch 78: 12–30

71. Rajewsky MF (1974) Proliferative properties of malignant cell systems. In: Altmann HW et al. (eds) Handbuch der Allgem Pathologie, Tumors I, vol VI/5. Springer, Berlin Heidelberg New York, pp 289–325

72. Rajewsky MF (1975) Proliferative parameters relevant to cancer therapy. Rec Res Cancer Res 52: 156–171

73. Rajewsky MF, Goth R, Laerum OD, Biesmann H, Hülser DF (1976) Molecular and cellular mechanisms in nervous system-specific carcinogenesis by N-ethyl-N-nitrosourea. In: Magee PN, Takayama S, Sugimura T, Matsushima T (eds) Fundamentals of cancer prevention. University of Tokyo Press, Tokyo, pp 313–334

74. Rajewsky MF (1980) Specificity of DNA damage in chemical carcinogenesis. In: Montesano R, Bartsch H, Tomatis L (eds) Molecular and cellular aspects of carcinogen screening tests. IARC Scientific Publ No. 27. Internat Agency for Res on Cancer, Lyon, pp 41–54

75. Rajewsky MF (1983) Structural modifications and repair of DNA in neuro-oncogenesis by N-ethyl-N-nitrosourea. Recent Results Cancer Res 42: 5236–5239

76. Rajewsky MF, Adamkiewicz J, Drosdziok W, Eberhardt W, Langenberg U (1983) High-affinity monoclonal antibodies directed against DNA components structurally modified by alkylating N-nitroso compounds. In: Milman HA, Sell S (eds) Application of biological markers to carcinogen testing. Plenum, New York, pp 373–385

77. Riggs AD, Jones PA (1983) 5-Methylcytosine, gene regulation, and cancer. Adv Cancer Res 40: 1–30

78. Roberts JM, Buck B, Axel R (1983) A structure for amplified DNA. Cell 33: 53–63

79. Rowley JD, Ultman J (eds) (1983) Chromosomes and cancer: From molecules to man. Academic, New York

80. Samson L, Schwartz JL (1980) Evidence for an adaptive DNA repair pathway in CHO and human skin fibroblast cell lines. Nature 287: 861–863

81. Sandberg AA (ed) (1980) The chromosomes in human cancer and leukemia. Elsevier/North-Holland, Amsterdam

82. Schimke RT (1980) Gene amplification and drug resistance. Sci Am 243: 50–59

83. Schimke RT (ed) (1982) Gene amplification. Cold Spring Harbor Laboratory, Cold Spring Harbor, New York

84. Schwartz EL, Sartorelli AC (1982) Structure-activity relationships for the induction of differentiation of HL-60 human acute promyelocytic leukemia cells by anthracyclines. Cancer Res 42: 2651–2655

85. Scudiero DA, Meyer SA, Clatterbuck BE, Mattern MR, Ziolkowski CHJ, Day RS III (1984) Relationship of DNA repair phenotypes of human fibroblast and tumor strains to killing by N-methyl-N'-nitro-N-nitrosoguanidine. Cancer Res 44: 961–969

86. Seeber S, Osieka R, Schmidt CG, Achterrath W, Crooke ST (1982) In vivo resistance towards anthracyclines, etoposide, and cis-diamminedichloroplatinum (II). Cancer Res 42: 4719–4725

87. Setlow RB (1983) Variations in DNA repair among humans. In: Harris CC, Autrup H (eds) Human carcinogenesis. Academic, New York, pp 231–254

88. Singer B, Kuśmierek JT (1982) Chemical mutagenesis. Ann Rev Biochem 52: 655–693

89. Siracký J (1979) An approach to the problem of heterogeneity of human tumour cell populations. Br J Cancer 39: 570–577

90. Skipper H (1983) The forty-year-old mutation theory of Luria and Delbrück and its pertinence to cancer chemotherapy. Adv Cancer Res 40: 331–363

91. Sklar RM, Strauss BS (1983) O^6-methylguanine removal by competent and incompetent human lymphoblastoid lines from the same male individual. Cancer Res 43: 3316–3320

92. Skovsgaard T (1978) Mechanisms of resistance to daunorubicin in Ehrlich ascites tumor cells. Cancer Res 38: 1785−1791
93. Steel GC (1977) Growth kinetics of tumours. Cell population kinetics in relation to the growth and treatment of cancer. Clarendon, Oxford
94. Steuart CD, Burke PJ (1971) Cytidine deaminase and the development of resistance to arabinosyl cytisine. Nature (New Biol) 233: 109−110
95. Su TS, Bock H-GO, O'Brien WE, Beaudet AL (1981) Cloning of cDNA for argininosuccinate synthetase mRNA and study of enzyme overproduction in a human cell line. J Biol Chem 256: 11826−11831
96. Symonds G, Sachs L (1982) Autoinduction of differentiation in myeloid leukemic cells: Restoration of normal coupling between growth and differentiation in leukemic cells that constitutively produce their own growth-inducing protein. EMBO J 1: 1343−1346
97. Tartoff K (1975) Redundant genes. Ann Rev. Genet 9: 355−387
98. Tong WP, Kirk MP, Ludlum DB (1981) Formation of the crosslink 1-[N^3-deoxycyti-dyl]-2-[N^1-deoxyguanosinyl]-ethane in DNA treated with N-N-bis(2-chloroethyl)-N-nitroso-urea. Cancer Res 42: 3102−3105
99. Ursprung H (ed) (1968) The stability of the differentiated state. Springer, Berlin
100. Vahakangas K, Autrup H, Harris CC (1984) Interindividual variation in carcinogen metabolism, DNA damage, and DNA repair. In: Methods of monitoring human exposure to carcinogenic and mutagenic agents. IARC Scientific Publ, Internat Agency for Res on Cancer, Lyon (in press)
101. Valeriote F, van Putten L (1975) Proliferation-dependent cytotoxicity of anticancer agents: A review. Cancer Res 35: 2619−2630
102. Varshavsky A (1981) On the possibility of metabolic control of replicon "misfiring": Relationship to emergence of malignant phenotypes in mammalian cell lineages. Proc Natl Acad Sci USA 76: 3673−3677
103. Vitetta ES, Krolick KA, Miyama-Inaba M, Cushley W, Uhr JW (1983) Immunotoxins: A new approach to cancer therapy. Science 219: 644−650
104. Wahl GM, Padgett RA, Stark GR (1979) Gene amplification causes overproduction of the first three enzymes of UMP synthesis in N-(phosphonacetyl)-L-aspartate-resistant hamster cells. J Biol Chem 254: 8679−8689
105. Wahl GM, de Saint Vincent BR, DeRose ML (1984) Effect of chromosomal position on amplification of transfected genes in animal cells. Nature 307: 516−520
106. Wallen CA, Higashikubo R, Dethlefsen LA (1984a) Murine mammary tumour cells in vitro. I. The development of a quiescent state. Cell Tissue Kinet 17: 65−77
107. Wallen CA, Higashikubo R, Dethlefsen LA (1984b) Murine mammary tumour cells in vitro. II. Recruitment of quiescent cells. Cell Tissue Kinet 17: 79−89
108. Waring MJ (1981) DNA modification and cancer. Ann Rev Biochem 50: 159−192
109. Weichselbaum RR, Schmidt A, Little JB (1982) Cellular repair factors influencing radio-curability of human malignant tumours. Br J Cancer 45: 10−16
110. Wiestler O, Kleihues P, Pegg AE (1984) O^6-alkylguanine-DNA alkyltransferase activity in human brain and brain tumors. Carcinogenesis 5: 121−124
111. Woodcock DM, Cooper IA (1981) Evidence for double replication of chromosomal DNA segments as a general consequence of DNA replication inhibition. Cancer Res 41: 2483−2490
112. Yarosh DB, Rice M, Day RS III, Foote RS, Mitra S (1984) O^6-methylguanine-DNA methyltransferase in human cells. Mutat Res 131: 27−36
113. Yunis JJ (1983) The chromosomal basis of human neoplasia. Science 221: 227−236
114. Zlotogorski C, Erickson LC (1983) Pretreatment of normal human fibroblasts and human colon carcinoma cells with MNNG allows chloroethylnitrosourea to produce NA interstrand cross-links not observed in cells treated with chloroethylnitrosourea alone. Carcinogenesis 4: 759−764

Impact of Early Detection of Breast Cancer on Adjuvant Chemotherapy

W. H. Hartmann

Department of Pathology, Vanderbildt University, School of Medicine, Nashville, TX 37232, USA

It has only been since the late 1940s that chemotherapy emerged as part of the therapeutic armamentarium for treating patients with disseminated breast cancer. Recently, however, the role of chemotherapeutic agents in prolonging life and disease-free interval in patients with breast cancer has come to be questioned.

All of us who are interested in the medical and biological problems of mammary carcinoma have one clearly stated goal: to eliminate the disease. To eliminate cancer! To do so would, of course, eliminate the need for chemotherapy and chemotherapists. I would like to discuss some strategies to hasten that day.

Human breast cancer, as a patient-care and biological problem can, for convenience, be thought of as having five phases: prevention, detection, diagnosis, treatment, and rehabilitation. Over the past 100 years, our attention has been focused on treatment, diagnosis and, more recently, rehabilitation.

Of these, treatment has occupied center stage since the turn of the century, with surgery the leading and most commonly employed modality to be supplemented by and complemented with radiotherapy and chemotherapy in certain defined situations. The arguments as to what is most appropriate in which situation need not concern us here.

As survival and morbidity data accumulated, the need for precision in diagnosis stimulated many studies, and at present there is reason to believe that diagnostic credibility among pathologists is quite good, and further reason to suggest that subclassification beyond invasive carcinoma is appropriate and necessary in the statistical analysis of large series [3]. Having the carcinoma subclassified [3] is significant in deciding on treatment of a patient.

Rehabilitation received its impetus beginning in the 1950s, in part due to the Reach to Recovery Program of the American Cancer Society – now a worldwide program.

It is my contention that treatment, diagnosis, and rehabilitation have been, at this time, fully exploited but do remain as areas where improvement can be made when further scientific breakthroughs have occurred.

That leaves detection and prevention as the two possible areas for aggressive study. Advances in X-ray technology have made breast cancer screening not only possible, but safe. In 1973, the American Cancer Society and the National Cancer Institute (US) initiated a breast cancer detection and demonstration project (BCDDP), stimulated by the results of the breast study of the health Insurance Plan of New York. The BCDDP was conceived of as demonstrating to both the American public and American physicians that screening for breast carcinoma was feasible. The incidence of breast cancer in the United

Table 1. Subclassification of breast carcinomas (modified from Baker [1], Table 16)

Lymph nodes	Noninfiltrating carcinoma	Infiltrating carcinoma < 1 cm	Other infiltrating carcinomas	Total
+	15	53	631	699
−	422	268	1,376	2,066
Unknown/unreported	345	50	397	792
Total	782	371	2,404	3,557

States is 75/100,000 population, with a death rate of 24/100,000 population. The data for Switzerland are almost identical making it a common disease and a serious disease for women and physicians of both countries [6]. The details of the project have been the subject of other reports [2]. Briefly, 280,000 women aged 35−74 were to have a history taken and a physical examination, be taught breast selfexamination, have X-ray studies done of their breasts, have recommendations made for further investigation based on these studies, and, be followed up. A quality-control program for pathology (PQCP) was established and began to function in 1978. Although a 5-year summary report of the BCDDP has appeared [1], review of the pathology material for precise classification continues. Follow-up data have not yet been reported even though, as noted, the program began in 1973.

There were 4,443 breast carcinoma recorded at the Data Management Center as of September 1981 (3,557 carcinomas were detected by the BCDDP and 886 were detected outside the project). Carcinomas were detected in 1,082 (32%) women who had not reached the age of 50. Of the cancers detected, 782 were noninfiltrating (in situ carcinoma); 371 were infiltrating and measured less than 1 cm in diameter. The rest were infiltrating carcinomas equal to or greater than 1 cm in diameter, or their size was not recorded.

Physical examination alone was able to detect only 8.7% (308 of 3,557) of the carcinomas, while mammography alone or in combination with physical examination was able to detect 88.9%.

The patients were treated at many hospitals and by various procedures. Nodal status is known for 2,765 of the breast carcinoma patients; 576 patients did not have nodes examined, and there is no information on 216. Of all the BCDDP-detected carcinomas whose lymph node status is known, 2,066 (75%) had negative lymph nodes (see Table 1). This is a number much smaller than that usually seen in unscreened populations [4]. Of significance is the fact that 53 of 321 (16.5%) invasive carcinomas of less than 1 cm in diameter have positive axillary lymph nodes. Only 631 of 2,007 (31.4%) carcinomas, all larger than 1 cm in diameter and for which information about the states of lymph nodes is known, had positive lymph nodes.

Cody et al. [3] reported a series of 544 patients who were operated on, not as a result of a screening procedure (as near as I can determine), and 41% of them had axillary lymph node metastasis. The data presented do not allow correlation with size.

The PQCP has material available on almost 500 of the 782 BCDDP patients with in situ carcinomas. To date, all cases of in situ carcinoma with lymph node metastasis are intraductal carcinoma. No case of in situ lobular carcinoma has lymph node metastasis.

My purpose is to establish the fact that screening can detect mammary carcinoma at a stage when the disease is localized and more amenable to simpler therapeutic strategies. Although I have focused on data from the American studies, similar data are available from other screening projects; what is lacking, to date, is significant follow-up information.

If we were to focus detection strategies on high-risk populations, would there be further improvement? Probably not! This also has implications for prevention.

In 1959, the American Cancer Society began a large-scale prospective study on cancer incidence. Seidman and associates [5] have recently published an analysis of these data as they apply to breast carcinoma. Participation was restricted to persons 30 years or older who lived in a household in which at least one person 45 or older was also involved in the study. Follow-up information was available on 98% of the study population of 365,812 white women out of a total population of 571,716) over a 12-year period. These women developed 3,130 new cases of breast carcinoma during the 6-year study period. Of the risk factors believed to be operative in breast cancer patients, the following ten were subjected to review:

1. History of breast cancer in mother and/or sister.
2. History of breast surgery for a benign condition.
3. Being Jewish.
4. Menopause at age 50 or older.
5. Menarche before age 12.
6. Never married.
7. First live birth at age 30 or nulliparity.
8. College degree.
9. Daily alcohol consumption.
10. A relative weight index of 110 or more.

The absence of these 10 risk factors.

"When we considered the risk factors alone or in combination, they explained only 21% of the breast cancer risk among women aged 30–54 and 29% among women aged 55–84" [5]. Only 21%–29% of all subsequent mammary carcinomas could be attributed to these risk factors! The obverse is both depressing and significant for everyday practice: It is that risk factors for mammary carcinoma, as we know them today, will not explain the occurrence of 71%–79% of all breast carcinomas; i.e., 71%–79% of mammary carcinomas occurring in American white women are associated with no known risk factors! It is clear that although strategies for prevention are both desperately needed and appropriate, known risk factors will not serve to readily identify a high-risk population. The physician treating female patients will still have to assume that the presence of breasts is a necessary and sufficient risk factor and examine and further study the patient. Screening remains our most effective and productive strategy for the successful eradication of breast carcinoma.

Available data lead to the following conclusions:
1. Breast carcinoma is a very common disease in women.
2. Incidence and mortality of breast carcinoma remain high in the United States and Switzerland.
3. Our common goal is the elimination of the disease.
4. To achieve this goal, strategies will have to be directed at detection.
5. Mammography remains the most readily available means of detection at the present time.

6. Breast selfexamination, although far cheaper and easier to utilize as a detection strategy, remains to be proven as effective.
7. Chemotherapists should join with other physicians and direct their efforts at effectively screening all adult women for breast cancer.

References

1. Baker LM (1982) Breast cancer detection demonstration project: Five-year summary report. CA 32: 194–225
2. Byrd BF Jr (1981) Breast cancer detection center projects in breast cancer, vol 4. Plenum, New York
3. Cody HS III et al. (1982) The continuing importance of adequate surgery for operable breast cancer: significant salvage of node positive patients in that adjuvant chemotherapy. CA 32: 242–252
4. Fisher B et al. (1969) Cancer of the breast. Size of neoplasm and prognosis. Cancer 24: 1071–1080
5. Seidman H et al. (1982) A different perspective on breast cancer risk factors: some implications of the non-attributable risk. CA 32: 301–313
6. Silverberg E (1984) Cancer statistics, 1984. CA 34: 7–23

Contribution of Prognostic Factors to Adjuvant Chemotherapy in Breast Cancer*

G. Bonadonna and P. Valagussa

Istituto Nazionale per lo Studio e la Cura dei Tumori, Via Venezian 1, 20133 Milano, Italy

Introduction

The prognostic factors in women with primary breast cancer are numerous [32]. In most reports published over the past 20 years they were assessed on retrospective evaluation of series whose staging, treatment and follow-up were often not homogeneous. However, in recent years prospective randomized clinical trials undertaken in patients with resectable breast cancer provided the opportunity to reassess the adequacy of given prognostic subgroups. In particular, through the analysis of large case series, the National Surgical Adjuvant Breast Project (NSABP) has contributed more than any other research group in systematically assessing and comparing the value of different prognostic variables [12–18].

In this report we briefly review and discuss the prognostic discriminants which may be utilized in the selection of women for adjuvant chemotherapy (Table 1).

Axillary Node Metastases

Number of Positive Nodes

Numerous reports have emphasized that in resectable breast cancer the probability of distant relapse and mortality is related to the pathological status of axillary lymph nodes, and the degree of nodal involvement remains the predominant indicator of patient outcome (Table 2).

More recently, the NSABP [12] and the Milan [7] groups have stressed the need for further subdivision of women with > 3 positive nodes, an observation made a few years ago by the M.D. Anderson group [9]. Figure 1 shows the probability of relapse-free survival (RFS) and of total survival at 9 years after mastectomy related to the degree of nodal involvement of 845 women enrolled in the first two Milan randomized adjuvant programs [7]. Irrespective of primary treatment (surgery alone or surgery plus CMF [cyclophosphamide + methotrexate + 5-fluorouracil] 12 or 6 cycles), there was little difference between patients having one, two, or three positive nodes. In contrast, women with 4–10 nodes

---

* Supported in part by Contract N01-CM-07338 with the Division of Cancer Treatment, National Cancer Institute, National Institutes of Health

Table 1. Main discriminants to be considered for adjuvant chemotherapy

- Axillary nodal metastases
  1−3 vs > 4 vs > 10 nodes
  Micro- vs macrometastases
- In the absence of nodal metastases:
  Receptor status
  Histologic grade
  Tumor necrosis
  Vascular invasion
  Labeling index
- Stage III (T_{3b}−T_4)

Table 2. Influence of axillary lymph node involvement on recurrence of breast cancer after primary surgery

Nodal status	Relapse rate (%)			
	18 months	3 years	5 years	10 years
All patients	18	35	42	51
Negative	5	15	20	25
1−3 positive	16	40	52	66
≥ 4 positive	44	65	75	85

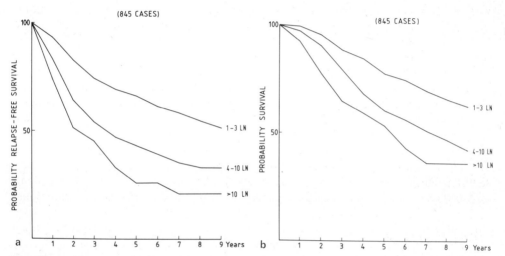

Fig. 1a, b. Nine-year results as function of number of axillary nodes. **a** relapse-free survival; **b** overall survival

fared significantly better compared with those having more than 10 nodes infiltrated ($P = 0.02$ for RFS and $P = 0.03$ for survival). It is important to mention that in the Milan series, where clinical T_{2a} primaries were predominant (72%) compared with T_{1a} (13%) and T_{3a} (15%), women having 1−3 positive nodes accounted for 65% of all patients with axillary involvement, 4−10 for 27%, and > 10 for 8%.

The NSABP group has recently reported a similar, but more detailed, analysis on 505 women participating in one or the other of two prospective randomized clinical trials coded as B-04 and B-05 [12]. The 5-year results, related to nodal subgroups, showed findings similar to those reported by the Milan group relative to the subset with 1−3 involved nodes. Furthermore, while little difference existed in RFS between women with four, five, or six positive nodes, greater numbers of involved nodes were associated with a progressively worse prognosis. Whereas patients having four nodes involved had a 40% RFS, only 16% of those with ≤ 13 positive nodes were free of disease at 5 years. The findings related to overall survival were concordant with those observed for RFS, i.e., subdivision of the > 3 positive node subgroup indicated an increasing mortality with increasing numbers of involved axillary nodes. All findings were similar between the two major age groups, i.e., ≤ 49 and ≥ 50 years of age.

The above-mentioned results from two independent research institutions reaffirm the effectiveness of the conventional nodal grouping of patients into negative, 1−3, and > 3 positive nodes but indicate that for higher prognostic precision there is need for further subdivision of those with > 3 positive nodes. Combining all women with > 3 positive nodes into a single group may provide misleading information also about the relative merit of given adjuvant regimens. Most adjuvant results are inversely related to the number of involved axillary nodes, and none of the drug combinations tested so far were reported to substantially improve the RFS in women with > 10 positive nodes [7]. For this reason, failure to ensure proper balance relative to nodal groups and subgroups between two treatment regimens in a given randomized study "may result in ineffective therapies appearing effective and effectual therapies being judged worthless" [12]. The risk would be even greater when comparing the value of identical or different treatments administered in various institutions that appear to have utilized putatively similar patient populations.

Micro- vs Macrometastases

Since, as previously mentioned, little difference in RFS and survival existed between patients having one, two, or three positive axillary nodes, it appears worthwhile to correlate prognosis with nodal micro- vs macrometastases. Nodal micrometastases are designated as neoplastic infiltrations < 2 mm in diameter. They account for $\leq 10\%$ of the cases with positive nodes and are significantly more frequent with primary cancers < 2 cm in diameter and with patients in whom only 1−3 axillary nodes are involved. It is worth recalling that minute "occult" micrometastases may be detected in up to 25% of patients with invasive pathological stage-I breast carcinoma by serial sectioning of lymph nodes [17].

The initial observations [2, 22] were based on rather small series of patients; they often failed to take tumor size into consideration, and the follow-up period was less than 10 years. The studies concluded that prognosis was less favorable in women with macrometastases than in those with negative nodes or micrometastases, regardless of the tumor size or the number of involved lymph nodes or the length of follow-up period. In particular, the NSABP group [17] reported that there was no significant 4-year survival difference between patients with micrometastases (21 cases) and those without nodal metastases (N−) although both groups exhibited significantly longer survival than patients with macrometastases. However, the RFS of women with micro- or macrometastases was not statistically different and inferior to that of N− women. The authors emphasized that prognosis was more directly related to the number of positive nodes than to the size of metastases. In fact, within each of the subgroups having 1−3 and > 3 positive nodes the RFS was similar for patients with micro- and macrometastases, while patients with 1−3 nodes and metastases ≥ 2 mm exhibited significantly greater treatment failure rates than those with N− but less than those with > 3 involved nodes. A similar trend was observed in women with metastases < 2 mm. The NSABP group also identified a very small subset of patients with micrometastases measuring ≤ 1.3 mm, whose RFS and survival rates were similar to those of N− patients.

The more recent series of Memorial Hospital [30] included 147 women with single axillary lymph node metastasis who were followed up for ≥ 10 years. In the entire series, there was

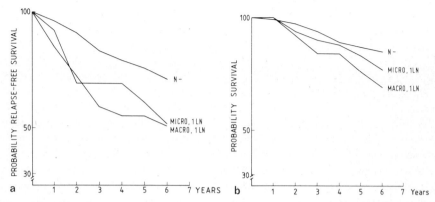

Fig. 2a, b. Six-year results as function of absence ($N-$) and presence ($N+$) of positive axillary nodes (micro- vs macrometastasis). **a** Relapse-free survival; **b** overall survival

Table 3. Micro- vs macrometastases in T_1 breast cancer (10-year results) (Courtesy of U. Veronesi)

Nodal status	No. of patients	RFS (%)	Survival (%)
N−	520	80.1	85.8
N+ micro	32	90.9	91.8
N+ macro	68	72.3	82.7

a significantly higher recurrence rate between the group with single macrometastases (30 of 77 cases, or 39%) compared with the group having single micrometastases (17 of 70, or 24%). A major prognostic differerence emerged after stratification by tumor size. In T_1 tumors the 12-year RFS of patients with either micro- or macrometastasis were nearly identical, and significantly worse than for those patients with N−. On the other hand, among T_2 women, those with single micrometastases or N− had RFS curves that did not differ significantly throughout the course of the follow-up period, and both groups had an outcome significantly better than that observed for patients with macrometastases.

Figure 2 shows the RFS and total survival curves of 68 women with a single micro- (13 cases) and macrometastasis (55 cases) enrolled as controls in the first Milan adjuvant trial. Most patients had T_2 primary breast cancer. The 6-year RFS was superimposable between the two metastatic nodal groups. The figure also includes, for comparison, the curve of 464 patients without pathological nodal metastases for whom the incidence of T_2 lesions was comparable to that of N+ patients, i.e., about 70%. The comparative findings clearly indicate that N− women have a more favorable prognosis than women with a single micrometastasis. In our T_1 series, including 701 patients randomized between Halsted's radical mastectomy and a breast-saving procedure [35], a single micrometastasis was observed in 32% of women with one positive lymph node. Patients with micrometastases exhibited the best 10-year RFS and survival slightly superior to that for N− women (Table 3). However, it should be stressed that all women with micrometastases and most with macrometastases in this series received postoperative adjuvant chemotherapy with CMF. The 10-year results reported by Gest et al. [21] on 35 patients with T_1 tumors confirmed that prognosis was significantly affected by the presence of one micrometastatic lymph node as compared with the absence of invasion, but it was not statistically different from that observed in the group with macrometastases.

Other Pathological Features

Within major nodal subgroups, some histopathological features further adversely influence prognosis. For instance, the NSABP group [18] has noticed in a multivariate analysis that in women with > 3 involved nodes, tumor necrosis, tumor size (≥ 4 cm vs ≤ 2 cm), infiltrating ductal type without specific features (NOS), and histological grade were significantly related to treatment failure. In contrast, none of the above-mentioned characteristics was significant in the subset having 1−3 involved nodes. Blood vessel invasion and ≥ 2 positive nodes were found by Weigand et al. [36] to exhibit a 70% recurrence by 2 years. However, blood vessel and lymphatic invasion were not observed to represent significant discriminants by the NSABP group [18].

In patients with positive axillary nodes, the estrogen receptor (ER) status was found to correlate negatively with morphological features which are associated with the degree of differentiation, i.e., histological and nuclear grade, and with the extent of necrosis, elastosis, and lymphoid cell infiltration into the tumor [16]. In particular, a highly significant relationship between receptor status and histological grade was observed [33].

Absence of Nodal Metastases

In the absence of pathological involvement of axillary lymph nodes the prognostic variables affecting treatment failure in patients subjected to local-regional therapy are probably numerous, but their relative merits are not yet well defined. Therefore, the prognostic discriminants to be utilized in the selection of high-risk groups for adjuvant chemotherapy remain, in part, controversial.

Receptor Status

The prognostic importance of ER status has been evaluated by a number of investigators. Table 4 summarizes the essential results observed in representative series. They are often difficult to compare, particularly as far as subgroups are concerned, because of differences in the size and characteristics of patient samples, receptor determination, and cutoff point, as well as differences in the follow-up times. However, a common denominator is represented by the authors' conclusion that women with ER-positive tumors exhibited RFS and survival rates which were significantly superior to those with ER negative tumors. An example of such retrospective study is reproduced in Fig. 3, which displays the 5-year results of 464 women with N− tumors treated in Milan with primary surgery alone. In other words, Hormone-dependent tumors have a better prognosis than their hormone-independent counterparts.

More recently, the prognostic value of progesterone receptor (PgR), the end product of estrogen action, was also evaluated in patients with resectable breast cancer. In an adjuvant study, which was essentially negative from the therapeutic point of view, involving 318

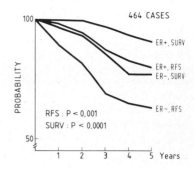

Fig. 3. Five-year results as function of estrogen receptor status in node negative patients

Table 4. Relapse-free survival related to ER+ vs ER− tumors (adapted and updated from Bonadonna and Valagussa [6][a]

Reference	Stage	Patients (n)	Significant difference
Knight	I−II	145	Yes
Allegra	I−II	292	Yes
Cooke	I−II	144	Yes
Maynard	I−II	232	Yes
Ryden	II	378	Yes
Harland	I−II	655	No
Valagussa	I	464	Yes (pre)
Crowe	I	510	Yes (post)

[a] Details of references cited in Bonadonna and Valagussa [6]

women with stage-II and treated with low dose CMF ± tamoxifen ± BCG [10], both ER and PgR were significant predictors of the 5-year RFS. However, when both receptors were analyzed together in multivariate models, PgR was more significant than ER for predicting time to recurrence. The findings were directly related to PgR levels, and the highest RFS was observed in women with ER+ and PgR+ tumors. The authors concluded that only the number of positive nodes and the presence of PgR significantly predicted longer RFS. The above-mentioned result, that PgR assay in primary breast cancer improves the prognostic value attributed to ER content, was supported by the findings of the Milan Cancer Institute in N− patients [4], as well as by the NSABP group [13] and Saez et al. in France [31]. However, the Guy's Hospital group [33] failed to detect any significant difference in the 5-year RFS of stages I and II between ER+ and ER− tumors or PgR+ and PgR− tumors, although there was a trend to longer RFS for ER+ and PgR+. Survival in receptor-positive tumors was significantly longer in ER+ than ER− tumors and when both ER+ and PgR+ tumors were compared with ER− and PgR− tumors. The conclusion was that steroid receptors significantly affected total survival but not RFS.

Pathological Features

Besides nodal status, a number of histopathological features were also recently reconsidered in the attempt to rank the prognostic significance of various discriminants in women without nodal involvement.

Table 5. Pathological features which adversely influence prognosis in node-negative breast cancer

NSABP [18] (266 cases)	Johns Hopkins [3] (74 cases)
Tumor necrosis	Extensive necrosis
Histological grade	Nuclear grade
Germinal center predominance	Germinal center hyperplasia
Tumor size (> 4 cm vs ≤ 2 cm)	Age ≤ 40 years

Table 5 lists the characteristics significantly related to the treatment failure of 266 N− women studied by the NSABP group [18] and of 74 women with N− and ER− tumors analyzed by the Johns Hopkins Hospital [3]. In the NSABP series, all four characteristics had a somewhat independent adverse effect upon treatment. As previously mentioned, ER− status was significantly associated with a high incidence of three or more unfavorable histological features [16]. However, other clinical and pathological characteristics such as age, lymphatic and blood vessel invasion, cell reaction to tumor, absent or mild elastosis, and the NOS tumor type were not found by contingency-table analysis to be significantly related to treatment failure. The investigators at Johns Hopkins Hospital [3] found significant correlations between 2-year recurrence and extensive necrosis, anaplastic tumor nuclear morphology, diffuse hyperplasia of axillary nodes, and age ≤ 40 years. With stepwise discriminant analysis, the single feature which best correlated with recurrence was tumor necrosis. The above-mentioned research groups failed to confirm that the presence of sinus histiocytosis had a significant correlation with treatment failure.

During the past few years, increasing attention has been paid by pathologists to the possible significance of lymphatic vessels invasion by neoplastic tissue in resectable breast cancer. The NSABP [15] reported that 33% of 1,000 cases exhibited unequivocal intralymphatic invasion within the dominant mass and 22% questionable invasion, regardless of concurrent nodal invasion. The finding was considered prognostically unfavorable in view of its strong association with other ominous events (nodal metastases, large size of primaries, high histological grading, etc.). A report on two small groups [24, 25] of selected patients with N− invasive and predominantly ductal carcinomas showed that tumor emboli in intramammary lymphatic vessels were fairly constant (8%−9%) and carried a high risk of early recurrence in distant sites. The negative influence on RFS of endolymphatic tumor emboli was recently confirmed by some American and British investigators [5, 29] as well as by our own institute [27] and, in the absence of nodal involvement, it appears to be the most valuable histopathological indicator of poor prognosis. However, it should be recalled that the recent reports of NSABP [18] and of Johns Hopkins Hospital [3] have failed to observe that both lymphatic and blood vessel invasion represented significant discriminants in their group of patients.

Blood vessel invasion in resectable carcinoma of the breast has been reported to vary from 5% to more than 40%, and its association with an unfavorable prognosis has always been stressed [27]. The recent analysis by Weigand et al. [36] of 175 cases has indicated that the presence of blood vessel invasion was highly associated with early disease recurrence only in patients with more than two positive nodes. In contrast, women with blood vessel invasion but one or no involved nodes experienced recurrence at a rate not significantly different from those without blood vessel invasion.

Kinetic Features

Kinetic characteristics of breast cancers have been studied more than those of any other human neoplasm. However, trends or significant correlations between the kinetic and the clinical and pathological features have been proposed and subsequently contradicted by different, and also by the same authors, using standardized techniques. The heterogeneity of breast cancer probably accounts for the controversial results. Recently, the Milan group [20] has studied the thymidine-^{3}H labelling index (LI) in 541 women with primary breast cancer. The only significant correlation between LI and the 4-year RFS was observed in 145 N− premenopausal women (low LI 100%, high LI 32.6%). In other words, the proliferative activity of the primary tumor appears to be a potentially useful indicator of biological aggressiveness in a given subset with no involved axillary nodes.

Tumor Size

Clinical measurements are obviously not superimposable on those of the surgical specimen. In general, clinicians have a tendency to overestimate the size of small tumors and to underestimate the size of large tumors. The difference between clinical and pathological dimensions of primary breast neoplasms is probably the main reason for some controversial results found in the literature regarding tumor sizes and recurrence rates. In general, tumor size has always been correlated with RFS and total survival particularly because tumor size influences the likelihood of nodal involvement, which in turn influences curability by surgery [12].

A direct relation of tumor size to 5- and 10-year RFS was found for carcinomas without axillary node metastases [19, 29]. Figure 4 shows the RFS and survival of 464 women with N− and 845 women with N+ treated in Milan. The results essentially confirmed the prognostic importance of the size of primary tumor for N+ patients, while correlation was of borderline significance for N− patients.

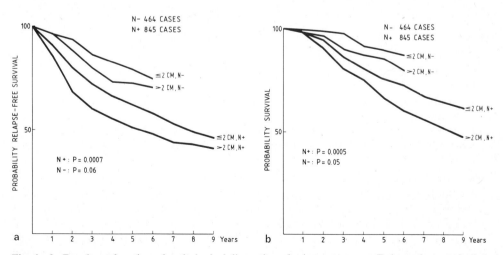

Fig. 4a, b. Results as function of pathological dimension of primary tumor. **a** Relapse-free survival; **b** overall survival

Biological Tumor Markers

The past decade has seen an explosion of biological and clincial interest in tumor markers [11]. Initially, the measurement of urinary or blood marker levels was viewed as the clinicians' panacea to the earlier diagnosis and monitoring of a variety of neoplasms. "Further studies, fortunately, resulted in a more rational approach to their use and the realization, at least as far as human mammary cancer is concerned, that their clinical role is limited" [8]. We will summarize some of the recent advances in establishing biological markers for breast cancer and their usefulness in the detection of recurrence in high-risk groups.

Table 6 lists the biochemical markers that have been correlated with the presence of breast cancer. Considering that the ideal marker [1] must be (a) sensitive enough to detect a very small tumor cell burden, (b) specific for breast cancer, and (c) easy and economical, we have to admit that work in the last decade has failed to provide realistic prognostic indexes. Therefore, none of the markers listed can today be utilized on a routine basis to identify high-risk subsets for adjuvant chemotherapy. However, two recent studies [23, 28] have reemphasized the potential usefulness of positive immunohistochemical staining for CEA.

The use of monoclonal antibodies as probes in the search for breast cancer antigens is producing a gamut of new findings that are changing our understanding of this field. The recent paper of Redding et al. [26] is an example of a new phase in the development of monoclonal antibody technology. The investigators used an immunocytochemical method to screen smears obtained at the time of primary surgery from multiple bone marrow sites in 110 patients with breast cancer. While no other techniques, including conventionally stained smears, had revealed metastases, the use of an antibody probe to the epithelial membrane antigen (EMA), a breast cell surface component, allowed detection of bone marrow tumor cells in a total of 31 (28%) patients. Furthermore, 83% of patients with conventional unfavorable prognostic variables showed micrometastases, compared with 11% of patients classified in a good prognosis category. Of particular importance was the presence of micrometastases in 24% of node-negative patients, since this finding correlates very well with the 10-year recurrence rate for N− women [34].

Table 6. Biochemical tumor markers for breast cancer

Tumor-derived
    Breast tissue protein (casein, lactalbumin)
    Oncofetal protein (carcinoembryonic antigen, ferritin, isoferritins)
    Hormones (calcitonin, human chorionic gonadotropin)
    Enzymes (γGT, AF)
    Receptors (ER, PR)
    Cell turnover products (urinary polyamines)
    Immune response markers

Tumor-associated
    Plasma proteins
    Hydroxyproline
    Miscellaneous (TPA, etc.)

Conclusion

The prognostic findings we have briefly reviewed indicate that a number of concomitant variables affect the prognosis of a highly heterogeneous disease such as breast cancer. Theoretically, they should all be taken into consideration in the selection of candidates for adjuvant therapy. However, from the practical point of view, for women with resectable tumors and for these in whom axillary node dissection or sampling has been performed, nodal status remains the predominant indicator for adjuvant chemotherapy.

In the presence of histologically positive nodes, regardless of their number and the extent of primary tumor, the RFS is invariably inferior to that of a comparable series of patients with absence of nodal involvement. The coexistence of other histopathological features such as tumor anaplasia, necrosis, or vascular invasion may further reinforce the need for an effective systemic treatment. Present data on single micrometastatic involvement and on positive estrogen and progesterone receptors are still too scanty or preliminary to separate out from the node-positive group a favorable prognostic subset of patients who can be spared adjuvant chemotherapy. It is quite possible that the systematic reevaluation of ongoing prospective series will allow a more precise reassessment of subsets for whom adjuvant chemotherapy may not be required. Recent studies emphasize the need for subdivision of patients with > 3 involved nodes into at least two subsets, i.e., 4–10 and > 10 nodes. This latter group, which accounts for about 10% of women with positive nodes, carries a very poor prognosis, and to our knowledge it has not been shown to be consistently or substantially affected by current adjuvant regimens. For these reasons, prospective randomized trials should properly balance this nodal subset for which new forms of drug therapy should be tested.

In node-negative women, many unfavorable prognostic variables were evaluated to explain the 20%–25% recurrence rate at 10 years following local-regional treatment alone. Unfortunately, in this patient group there is as yet no easily reproducible predominant indicator of treatment failure. However, two prognostic factors appear most consistent and applicable in clinical practice: the absence of both estrogen and progesterone receptors and/or the presence of intralymphatic tumor emboli. If confirmed on a larger series of patients, the detection of bone marrow infiltration using monoclonal antibodies [26] will certainly represent a new avenue for better assessing prognosis and selecting patients for adjuvant chemotherapy.

References

1. Andersen JA, Mattheiem WH (1983) Markers and prognostic factors in breast cancer disease. Workshop report. Eur J Cancer Clin Oncol 19: 1699–1707
2. Attiyeh FF, Jensen M, Huvos AG, Fracchia A (1977) Axillary micrometastases and macrometastases in carcinoma of the breast. Surg Gynecol Obstet 144: 839–842
3. Bauer TW, O'Ceallaigh D, Eggleston JC, Moore GW, Baker RR (1983) Prognostic factors in patients with stage I, estrogen receptor-negative carcinoma of the breast. A clinicopathologic study. Cancer 52: 1423–1431
4. Bertuzzi A, Vezzoni P, Ronchi E (1981) Prognostic importance of progesterone receptors alone or in combination with estrogen receptors in node negative breast cancer (Abstr). Proc Am Soc Clin Oncol 22: 447
5. Bettelheim R, Neville AM (1981) Lymphatic and vascular channel involvement within infiltrative breast carcinomas as a guide to prognosis at the time of primary surgical treatment. Lancet 2: 631

6. Bonadonna G, Valagussa P (1983) Chemotherapy of breast cancer: current views and results. Int J Radiat Oncol Biol Phys 9:279–297
7. Bonadonna G, Valagussa P (to be published) Adjuvant systemic therapy for resectable breast cancer
8. Buckman R, Coombes RC, Dearnaley DP, Gore M, Gusterson B, Neville AM (to be published) Some clinical uses of biological markers. In: Bonadonna G (ed) Breast cancer: diagnosis and management. Wiley, London
9. Buzdar A, Smith T, Blumenschein G, Hortobagyi G, Hersh E, Gehan E (1981) Adjuvant chemotherapy with fluorouracil, doxorubicin, and cyclophosphamide (FAC) for stage II or III breast cancer: 5-year results. In: Salmon SE, Jones SE (eds) Adjuvant therapy of cancer III. Grune and Stratton, New York, pp 419–426
10. Clark GM, McGuire WL, Hubay CA, Pearson OH, Marshall JS (1983) Progesterone receptor as a prognostic factor in Stage II breast cancer. N Engl J Med 309:1343–1347
11. Colnaghi MI, Buraggi GL, Ghione M (eds) (1982) Markers for diagnosis and monitoring of human cancer. Academic, London (Proceedings of the Serono symposia, no 46)
12. Fisher B, Bauer M, Wickerham DL, Redmond CK, Fisher ER, Cruz AB, Foster R, Gardner B, Lerner H, Margolese R, Poisson R, Shibata H, Volk H et al. (1983) Relation of number of positive axillary nodes to the prognosis of patients with primary breast cancer. An NSABP update. Cancer 52:1551–1557
13. Fisher B, Redmond CK, Wickerham L, Rockette HE, Brown A, Allegra J, Bowman D, Plotkin D, Wolter J et al. (1983) Relation of estrogen and/or progesterone receptor content of breast cancer to patient outcome following adjuvant chemotherapy. Breast Cancer Res Treat 3:355–364
14. Fisher B, Slack NH, Bross IDJ (1969) Cancer of the breast: size of neoplasm and prognosis. Cancer 24:1071–1080
15. Fisher ER, Gregorio RM, Fisher B (1975) The pathology of invasive breast cancer. A syllabus derived from findings of the National Surgical Adjuvant Breast Project (protocol no 4). Cancer 36:1–85
16. Fisher ER, Osborne CK, McGuire WL, Redmond C, Knight WA III, Fisher B, Bannayan G, Walder A, Gregory EJ, Jacobsen A, Queen DM, Bennet DE, Ford HC (1981) Correlation of primary breast cancer histopathology and estrogen receptor content. Breast Cancer Res Treat 1:37–41
17. Fisher ER, Palekar AS, Rockette H, Redmond C, Fisher B (1978) Pathologic findings from the National Surgical Adjuvant Breast Project (protocol no 4). V. Significance of axillary nodal micro- and macrometastases. Cancer 42:2032–2038
18. Fisher ER, Redmond C, Fisher B (1980) Pathologic findings from the National Surgical Adjuvant Breast Project (protocol no 4). VI. Discriminants for five-year treatment failure. Cancer 46:908–918
19. Fracchia AA, Rosen PP, Ashikari R (1980) Primary carcinoma of the breast without axillary lymph node metastases. Surg Gynecol Obstet 151:375–378
20. Gentili C, Sanfilippo O, Silvestrini R (1981) Cell proliferation and its relationship to clinical features and relapse in breast cancer. Cancer 48:974–979
21. Gest J, Brunet M, Hebert H, Pallud C, Tubiana M (1982) Prognostic significance of axillary micro and macrometastasis in breast cancer (T_1 and T_2). Preliminary results. Int J Breast Mammary Pathol Senologia 1:49–52
22. Huvos AG, Hutter RVP, Berg JW (1971) Significance of axillary macrometastases and micrometastases in mammary cancer. Ann Surg 173:44–46
23. Mansour EG, Hastert M, Park CH, Koehler KA, Petrelli M (1983) Tissue and plasma carcinoembryonic antigen in early breast cancer. A prognostic factor. Cancer 51:1243–1248
24. Merlin C, Gloor F, Hardmeier T, Senn HJ (1980) Hat die intramammäre Lymphangiosis carcinomatosa beim nodal-negativen Mammakarzinom eine prognostische Bedeutung? Schweiz Med Wochenschr 110:605–609

25. Nime FA, Rosen PP, Thaler HT, Ashikari R, Urban JA (1977) Prognostic significance of tumor emboli in intramammary lymphatics in patients with mammary carcinoma. Am J Surg Pathol 1: 25−30
26. Redding WH, Coombes RC, Monaghan P, Clink HM, Imrie SF, Dearnaley DP, Ormerod MG, Sloane JP, Gozet JC, Powles TJ, Neville AM (1983) Detection of micrometastases in patients with primary breast cancer. Lancet 2: 1271−1273
27. Rilke F (to be published) Influence of pathologic factors on management. In: Bonadonna G (ed) Breast cancer: diagnosis and management. Wiley, London
28. Rolf Smith S, Howell A, Minawa A, Morrison JM (1982) The clinical value of immunohistochemically demonstrable CEA in breast cancer: a possible method of selecting patients for adjuvant chemotherapy. Br J Cancer 46: 757−764
29. Rosen PP, Saigo PE, Braun DW, Weathers E, De Palo A (1981) Precitors of recurrence in stage I (T1NOMO) breast carcinoma. Ann Surg 193: 15−25
30. Rosen PP, Saigo PE, Braun DW, Weathers E, Fracchia AA, Kinne DW (1981) Axillary micro- and macrometastases in breast cancer. Prognostic significance of tumor size. Ann Surg 194: 585−591
31. Saez S, Cheix F, Asselain B (1983) Prognostic value of estrogen and progesterone receptors in primary breast cancer. Breast Cancer Res Treat 3: 345−354
32. Stewart JF, Rubens RD (to be published) General prognostic factors. In: Bonadonna G (ed) Breast cancer: diagnosis and management. Wiley, London
33. Stewart JF, Rubens RD, Millis RR, King RJ, Hayward JL (1983) Steroid receptors and prognosis in operable (stage I and II) breast cancer. Eur J Cancer Clin Oncol 19: 1381−1387
34. Valagussa P, Bonadonna G, Veronesi U (1978) Patterns of relapse and survival following radical mastectomy. Analysis of 716 consecutive patients. Cancer 41: 1171−1178
35. Veronesi U, Saccozzi R, Del Vecchio M, Banfi A, Clemente C, De Lena M, Gallus G, Greco M, Luini A, Marubini E, Muscolino G, Rilke F, Salvadori B, Zecchini A, Zucali R (1981) Comparing radical mastectomy with quadrantectomy, axillary dissection and radiotherapy in patients with small cancer of the breast. N Engl J Med 305: 6−11
36. Weigand RA, Isenberg WM, Russo J, Brennan MJ, Rich MA, and Breast Cancer Prognostic Study Associates (1982) Blood vessel invasion and axillary lymph node involvement as prognostic indicators for human breast cancer. Cancer 50: 962−969

Review: Scientific Basis of Adjuvant Chemotherapy in Breast Cancer

D. P. Griswold

Southern Research Institute, 2000 Ninth Avenue, South, P.O. Box 55305, Birmingham, AL 35255-5305/USA

This group of papers centers on preclinical and clinical observations, their impact on recent achievements in adjuvant chemotherapy, and conceptual changes that may further alter the course of breast cancer. The overtone ranges from pessimism to guarded optimism with a general feeling that progress, at least for the time being, has plateaued. Nevertheless, several observations critical to further progress in disease detection and management are brought to light.

Through the Breast Cancer Detection and Demonstration Project and the Pathology Quality Control Project more than 19,000 cases have been reviewed in the past decade. Several critical findings have resulted from these studies, two of the most important being that the detection of in situ carcinoma has improved about twofold and the lymph node-negative patient group is approaching 90%. These diagnostic improvements are expected to have a favorable effect on the outcome of treatment, an effect that remains to be realized. The need for early diagnosis, stressed by all of the contributors, correlates with earlier preclinical observations in that there it an inverse relationship between tumor burden and cure, and with more recent observations in that there is a direct relationship between the size of a tumor-cell population and the presence of specifically drug-resistant tumor cells.

Although there is a strong correlation between early detection and the use of mammography, self-diagnosis has had a disappointingly small effect; the reasons for this are not entirely clear. Similarly, identification of risk factors associated with breast cancer has not been markedly productive: age remains the most meaningful factor.

The identification and use of prognostic factors require further improvement, particularly for purposes of staging subgroups; this is substantiated by preclinical studies demonstrating the random nature of metastasis, as well as by the retrospective study of clinical surgical control arms. It is noted that where axillary-node metastasis was clinically absent, little difference in relapse-free survival was discerned between patients with one, two, or three positive nodes. Similarly, there is little difference in benefit between negative-node patients and those who are node positive but with micrometastases, the latter defined as being < 2 mm. Although nodal status is an important prognostic factor, albeit with certain limitations, tumor size is far less significant, except in negative-node patients. Improved response is associated with a positive estrogen receptor and estrogen/progesterone receptor status and, in some cases, with blood vessel invasion and vascularity. Clearly, it would be of great help if patient subgroups could be identified on the basis of narrower ranges of the extent of metastatic tumor burden. If it is indeed true that "cure" is presently limited by tumor burden, then it is imperative that those patients beyond likely hope of curability by adjuvant therapy be excluded from the patient population whose probability of cure by currently available means is reasonable. This is not meant to imply that *any* patient should be denied treatment. It is simply that better definition of subgroups will provide a better basis for staging, improved interpretation of results, and perhaps different treatment strategies for each subgroup.

This leads to another problem area identified that has to do with the imprecise quantitative techniques which are available for the measurement of residual disease. This becomes increasingly important as a growing percentage of patients with minimal disease become available for adjuvant therapy. In such cases, not only can the metastatic burden at the onset of treatment not be accurately defined, but treatment success, if any, cannot be followed progressively. Commonly used parameters such as relapse-free survival or time to treatment failure may misleadingly suggest improvement when there will ultimately be no overall benefit. It has long been known that tumor volume changes often correlate poorly with the *net* tumor cell kill achieved with radiation or chemotherapy. Unfortunately, the endpoints used clinically and often preclinically for determination of treatment efficacy are based on changes in volume or mass. The quantitative assays that are sometimes used in animal models for determination of the number of clonogenic tumor cells surviving treatment cannot be used in man. Neither are biochemical markers available that have the precision necessary to make such estimates.

It is suggested that some of the hypotheses, related to tumor growth and response to treatment, developed during the 1960s and may not have been tested adequately later in a clinical situation, and that more recently developed concepts may require clinical evaluation. For example, do differences, even if subtle, in the manner of tumor growth affect the design and results of adjuvant therapy regimens? Which model best describes tumor growth: Gompertzian, Norton-Simon, Speer-Retsky, or others? Has perioperative chemotherapy been adequately evaluated? Should the Goldie-Coldman hypothesis (every minute counts) be subjected to controlled clinical trial? These and other conceptual questions have drawn considerable discussion, but no firm answers.

A number of obstacles to further progress with adjuvant chemotherapy have been defined. These include the presence in some patients of a metastatic burden beyond the curative potential of currently available drugs, recognizing the narrow range from minimal effective dose to maximum tolerated dose; the selection and overgrowth of drug-resistant tumor cells; and pharmacological and/or population kinetic barriers. The latter may be related to a variety of cellular and molecular phenomena, including tumor architecture and vascularity, phenotypic plasticity, and heterogeneity, not only in growth kinetics but in terms of drug uptake, activation and inactivation, and cellular repair. Some of these obstacles may be overcome by further refinement of presently available techniques; others will obviously require the development of new and/or improved methodology.

This section is intended to serve as an uptdate on breast cancer adjuvant chemotherapy with regard to the application of concepts put to test in preclinical and clinical trial. It is obvious that some concepts have not been properly evaluated, while with others the trial results may require reanalysis. Certainly, several problem areas remain − e.g., prognostic factors, quantitative measures, and therapeutic strategies aimed at breaking the cure barrier. Improvement in any of these areas offers hope for further progress with adjuvant chemotherapy.

Clinical Results I:
Experience of Randomized Trials with Surgical Controls

Scandinavian Trials with a Short Postoperative Course Versus a 12-Cycle Course

R. Nissen-Meyer, H. Høst, K. Kjellgren, B. Månsson, and T. Norin

Tyribakken 10, Oslo 2, Norway

Introduction

Adjuvant chemotherapy for 1 year after mastectomy has for some years now been the standard treatment for breast cancer in many centers. The results have perhaps not been quite as good as many hoped some 5 years ago. In addition, it has become increasingly clear that the side effects of intense chemotherapy may seriously impair the quality of life during the year of administration.

Clinical trials are now being performed to ascertain whether the duration of adjuvant chemotherapy may be reduced without losing too much of the effect. We report here the

Table 1. Members of the Scandinavian Adjuvant Chemotherapy Study Group

Finland

Helsinki: AA. Järvinen[†], L. Holsti, K. Malmio[†]
Oulu: G. Blanco, T. Larmi
Vasa: P.-O. Grönblom

Norway

Akershus: T. Brøyn, N. Helsingen, F. W. Vaagenes
Bergen: L. Kolsaker, B. Rosengren, M. Tangen
Bodø: R. Capoferro, S. M. Sivertsen
Lillehammer: I. Hareide, S. K. Hjort
Oslo: I. O. Brennhovd, S. Gundersen, S. Hagen, T. Harbitz, H. Høst, O. G. Jørgensen, S. Kvaløy, H. O. Myhre, R. Nissen-Meyer (coordinator)

Sweden

Borås: S. Ahlström, C.-A. Ekman, B. Månsson
Gävle: G. Hellström, T. Norin, G. Odén
Jönköping: I. Iacobaeus, B. Mårtensson
Kalmar: B. Pallin
Linköping: J. Sääf, D. Turesson
Norrköping: H. O. Ahnlund, K. Kjellgren, R. Peterhoff
Västervik: K. Wiegner

Recent Results in Cancer Research. Vol. 96
© Springer-Verlag Berlin · Heidelberg 1984

contribution of the Scandinavian Adjuvant Chemotherapy Study Group to the solution of the problem of the optimal duration of adjuvant chemotherapy, approaching the problem from the other end. Study 1 started January 1965, with the aim of assessing the effectiveness, side effects, and risk of a single, short adjuvant course. Study 2 started March 1977 and was a cost-benefit analysis of the results of prolonging the adjuvant chemotherapy from 1 week to 1 year.

Summary

In *study 1* Cyclophosphamide 5 mg/kg/day i.v. for six days, one single course, was given to 559 patients, with 577 randomized controls. Followup up to $18^1/_2$ years. A longlasting crude survival benefit was observed. The difference was 49 deaths ($P < 0.02$) in 1980, in 1983 reduced to 40, as the number of deaths unrelated to breast cancer increased.

In 1,026 cases randomization and start of chemotherapy immediately after mastectomy. Effect of the immediate course was a highly significant relapse benefit, increasing to 12.8% after 17 years.

In 110 cases randomization and start of chemotherapy was 2–4 weeks delayed. No effect of the delayed course was seen.

In *study 2* one short multidrug course was given immediately after mastectomy to all 1,025 patients. One half of the 345 histologic node positive patients were randomized to continue with CMF for one year. Effect of the prolonged treatment was an increase of the relapsefree rate with 16% after $2^1/_2$ years, but this difference was reduced to 6% after 6 years. These results are preliminary.

Side effects of the single short courses were almost negligible, side effects of the one-year treatment severe.

Material and Methods

Study 1. A total of 1,136 routine patients were treated by mastectomy and postoperative local radiotherapy. They were randomized into a chemotherapy group (559 cases) and a control group (577 cases). The chemotherapy group received cyclophosphamide i.v. 5 mg/kg/day for 6 days. In 10 surgical clinics the patients were randomized by telephone from the operating theater, and the chemotherapy course started immediately. In one radiotherapy institute the patients arrived 2–4 weeks after surgery and were randomized after arrival. Here the chemotherapy course started 21 days (mean) after mastectomy. Detailed description of the case material and the methods used in study 1 may be found in a previous paper [1].

Study 2. All routine patients received a single, short chemotherapy course immediately after mastectomy. In light of the general development in cancer chemotherapy between 1965 and 1977 we changed our monodrug course to a multidrug course.

The 680 node-negative patients received no more adjuvant chemotherapy.

The 345 histologically node-positive patients were randomized into a control group and a group supposed to continue with adjuvant chemotherapy for 1 year. These latter patients were strongly encouraged to continue the treatment, but were told that it was a clinical trial and that if they considered the side effects intolerable, they could stop at any time.

Table 2. Chemotherapy schedules in study 2

Drug	Single, short perioperative course		CMF course	
	Day 0	Day 7	Day 1	Day 8
Cyclophosphamide	500	500	500	500
Vincristine	1	1	–	–
5-FU	750	–	750	750
Methotrexate	–	50	50	50

The single course after mastectomy was cyclophosphamide, 5-fluorouracil (5-FU), and vincristine immediately after mastectomy, and cyclophosphamide, methotrexate, and vincristine 7 days later. The long-term chemotherapy, which was offered to half of the node-positive patients, was cyclophosphamide, methotrexate, and 5-FU (CMF) on days 1 and 8 in each 4-week cycle, for 12 cycles. The doses shown in Table 2 are for a patient of 70 kg, and are the maximum we gave. If the patient weights less than 70 kg, the doses are reduced accordingly. All drugs are given intravenously.

Half the patients in study 2 were also randomized to receive immunotherapy with *Corynebacterium parvum,* given subcutaneously around the mastectomy scar. This treatment has shown no effect on the overall results so far, and will not be published until we have a reasonable number of patients followed up for 5 years in the various subgroups.

Results

Table 3 shows the total number of deaths reported in study 1 by March 1980 [2], and by August 1983. In 1980 there was a significant difference of 49 deaths in favor of the cyclophosphamide group. This difference was reduced by 1983 to 40, which is not significant at the 5% level.

The median age at mastectomy was 55 years. The follow-up is not until death or for a median time of 13 years. A large proportion of the patients have reached a very advanced age, and there are many deaths from causes unrelated to breast cancer. In the cyclophosphamide group 61 patients died from specified causes without any indication of residual breast cancer tissue; in the control group the corresponding figure was 55.

Figure 1 shows the proportion of relapse-free patients at the 10 clinics using a single immediate cyclophosphamide course. The difference in favour of the 507 treatment cases was small in the beginning, highly significant after 4 years, and remained at a level of about 12% for at least 17 years thereafter.

By means of retrospective stratification according to lymph node status and menopausal status the same effect was found in all strata.

Figure 2 shows the proportion of relapse-free patients at the clinic with the delayed randomization. For the sake of comparision the curves from the 10 clinics with the immediate course are plotted again. At no point is there any significant difference between the two curves from the clinic with the delayed course; they both follow closely the control curve from the 10 clinics with the immediate course. The chance fluctuations must necessarily be greater in the much smaller groups (52 vs 58).

Table 3. Total number of deaths reported in study 1

	Control group	Cyclophosphamide group
March 1980	283	234 $(P < 0.02)$
August 1983	307	267

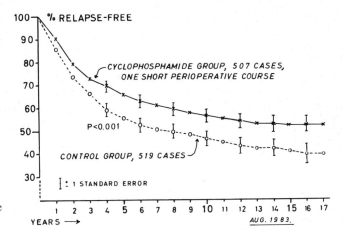

Fig. 1. Effect of the short immediate cyclophosphamide course in study 1

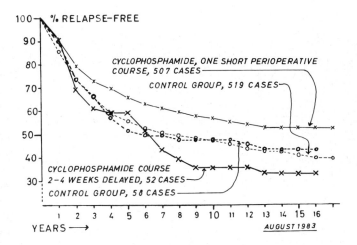

Fig. 2. Comparison of the immediate and the delayed short course in study 1

Figure 3 shows the node-negative cases in both studies. The results in study 2 seem to be slightly better than the results in the experimental group of study 1.

Figure 4 shows the node-positive cases in both studies. The performance of the control group in study 2 seems to be slightly better than the experimental group in study 1. The effect of prolonging adjuvant chemotherapy from 1 week to 1 year is reflected in the difference between the two randomized groups of study 2 − rather, this is the effect of our intention to continue chemotherapy for 1 year. A clear decision by the patient to terminate the treatment earlier had to be respected (see Side Effects).

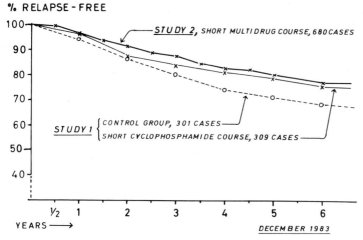

Fig. 3. Comparison of the short multidrug course and the short cyclophosphamide course in node-negative cases

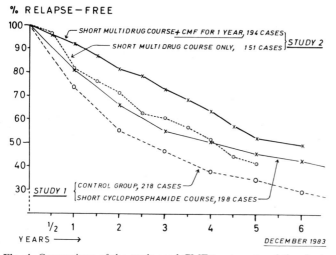

Fig. 4. Comparison of the prolonged CMF treatment and the single, short courses in node-positive cases

During the first few years after mastectomy the difference between the group with long-term treatment and the two groups with one single course increased to 16%, but after 6 years it was reduced to 6%.

Side Effects

The immediate side effects of the short cyclophosphamide course were reported in detail in a previous paper [1]. It may be concluded that they were very moderate and, above all, of short duration. They were easy to palliate since the patients during the treatment period

Table 4. Second malignant disease observed in study 1 (excluding carcinoma basocellulare and new primary tumors in the second breast)

	Control group	Cyclophosphamide group
Leukemia/lymphoma	4	1
Gynecological cancer	6	3
Gastrointestinal cancer	6	8
Other neoplasms	6	5
Total	22	17

were still in hospital after the mastectomy. They did not affect the recovery after surgery or the wound healing, and radiotherapy to lymph node regions could start as usual 4−6 days after mastecomy.

With more than 550 cases in each of the two randomized groups and up to 18 years follow-up, we may now evaluate the potential risk of a carcinogenic effect. As seen from Table 4, there is no indication that the single, short cyclophosphamide course carries such a risk.

The short multidrug course has been as easily tolerated as the short cyclophosphamide course. It has now been used in 1,025 cases, and has caused no problems.

The side effects from the long-term i.v. CMF treatment, however, have been a major problem, for the patients and for us. Only 63/173 (36%) of the patients managed to complete this treatment with at least 90% of the scheduled dose. The side effects were considered mild in 14, moderate in 19, and severe in 30 patients. In the rest of the patients the dose had to be reduced due to the side effects, 38% received 50%−90% of the scheduled dose, 20% less than 50%. Nine patients (5%) refused to start the CMF treatment they were allotted to.

Nausea and vomiting tended to increase in severity with increasing number of courses, and could continue for a whole week after each injection. A reduction of the doses usually had little effect on this pattern of side effects, when it was first established. As a consequence of this, 68/164 (41%) eventually insisted that the CMF treatment should be terminated, after a median of 14 injections (7 courses).

Discussion and Conclusions

With one single, short chemotherapy course given immediately after mastectomy we have observed a highly significant benefit in relapse-free rates, increasing to 12.8% by 17 years after mastectomy. We have also observed a significant, long-lasting crude survival benefit (although the increasing number of deaths due to old age now tends to obscure this benefit).

This pattern cannot be explained only by a delaying influence on the course of the disease; the effect observed must be due to an increased cure rate.

There was no major difference in results between the short cyclophosphamide course and the short multidrug course, but this was not a randomized comparison. However, the observations may indicate that the new multidrug course was at least as effective as the old monodrug course, and it was at least as easily tolerated.

The comparison of the effects obtained in the clinic with the delayed course and the 10 clinics with the immediate course indicates that by 2−4 weeks after mastectomy the optimal time for start of adjuvant chemotherapy may have passed.

The immediate side effects of the short, single chemotherapy courses were almost negligible, and we found no indication of late complications. The number of second malignancies was not higher in the cyclophosphamide gorup than in the randomized control group, and represents only the general tendency for patients surviving one cancer to develop another malignant disease.

On the other hand, the side effects from the long-term chemotherapy were very distressing, and it was not possible to persuade more than 59% of the patients to continue treatment for a whole year. The first few courses were usually not so bad, but nausea and vomiting tended to increase with time, and severely impaired the quality of life. The patients insisting that the treatment should be terminated did so after a median of 7 courses. The learned aversion to cytotoxic drugs must necessarily have a negative influence upon the chance of successful treatment of recurrent disease later.

Our observation time in study 2 is still too short to evaluate the possible risk of second malignancies due to long-term chemotherapy.

It is also too early to obtain a reliable evaluation of the beneficial effects of our attempt to prolong chemotherapy from 1 week to 1 year. We have observed an additional relapse-free rate of up to 16% during the first $2^1/_2$ years after mastectomy, but this difference seems to be reduced considerably during the next 2−4 years. If this trend is supported when a larger number of cases have been followed up for a sufficient time, it will mean that the prolonged treatment mainly adds a disease-delaying effect to the effect on the ultimate cure rate which we have obtained with the first short course.

We may conclude that one short, immediate chemotherapy course may be recommended to all patients after mastectomy. But we are still in doubt regarding the 1-year treatment. Many more trials are needed to define the optimal duration of adjuvant chemotherapy for the various prognostic groups, taking into account benefit, side effects, and risk.

References

1. Nissen-Meyer R, Kjellgren K, Malmio K, Månsson B, Norin T (1978) Surgical adjuvant chemotherapy. Results with one short course with cyclophosphamide after mastectomy for breast cancer. Cancer 39: 2875−2882
2. Nissen-Meyer R, Kjellgren K, Månsson B (1982) Adjuvant chemotherapy in breast cancer. In: Mathé G, Bonadonna G, Salmon S (eds) Adjuvant therapies of cancer. Springer, Berlin Heidelberg New York, pp 142−148 (Recent results in cancer research, vol 80)

A Brief Overview of Findings from NSABP Trials of Adjuvant Therapy

B. Fisher, E. R. Fisher, C. Redmond,
and Participating NSABP Investigators*

NSABP National Surgical Adjuvant Project for Breast and Bowel Cancers,
Biostatistical Center, Suite 730, 3515 Fifth Avenue, Pittsburgh, PA 15213, USA

Introduction

Since 1972 the National Surgical Adjuvant Breast and Bowel Project (NSABP) has initiated nine major trials to determine the value of adjuvant therapy in the management of patients with primary breast cancer (Table 1). Seven of the trials involved patients with one or more histologically positive axillary nodes and the other two employed negative-node patients.

More than 6,000 patients who were entered into the various protocols met the same specific criteria of eligibility. Beginning with Protocol B-09, but excluding B-10, estrogen and progesterone receptor analyses of the tumor were required. All patients were treated at NSABP member institutions in the United States and Canada. The rationale for the first three trials using adjuvant chemotherapy (ACT) related to the kinetic principles promulgated by Skipper and Schabel which suggested that certain patients might benefit from the use of a single chemotherapeutic agent and that others would require more complex regimens. Thus, those studies were planned to be carried out in a stepwise sequential manner in order to identify subsets of patients who were likely to respond to one, two, or three chemotherapeutic agents. It was recognized at the time that the first protocol was initiated that L-PAM (P) given as a single drug did not represent the most effective regimen in advanced disease and the superiority of combination chemotherapy in that setting was suggested. Despite that consideration, the initial trial compared single-agent P with a placebo with the intention of providing the preliminary framework upon which the efficacy of more complex therapeutic regimens could be implemented. At the time of protocol commencement, it was neither anticipated nor believed that P would represent the ideal in adjuvant therapy; on the contrary, it was hoped that the results obtained with P would be improved upon by subsequent regimens with the resultant characterization of patient subsets likely to benefit from two or three chemotherapy agents. In the initial investigation, (B-05) one-half of the patients received P and the other half were administered a placebo. The P was given on 5 successive days of a 6-week cycle. This study as well as *all* subsequent NSABP adjuvant therapy protocols for stage II disease required that the therapy be given for 2 years.

---

* Refer to papers in References for listing in NSABP investigators and institutions contributing to these studies

Table 1. NSABP protocols evaluating systemic therapy

Protocol	Nodal status	Randomization		# Patients randomized (6409)	Average time on study (months)[a]
		Begun	Terminated		
05 Placebo vs P	+	9-22-72	2-5-75	380	114 (103−133)
07 P vs PF	+	2-5-75	5-15-76	741	95 (88−106)
08 PF vs PMF	+	4-12-76	4-29-77	737	82 (76−89)
09 PF vs PFT	+	1-1-77	5-16-80	1,891	58 (40−81)
10 PF vs PF + CP	+	5-1-77	5-31-81	265	58 (30−76)
11 PF vs PAF (ER and/or PR neg.)	+	6-1-81	Open	623	−
12 PFT vs PAFT (ER and/or PR pos.)	+	6-1-81	Open	949	−
13 Untreated vs M → F (ER neg.)	−	−	Open	227	−
14 Placebo vs T (ER pos.)	−	1-4-82	Open	596	−

[a] As of 3-31-84

Following demonstration of early benefit from the single agent [1], and in keeping with our original strategy to proceed in stepwise fashion with protocols employing increasing numbers of drugs, a second study (B-07) which compared P with P + 5-fluorouracil (5-FU) (PF) was carried out. Next, the effect of three-drug therapy − PF + methotrexate (MTX) (PMF) − was compared with findings obtained with PF (Protocol B-08). When early findings indicated that the two-drug combination (PF) might be beneficial in more subsets of patients than the single agent [2, 3] and results were not yet available regarding the effectiveness of the three drugs, two additional studies were implemented. One (Protocol B-09) had as its objective the determination of whether the addition of tamoxifen (T) to PF would enhance disease-free survival and survival. The other (Protocol B-10) was carried out to determine whether the addition to PF of the nonspecific stimulating agent, C. parvum (CP), was more beneficial than PF alone.

With failure to observe that the addition of MTX enhanced the effectiveness of PF, two additional studies were conducted. They were carried out to determine the value of the addition of adriamycin to PF (B-11) or to PFT (B-12). As a result of early findings in B-09 [4, 5] indicating that the outcome of patients receiving T with PF was related both to age and to estrogen and progesterone receptor (ER and PR) content of the tumor, those discriminants were used to assign patients to the two trials (B-11 and B-12) (Table 2). With evidence indicating that node-negative, ER− patients have a high rate of recurrence, Protocol B-13 was designed to determine the worth of the sequential use of MTX and 5-FU

Table 2. Assignment of node-positive patients to protocols
B-11 or B-12

Age	ER level	PR level 0−9	(fmol) 10+
Up to 49	0−9	B-11	B-11
	10+	B-11	B-12
50−59	0−9	B-11	B-12
	10+	B-11	B-12
60−70	0−9	B-12	B-12
	10+	B-12	B-12

(M → F). Node-negative patients with ER+ tumors were recipients of either T or placebo in Protocol B-14. This report presents the more significant findings from those protocols which have progressed for a sufficient time to provide meaningful data.

Results

Effectiveness of the Single Agent L-PAM (P)

With the exception of a prior NSABP thiotepa study begun in 1958 [6], the early findings of Protocol B-05 provided the first evidence that adjuvant chemotherapy could alter the natural history of breast cancer. It also indicated that premenopausal and postmenopausal patients were affected differently by chemotherapy. It was the first study to emphasize the need for evaluating patients according to age and nodal status. The early findings gave a clue (unappreciated at the time) that patients 50 years old and older with one to three positive nodes were likely to be less responsive to chemotherapy than those with four or more positive nodes. The original report in 1975 [7] observed that all patients who received L-PAM survived disease free significantly longer than those receiving placebo ($P = 0.02$). Both premenopausal and postmenopausal women showed beneficial results. The benefit noted in premenopausal women in the early findings was maintained, whereas the benefit in older women was lost after 2 years.

The findings originally reported continue to be maintained after 10 years. Patients ≤ 49 years have a significantly better disease-free survival (DFS) ($P = 0.02$) and survival (S) ($P = 0.05$) than do patients receiving placebo. The effect, as previously noted is primarily due to the effect of P on patients ≤ 49 years with 1−3 positive nodes (Fig. 1). In that group after 10 years there is a 36% reduction in treatment failure (TF) and a 44% reduction in mortality.

Effectiveness of the L-PAM plus 5-FU Combination (PF)

Early on, patients receiving PF therapy had a significant advantage over those receiving P alone. It was consistently superior in patients under 50 years of age but the major differences in results were in those ≥ 50 years. In the latter group those having more than three positive nodes demonstrated a significant improvement in both DFS and S. When the

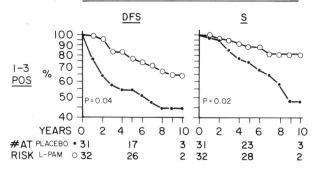

Fig. 1. Placebo vs L-PAM: DFS and S in patients ≤ 49 years with 1−3 positive nodes

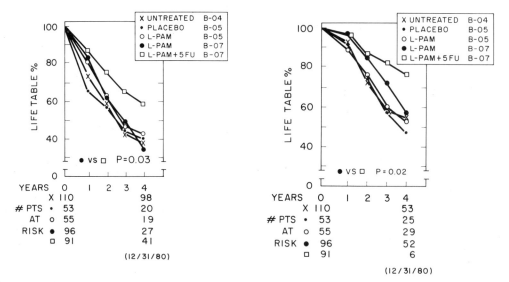

Fig. 2 *(left).* DFS following L-PAM + 5-FU in patients ≥ 50 years with ≥ 4 positive nodes

Fig. 3 *(right).* S following L-PAM + 5-FU in patients ≥ 50 years with ≥ 4 positive nodes

findings with PF in this group were compared not only with those of the L-PAM group in Protocol B-07, but with those of the L-PAM group in Protocol B-05, as well as with placebo patients in Protocol B-05 and untreated radical mastectomy patients in Protocol B-04, the effect of PF therapy on DFS (Fig. 2) and S (Fig. 3) during the first 4 postoperative years became even more evident.

Repetitive analyses carried out at approximately 6-month intervals (in compliance with funding requirements) provide insight into the onset, duration, and magnitude of difference between the two therapies. The data set analyzed 43 months from the onset of the trial, for example, indicated that there was a significant improvement in DFS ($P = 0.01$) and that subsequent analyses during the next several years continued to demonstrate that advantage (Table 3). Between the second and fourth years there was a reduction of between 30% and 40% in treatment failure. During the next 2 years the DFS advantage

Table 3. B-07: Patients $\geq$ 50 years with $\geq$ 4 positive nodes − disease-free survival at various times after operation

Data set (months from onset of trial)[a]	Life-table probability (%)				Treatment-failure reduction (%)
	Years	P 97 patients	PF 91 patients	P Value	
31	2	66	71	0.5	15
37	2	63	71	0.1	21
43	2	63	74	0.01	30
47	2	63	74	0.01	30
53	3	41	66	0.005	42
59	4	33	56	0.01	34
65	4	33	57	0.01	36
71	5	31	40	0.03	13
77	5	29	38	0.03	13
83	5	28	40	0.03	17
89	6	26	33	0.04	9
96	6	26	33	0.04	9
103	7	24	30	0.2	8

[a] Patient accrual 2-5-75 to 5-15-76

Table 4. B-07: Patients $\geq$ 50 years with $\geq$ 4 positive nodes − survival at various times after operation

Data set (months from onset of trial)[a]	Life-table probability (%)				Mortality reduction (%)
	Years	P 97 patients	PF 91 patients	P Value	
31	2	88	82	0.3	0
37	2	82	86	0.3	22
43	2	75	85	0.1	40
47	2	86	86	0.1	0
53	3	69	82	0.04	42
59	4	55	76	0.04	47
65	4	58	74	0.05	38
71	5	47	68	0.02	40
77	5	46	65	0.02	37
83	5	47	66	0.01	36
89	6	35	53	0.01	28
96	6	35	53	0.02	28
103	7	34	46	0.1	18

[a] Patient accrual 2-5-75 to 5-15-76

persisted but gradually lessened so that by the seventh year it was no longer significant. A survival advantage for those receiving PF made its appearance in the third and fourth postoperative years and continued to be significant for at least 6 years (Table 4). Five years after operation there was about a 40% reduction in mortality.

Table 5. B-09: Comparison of PE with PFT without regard for receptor status − disease-free survival and survival at 4 years

Study group	Life-table DES (%)			Treatment-failure reduction (%)	Life-table S (%)			Mortality reduction (%)
	PF	PFT	P		PE	PFT	P	
All patients	53	59	0.004	13	74	75	0.08	4
≤ 49 years	57	54	0.6	0	74	70	0.07	0
1−3 +	69	66	0.8	0	83	82	0.2	0
≥ 4 +	42	40	0.5	0	64	57	0.1	0
≥ 50 years	49	63	0.001	27	75	78	0.2	12
1−3 +	66	72	0.2	18	66	72	0.2	18
≥ 4 +	35	54	< 0.001	29	65	72	0.04	20

Effectiveness of the Three-Drug Combination; L-PAM plus 5-FU plus Methotrexate (PMF)

The final of this trilogy of protocols compared PF with PMF. Patients followed for as long as 6 years when considered overall, according to age, or to age and nodal status fail to demonstrate that PMF is superior to PF. Findings relative to both DFS and S support that conclusion. At no time in the follow-up was there evidence of a favorable effect with PMF. The failure of the three-drug combination to achieve a benefit over two drugs challenges the popular belief that the efficacy of a chemotherapeutic regimen is directly porportional to the number of agents employed.

Effectiveness of Tamoxifen Added to L-PAM + 5-FU (PFT)

The antitumor effect of tamoxifen (termed T), a synthetic nonsteroid compound having antiestrogenic activity, in patients with metastatic breast cancer suggested its possible value in women with primary disease. Consequently, a trial was undertaken to determine whether the addition of T to PF would enhance DFS.

When a comparison was made between PF- and PFT-treated patients *without regard* for tumor ER or PR, life-table analyses of information from nearly 2,000 patients indicated a significant decrease ($P = 0.004$) in DFS and to a lesser extent in S ($P = 0.08$) (Table 5). These differences were due to findings in patients ≥ 50 years with ≥ 4 positive nodes [4]. In that group, a significant survival differences exists ($P = 0.04$) at the present time. Previous analyses [5] have shown that outcome is related to tumor receptor status and age. Such findings are best exemplified by noting the effect of PFT in patients ≥ 50 years with increasing levels of tumor ER (Fig. 4) or PR (Fig. 5).

NSABP Protocol Comparisons

Since the sequential series of NSABP protocols utilized common eligibility criteria and were similar in all respects except in the therapy employed, it is of interest to compare the outcome of patients in the various protocols. The following exemplifies findings from such

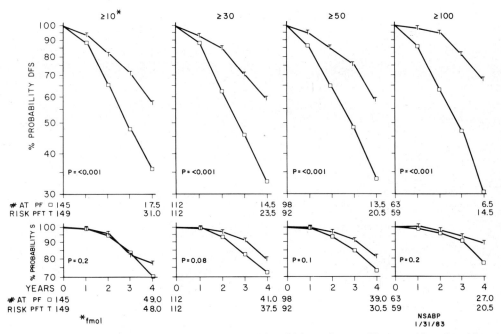

Fig. 4. Effect of increasing levels of tumor ER on DFS and S in patients ≥ 50 years with ≥ 4 positive nodes

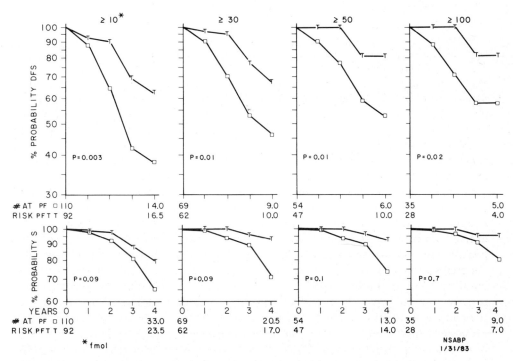

Fig. 5. Effect of increasing levels of tumor PR on DFS and S in patients ≥ 50 years with ≥ 4 positive nodes

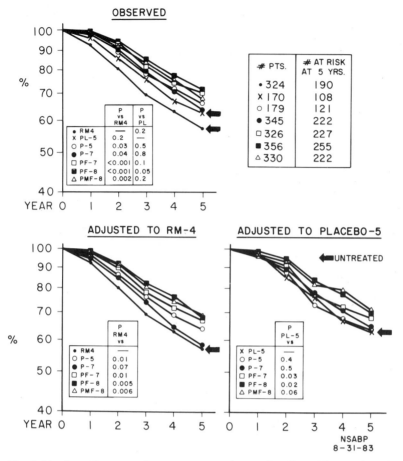

Fig. 6. S in chemotherapy regimens vs untreated controls: adjusted for number of positive nodes, age, nuclear grade, and clinical tumor size

comparisons. The survival of all patients receiving the various chemotherapy regimens was compared with the survival of patients in two NSABP untreated control groups (Fig. 6). First the treatment groups were compared with each of the controls just as was observed and it was found that while there was no significant difference between the two controls (all P values, 2-tailed) the survival of those treated was consistently and more significantly different from the untreated radical mastectomy patients of B-04 than from the placebo patients of B-05. Each of the treatment groups was then compared only after adjustment of the group to the control employed. The adjustment was made relative to the number of positive nodes, age, nuclear grade, and clinical tumor size. It was then observed that those receiving two- and three-drug chemotherapy had a significant difference in survival when compared with either of the controls. When S of patients ≥ 50 years was examined after making appropriate adjustments it was evident that for at least 5 years there was a survival benefit from the chemotherapy (Fig. 7). When the survival was related to nuclear grade, each of the chemotherapy regimens employed demonstrated a striking benefit when tumors were nuclear-grade poor (Fig. 8).

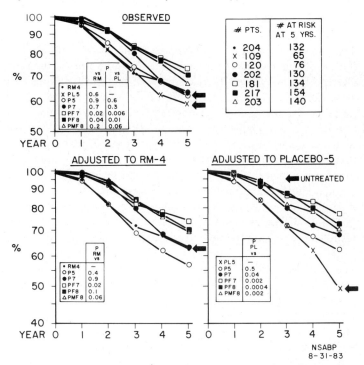

Fig. 7. S in chemotherapy regimens vs untreated controls in patients ≥ 50 years: adjusted for number of positive nodes, age, nuclear grade, and clinical tumor size

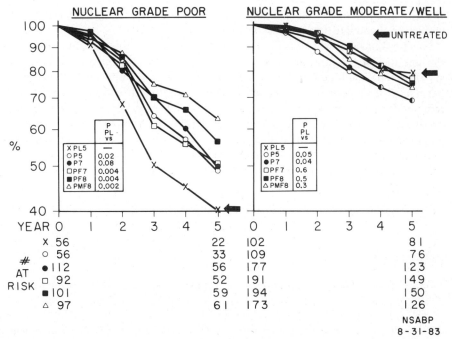

Fig. 8. S in chemotherapy regimens vs B-05 placebo by nuclear grade: adjusted for number of positive nodes, age, and clinical tumor size

Comment and Summary

The brief overview of NSABP findings demonstrates that we have achieved a benefit with the use of adjuvant chemotherapy. The natural history of breast cancer has been favorably altered. The heterogeneity of response to therapy in various patient subsets continues to attest to the biological complexity of the disease. In all NSABP regimens evaluated, differences in therapeutic response have been found to relate to such variables as number of positive axillary nodes, age, ER and PR content of tumors, and a variety of histological tumor characteristics. Of particular pertinence in that regard are our findings indicating that chemotherapeutic responsiveness is related to tumor differentiation. We have previously demonstrated [8] that those tumors with poor histologic grade (grade three) − a marker of differentiation − had a more favorable response to the regimens employed by us than did those with tumors considered to be histologic grade one and two. The present findings indicate, as might be expected, that those with poor nuclear grade (grade one) responded to chemotherapy to a greater degree than did those with a better nuclear grade.

The reported findings continue to substantiate the first findings reported in 1975 which indicated that L-PAM markedly benefited patients ≤ 49 years, particularly those with 1−3 positive nodes. After 10 years they demonstrate that there is a significant benefit in both DFS and S in that subset of patients.

Our results from two protocols (B-07 and B-09) clearly show an advantage in both DFS and S for those patients ≥ 50 years of age. They fail to support the contention that there is no value for adjuvant therapy in postmenopausal patients. Women in that age group with ≥ 4 positive nodes who received PF had a prolonged reduction in treatment failure and in mortality when compared with those receiving L-PAM. An even better outcome was observed in those ≥ 50 years with 1−3 and ≥ 4 positive nodes when T was given in combination with PF. In that subgroup patients whose tumors had increasing levels of ER and/or PR benefited the most from PFT.

It may be concluded from our findings and those of others that benefit has been achieved through the use of adjuvant chemotherapy. It is less clear which regimen of therapy is superior and should be used to the exclusion of others. The maximally effective regimen has not yet been defined. Consequently, since such therapy continues to be "evolving" it remains "experimental". The assumption that three- or five-drug combinations have produced significantly better results than those achieved with the two-drug regimen, PF, as employed by the NSABP, is challenged. The use of adjuvant therapy for the management of patients with histologically negative regional lymph nodes is difficult to justify unless it is carried out within the framework of a controlled clinical trial.

Acknowledgements. This work was supported by USPHS grants R-01-CA-12027, contract N01-CB-23876 and by American Cancer Society grant RC-13.

References

1. Fisher B, Carbone P, Economou SG et al. (1975) L-phenylalanine mustard (L-PAM) in the management of primary breast cancer: A report of early findings. N Engl J Med 292:117−122
2. Fisher B, Glass A, Redmond C et al. (1977) L-phenylalanine mustard (L-PAM) in the management of primary breast cancer: An update of earlier findings and a comparison with those utilizing L-PAM plus 5-fluorouracil (5-FU). Cancer 39:2883−3903

3. Fisher B, Redmond C, Fisher ER et al. (1980) The contribution of recent NSABP clinical trials of primary breast cancer therapy to an understanding of tumor biology — An overview of findings. Cancer 46: 1009–1025
4. Fisher B, Redmond C, Brown A et al. (1981) Treatment of primary breast cancer with chemotherapy and tamoxifen. New Engl J Med 305: 1–6
5. Fisher B, Redmond C, Brown A et al. (1983) Influence of tumor estrogen and progesterone receptor levels on the response to tamoxifen and chemotherapy in primary breast cancer. J Clin Onc 1: 227–241
6. Fisher B, Ravdin RG, Ausman RK et al. (1968) Surgical adjuvant chemotherapy in cancer of the breast: results of a decade of cooperative investigation. Ann Surg 168: 337–357
7. Fisher B, Carbone P, Economou SG et al. (1975) L-phenylalanine mustard (L-PAM) in the management of primary breast cancer: a report of early findings. N Engl J Med 292: 117–122
8. Fisher E, Redmond C, Fisher B et al. (1983) Pathologic findings from the National Surgical Adjuvant Breast Project: VIII. Relationship of chemotherapeutic responsiveness to tumor differentiation. Cancer 51: 181–191

CMF Adjuvant Programs at the Milan Cancer Institute

G. Bonadonna, A. Rossi, G. Tancini, P. Valagussa, and U. Veronesi

Istituto Nazionale per lo Studio e la Cura dei Tumori, Via Venezian 1, 20133 Milano, Italy

Introduction

We present here an uptdated report on the treatment results achieved with adjuvant CMF chemotherapy in two controlled studies at the Milan Cancer Institute. Readers are referred to some of our previous publications [1, 3, 7, 14] for details concerning patient selection, dose schedules, immediate toxic effects, and follow-up studies. For the purpose of this report, suffice it to recall that: (a) the first study (control vs 12 cycles of CMF) was undertaken to test the efficacy of combination chemotherapy on micrometastatic disease; (b) the aim of the second study (CMF 12 cycles vs 6 cycles) was to identify the optimal treatment duration; (c) both patient selection and drug treatment were uniform throughout the two adjuvant programs. Table 1 shows that the treatment arms were properly balanced for two of the major prognostic factors, such as size of primary tumor (T) and extent of axillary node involvement (N), thus ensuring adequate comparability.

As far as statistical evaluation was concerned, relapse-free survival (RFS) and total survival rates were plotted using the product-limit method. Probabilities represent comparison of the entire plots and were calculated using the log-rank test and values of significance [12].

RFS and Survival: Overall Results

RFS and total survival rates for both series of patients are reported in Figs 1 and 2. At 9 years from mastectomy, the difference in RFS between control and CMF remains

Table 1. Main patient characteristics in the two CMF adjuvant trials

Group	n	Pathologic extent			Lymph nodes			
		T1a (%)	T2a (%)	T3a (%)	1 (%)	1–3 (%)	4–10 (%)	> 10 (%)
Control	179	53	45	2	38	70	25	5
CMF 12 A	207	50	47	3	30	68	23	9
CMF 12 B	243	49	48	3	29	62	30	8
CMF 6	216	47	51	2	28	61	30	9

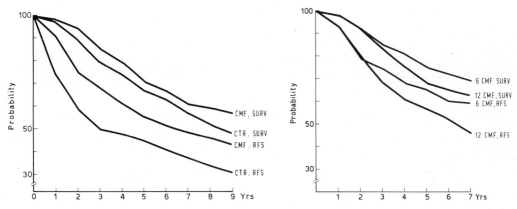

Fig. 1 *(left).* First CMF program (control vs CMF); 9-year results

Fig. 2 *(right).* Second CMF program (CMF 12 vs 6 cycles); 7-year results

statistically significant in favor of the chemotherapy group (31.6% vs 43.2%, $P < 0.001$). While there was a progressive decline over time in both curves, there was little difference in the comparative proportion of patients continuously disease-free at each interval. This would suggest that the percent difference of women benefiting from mastectomy alone vs mastectomy + CMF was already evident by the 3rd year, and the time of clinical manifestation of relapse was probably related only to the growth characteristics of micrometastases. Treatments applied at relapse were comparable between control and CMF groups [5], and included combination chemotherapy in 76% of patients subjected to surgery alone (CMF 84%, equivalent polydrug regimens 26%). Eventually, most relapsing women were subjected before their death to practically all forms of cytotoxic and hormonal treatments. The survival difference in Fig. 1 for the entire series showed only a trend in favor of CMF vs control (58.9% vs 47.9%, $P = 0.14$). It is important to emphasize that the median survival from first relapse was the same for control (30 months) and treated (28 months) groups, indicating that the observed survival difference between control and CMF was due to the effect of adjuvant chemotherapy and not to the treatments applied after relapse.

Figure 2 displays the comparative RFS and survival curves between women subjected to 12 vs 6 cycles of adjuvant CMF. Although at 7 years there was no significant difference between the two treatment groups, the trend was in favor of patients receiving 6 treatment cycles (RFS: 12 CMF 46.2% vs 6 CMF 59.4%, $P = 0.14$). The above-reported findings confirmed that the maximum tumor cell kill by drugs occurred during the first few cycles, while treatment failure was a consequence of progressive growth of specifically and permanently resistant neoplastic cells. Other investigators have observed the lack of significant therapeutic advantage by prolonged treatment with the same drug combination [10, 13, 15].

Results Related to Menopausal and Nodal Subsets

Due to considerable tumor cell heterogeneity, the term breast cancer involves a mosaic of prognostic factors. Using the overall findings may often provide misleading information

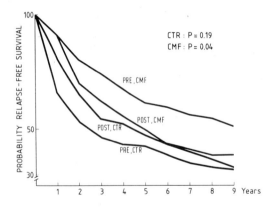

Fig. 3. First CMF program; relapse-free
survival as function of menopausal status

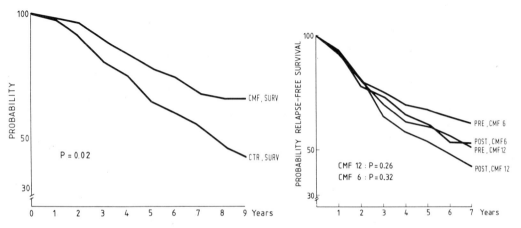

Fig. 4 *(left).* First CMF program; total survival in premenopausal women
Fig. 5 *(right).* Second CMF program; relapse-free survival as function of menopausal status

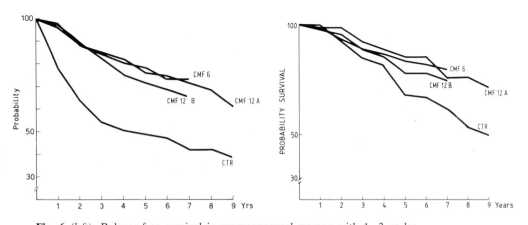

Fig. 6 *(left).* Relapse-free survival in premenopausal women with 1−3 nodes
Fig. 7 *(right).* Total survival in premenopausal women with 1−3 nodes

regarding prognosis and the worth of given treatment since it may obscure subsets benefiting from therapy. Thus, particularly in the evaluation and comparison of adjuvant treatments, analysis by subsets assumes critical importance. For instance, recent observations [6, 9] have strongly indicated the need to accurately quantify the degree of nodal involvement (e.g., in the group having > 3 nodes positive) "to avoid a situation where ineffective therapies appear useful and effective therapies are judged worthless" [9].

Figure 3 shows the comparative RFS of the first CMF study related to menopausal status. The findings confirmed our previous observations [2, 3, 7, 14]. Although a multivariate analysis [11] failed to show that menopausal status per se represented a significant variable between control groups, the impact of 12 CMF cycles, as given, was different in precompared with postmenopausal women. In premenopausal women given CMF total survival was significantly improved over control (65.9% vs 42.8%, $P = 0.02$) indicating that a marked improvement in RFS can be translated into a prolonged total survival advantage (Fig. 4).

Figure 5 compares RFS related to menopause between 12 and 6 cycles of CMF. The trend in favor of 6 cycles remains evident in both menopausal groups. Furthermore, this relatively short-term treatment yielded, at 7 years, superior results in postmenopausal women when findings were compared with those achieved after the first CMF treatment.

Figures 6−9 illustrate the results relative to nodal involvment. Briefly, it appears evident that: (a) the same drug regimen exhibited superior results in the presence of limited axillary node involvement; (b) in the postmenopausal subset with 1−3 positive nodes, the second CMF program yielded a superior RFS compared with the first CMF program, probably because in the former a smaller percentage of patients received dose reductions; (c) 6 cycles of CMF maintained their superiority compared with 12 cycles, particularly in the RFS of premenopausal women with 4−10 involved nodes. As for premenopausal women with higher nodal involvement, there were only 4 patients in the control group with > 10 nodes and all showed new disease manifestations within 6 months of mastectomy.

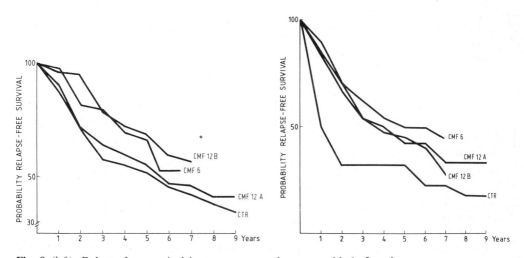

Fig. 8 *(left).* Relapse-free survival in postmenopausal women with 1−3 nodes

Fig. 9 *(right).* Relapse-free survival in premenopausal women with 4−10 nodes

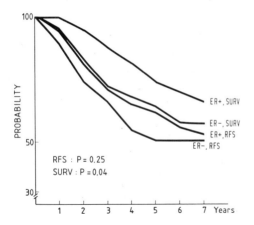

Fig. 10. Second CMF program; results as a function of estrogen receptor status

Similarly, 10 of 11 and 14 of 17 women given 12 CMF cycles (first and second program, respectively) showed relapse within 9 and 7 years. By contrast, only 9 of 18 patients treated with 6 cycles of CMF showed new disease manifestations within 7 years. The small number of patients in each subset, however, prevents a meaningful comparison.

Results Related to Estrogen Receptors

As mentioned in a previous publication [14], estrogen receptor (ER) status was determined only in 56% of patients enrolled in the second CMF adjuvant study. Figure 10 confirms our previous observation. In fact, there was no difference in RFS between women with ER+ and ER− tumors while ER+ tumor exhibited a significantly superior 7-year survival ($P = 0.04$) compared to ER− tumors.

Results Related to Dose Levels

Table 2 updates our previous findings [2, 4] and reiterates the importance of administering full or nearly full drug doses. The efficacy of full- vs low-dose regimen was recently confirmed by Cavalli et al. [8] through a prospective randomized study in advanced breast cancer. It is important to point out that dose-response effect does not apply in the usual sense after treatment has selected a cell subline that is resistant to the chemotherapy being employed. In fact, the treatment may continue to kill the sensitive tumor cells at the same rate, but this is of little clinical consequence after the resistant cells comprise the vast majority of neoplastic population. Therefore, one may anticipate a dose-response effect in the early part of therapy, while over a long period of treatment (e.g., 2 years), when compared with RFS or survival the relationship may be a confusing one.

Second Neoplasms

Table 3 reports the observed second neoplasms in the four treatment groups. A detailed analysis of this topic including our own data, is discussed elsewhere in this book (by Holdener and co-workers). For the purpose of this paper, suffice it to state that available

Table 2. Nine-year results as function of dose levels

	Relapse-free survival (%)	Total survival (%)
Level I	61.2	70.6
Level II	41.6	54.2
Level III	38.0.	48.8
Control	31.6	47.9
Significance		
Level I vs control	< 0.0002	0.02
Level I vs II	0.02	0.06
Level I vs III	0.02	< 0.05

Table 3. Frequency of second neoplasms other than contralateral breast cancer

	n	%
Control	4	2.2[a]
CMF 12 A	6	2.9[a]
CMF 12 B	4	1.6[b]
CMF 6	2	0.9[b]

[a] At 9 years
[b] At 7 years

results confirmed the absence of increased incidence of second neoplasms in the CMF-treated women compared with control women. In particular, no acute or chronic leukemia was observed. Obviously, a longer period of follow-up is required to properly assess the incidence of drug-induced canerogenesis.

Conclusions

The interpretation of our CMF adjuvant programs can be synthesized as follows:

1. CMF exhibited prolonged antitumor effect on a fraction of patients with micrometastases. Although it remains too early to determine cure rate, for none of the survival curves has yet reached a plateau, the consistent and prolonged clinical benefit achieved in given subsets is undeniable.
2. The efficacy of adjuvant treatment was consistently related to the number of positive nodes as well as to dose levels of CMF. As far as menopause was concerned, significant RFS and survival rates were observed in premenopausal and not in postmenopausal women. However, considering the results of both adjuvant programs, we do not have sufficient evidence to state that benefit from CMF chemotherapy, as given, was limited to premenopausal patients.
3. Six cycles of CMF achieved similar, if not better, results than 12 cycles. Although we are unable, at present, to explain the almost constant trend in favor of 6 cycles of chemotherapy, our findings, as well as those of other investigators [10, 13, 15], imply

that the maximum cell kill of sensitive tumor cells occurs within the first few treatment cycles.

4. Immediate and early toxicity related to CMF administration were acceptable, and patients also benefited psychologically from reduction of adjuvant therapy to 6 cycles.
5. Our adjuvant results confirm the heterogeneity of breast cancer and indicate the impropriety of always using overall findings rather than subsets.
6. The benefit from salvage chemotherapy in unselected consecutive patients with recurrent breast cancer was limited and did not influence total survival.
7. In high-risk groups, combined modality treatment is a correct new strategy. What may be considered a limited success should be translated into the total number of high-risk women who, today, can remain continuously disease-free fro 5 or more years following adjuvant treatments of relatively short duration. Therefore, drug combinations (such as 6 cycles of CMF) tested successfully and safely through randomized studies can have a judiciously wide application in women who may benefit from such therapy. The main goal of adjuvant therapy for breast cancer is to maximize RFS. To this end much remains to be elucidated in terms of optimal drug combinations, intervals, and treatment duration through more complex and pharmacologically correct drug regimens.

Acknowledgements. The research reported here was supported in part by contract N01-CM-33714, Department of Cancer Treatment, National Cancer Institute, National Institutes of Health, Bethesda, MD.

References

1. Bonadonna G, Brusamolino E, Valagussa P, Rossi A, Brugnatelli L, Brambilla C, De Lena M, Tancini G, Bajetta E, Musumeci R, Veronesi U (1976) Combination chemotherapy as an adjuvant treatment in operable breast cancer. N Engl J Med 294: 405–410
2. Bonadonna G, Valagussa P (1981) Dose-response effect of adjuvant chemotherapy in breast cancer. N Engl J Med 304: 10–15
3. Bonadonna G, Valagussa P (1983) Chemotherapy of breast cancer: Current views and results. Int J Radiat Oncol Biol Phys 9: 279–297
4. Bonadonna G, Valagussa P (1983) Comment on "The methodologic dilemma in retrospectively correlating the amount of chemotherapy received in adjuvant therapy protocols with disease-free survival." Cancer Treat Rep 67: 527–529
5. Bonadonna G, Valagussa P (to be published) Adjuvant chemotherapy of breast cancer (Letter to the editor). Int J Radiat Oncol Biol Phys
6. Bonadonna C, Valagussa P (1984) Contribution of prognostic factors to adjuvant chemotherapy in breast cancer. (In this volume)
7. Bonadonna G, Valagussa P, Rossi A, Tancini G, Brambilla C, Marchini S, Veronesi U (1981) Multimodal therapy with CMF in resectable breast cancer with positive axillary nodes. The Milan Institute experience. In: Salmon SE, Jones SE (eds) Adjuvant therapy of cancer III. Grune and Stratton, New York, pp 435–444
8. Cavalli F, Pedrazzini A, Martz G, Jungi WF, Brunner KW, Goldhirsch A, Mermillod B, Alberto P (1983) Randomized trial of 3 different regimens of combination chemotherapy in patients receiving simultaneously a hormonal treatment for advanced breast cancer. Eur J Cancer Clin Oncol 19: 1615–1624
9. Fisher B, Bauer M, Wickerham DL, Redmond CK, Fisher ER, Cruz AB, Foster R, Gardner B, Lerner H, Margolese R, Poisson R, Shibata H, Volk H et al. (1983) Relation of number of

positive axillary nodes to the prognosis of patients with primary breast cancer. An NSABP update. Cancer 52: 1551–1557

10. Henderson IC, Gelman R, Parker LM, Skarin AT, Mayer RJ, Garnick MB, Canellos GP (1982) 15 vs 30 weeks of adjuvant chemotherapy for breast cancer patients with a high risk of recurrence: a randomized trial. Proc Am Soc Clin Oncol 1: 75

11. Micciolo R, Valagussa P, Marubini E (to be published) An assessment on the use of historical controls in breast cancer trials

12. Peto R, Pike MC, Armitage P, Breslow NE, Cox DR, Howard SV, Mantel N, McPherson K, Peto J, Smith PG (1977) Design and analysis of randomized clinical trials requiring prolonged observation of each patient. II. Analysis and examples. Br J Cancer 35: 1–39

13. Senn HJ (1982) Current status and indication for adjuvant therapy in breast cancer. Cancer Chemother Pharmacol 8: 139–150

14. Tancini G, Bonadonna G, Valagussa P, Marchini S, Veronesi U (1983) Adjuvant CMF in breast cancer: comparative 5-year results of 12 versus 6 cycles. J Clin Oncol 1: 2–10

15. Vélez García E, Moore M, Marcial V, Vogel C, Bartolucci A, Lin C, Ketcham A, Smalley R (1983) Post-operative adjuvant chemotherapy with or without radiation therapy in patients with stage II breast cancer. A Southeastern Cancer Study Group (SECSG) study. Proc Soc Clin Oncol 2: 111

A Controlled Trial of Adjuvant Chemotherapy with Melphalan Versus Cyclophosphamide, Methotrexate, and Fluorouracil for Breast Cancer

A. Howell, R. D. Rubens, H. Bush, W. D. George, J. M. T. Howat, D. Crowther, R. A. Sellwood, J. L. Hayward, R. K. Knight, R. D. Bulbrook, I. S. Fentiman, and M. Chaudary

Departments of Medical Oncology and Surgery, University Hospital of South Manchester, Manchester and Imperial Cancer Research Fund, Breast Cancer Unit, Guy's Hospital, London, Great Britain

Introduction

The hypothesis that chemotherapy may be more effective when there is only a slight tumor burden has led to its use after mastectomy in patients at high risk of recurrence. The preliminary results of a trial of melphalan (L-PAM) as adjuvant therapy carried out by the National Surgical Adjuvant Breast Project (NSABP) [1], suggested that melphalan therapy could significantly prolong postoperative relapse-free survival (RFS). Because of the importance of these findings we decided, in March 1975, to repeat the trial at the breast unit at Guy's Hospital. Results from the Istituto Nationale Tumori in Milan on the use of a combination of cyclophosphamide, methotrexate, and fluorouracil (CMF) in patients with involved axillary nodes after mastectomy [2] suggested that postoperative RFS could be prolonged by chemotherapy. These findings led to the establishment, in March 1976, of a three-armed trial in the University Hospital of South Manchester comparing no adjuvant treatment, melphalan, and CMF. Because of the similarity of protocols and interests at Guy's Hospital and in Manchester, we decided in 1979 to amalgamate the trials. We now report the results of the combined randomised trial comparing adjuvant melphalan, adjuvant CMF, and no adjuvant therapy.

Patients and Methods

In each centre patients with operable breast cancer (TO-3; NO, 1; MO) were treated by total mastectomy and complete axillary clearance. Preoperative staging was clinical and confirmed after chest radiography, biochemical screening, and isotopic bone scan. All axillary lymph nodes found were examined histologically (mean ± SD nodes examined: melphalan study, 26.4 ± 9.4 per patient; CMF study, 23.6 ± 10.2 per patient). Patients aged less than 75 years (Guy's) or 70 years (Manchester) with involved axillary lymph nodes were allocated randomly either to no additional treatment or to melphalan. Patients aged less than 70 years were allocated randomly either to no additional treatment or to CMF. No patient received postoperative radiotherapy. Recruitment to the melphalan study was from March 1975 to September 1979 at Guy's (258 patients) and from March 1976 to November 1979 at Manchester (112 patients). Recruitment to the CMF study was from March 1976 to December 1981 in Manchester (186 patients) and from October 1979 to October 1983 at Guy's (141 patients). From October 1979 to May 1981 premenopausal patients only were entered at Guy's.

Recent Results in Cancer Research. Vol. 96
© Springer-Verlag Berlin · Heidelberg 1984

Melphalan was given by mouth at a dose of 6 mg/m² (max. 10 mg) daily for 5 days every 6 weeks for 16 cycles. Cyclophosphamide was given by mouth at a dose of 80 mg/m² on days 1–14 of each cycle, methotrexate was given i.v. at a dose of 32 mg/m² on day 1 and day 8 of each cycle, and fluorouracil was given i.v. at a dose of 480 mg/m² on day 1 and day 8 of each cycle. Chemotherapy was started usually within 2 weeks of mastectomy and repeated every 28 days for 12 cycles. Full doses were given provided the total WBC count was $> 4 \times 10^9$/l (Guy's) or $> 3.5 \times 10^9$/l (Manchester) and the platelet count was $> 100 \times 10^9$/l (Guy's) or $> 125 \times 10^9$/l (Manchester). For patients with grade 1 haematological toxicity [WBC count $2-3.9 \times 10^9$/l (Guy's) or $2.5-3.5 \times 10^9$/l (Manchester); platelets $70-99.9 \times 10^9$/l (Gy's), $100-125 \times 10^9$/l (Manchester)], the dose of melphalan was reduced to half. For grade 2 haematological toxicity [WBC count $> 1.9 \times 10^9$/l (Guy's) or $< 2.5 \times 10^9$/l (Manchester); platelets $< 70 \times 10^9$/l (Guy's) or $< 100 \times 10^9$/l (Manchester)], the drug was omitted until haematological toxicity fell to grade 1 and treatment was resumed with half doses. A similar dosage reduction schedule was used for the CMF study using Manchester criteria.

Follow-up included physical examination on day 1 of each treatment cycle and at precisely the same time in controls. WBC and platelet counts were made on day 1 and day 8 in the CMF study of each treatment cycle in patients randomised to receive adjuvant chemotherapy. For the first 2 years after mastectomy, biochemical screening and chest radiography were carried out every 3 months and isotopic bone scans were made every 6 months. Thereafter, follow-up was every 3 months by physical examination only with other investigations repeated as indicated. From 5 years onwards follow-up was annual.

The trial was assessed by postoperative RFS, overall survival, pattern of recurrent disease, and toxicity due to treatment. RFS was taken as the time from date of mastectomy to date of first relapse as defined by Hayward et al. [3]. Disease status was assessed annually by external review (Dr J. W. Meakin) and last verified in October 1983. RFS and overall survival are analysed by the log-rank method [4].

Oestrogen and progesterone receptors were measured by the dextran-coated charcoal technique and Scatchard analysis as previously described [5, 6]. Oestrogen receptors were taken to be present if > 5 fmol/mg of cytosol protein was detected and progesterone receptors were taken to be present if $\geqslant 15$ fmol/mg of cytosol protein was detected ($\geqslant 5$ in melphalan study). The results of a study reporting the effects of CMF on psychological function in patients in this trial and the results of the melphalan study have already been published [7, 8].

Results

The characteristics of the combined Manchester and Guy's patients are shown in Table 1. There were no significant differences in these characteristics between treatment and control groups for the melphalan study or the CMF study. In the CMF study there are proportionately more premenopausal patients because from October 1979 to May 1981 premenopausal patients only were admitted to the trial at Guy's.

Relapse Free Survival

Melphalan Study

In the melphalan study there were no significant differences in RFS for the treatment and control groups for all patients or within the strata of nodal and menopausal status. A

Table 1. Characteristics of patients in the three treatment groups

Age (years)	Controls $n = 162$	CMF $n = 165$	Controls $n = 183$	Melphalan $n = 187$
< 40	18	21	16	17
40−49	52	51	56	53
50−59	62	63	61	56
⩾ 60	30	30	50	61
Menopausal status				
Premenopausal	87	81	77	79
Postmenopausal	75	84	106	108
Axillary nodes involved				
⩽ 3	100	99	115	109
⩾ 4	62	66	68	78
Tumour stage				
T0	0	0	2	8
T1	26	34	37	40
T2	99	96	108	117
T3	24	30	34	20
Paget's disease	4	2	0	0
NK	9	3	2	2
Histology				
Ductal carcinoma	134	139	165	167
Lobular carcinoma	22	16	8	7
Other	6	10	10	13
Oestrogen receptor content[a]				
< 5	42	36	59	56
⩾ 5	93	102	113	108
NK	27	27	11	23
Progesterone receptor content[a]				
< 15	70	72	112	96
⩾ 15	64	69	56[b]	63[b]
NK	28	24	14	28

[a] In fmol/mg cytosol protein
[b] ⩾ 5 fmol/mg cytosol protein

comparison of the treatment and control groups is shown in Fig. 1a. Patients in the melphalan group had a marginally (5%−10%) better RFS, but the difference from the controls was not significant ($P = 0.11$).

Recurrence rates were compared for subsets of the pooled data. Premenopausal women treated with melphalan had a slightly greater RFS than premenopausal controls, but again the difference was not significant ($P = 0.14$). In postmenopausal women, the RFS curves were almost identical ($P = 0.39$). Melphalan-treated patients with 1−3 nodes involved had a 10% increase in RFS from 4 years after mastectomy, but the difference from the control experience was not significant ($P = 0.08$). In patients with heavy nodal involvement there was again no appreciable benefit from melphalan ($P = 0.33$).

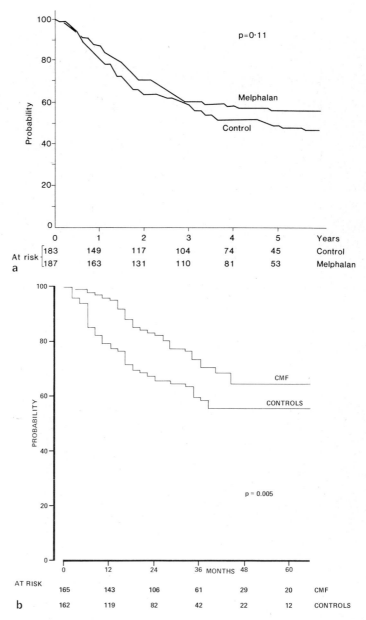

Fig. 1. a Postoperative RFS for all patients: melphalan vs control. **b** Postoperative RFS for all patients: CMF vs control

Fisher et al. found, when their original series of patients was followed up, that the most striking benefit from adjuvant therapy with melphalan was obtained in premenopausal women with 1−3 nodes involved. When we examined recurrence rates in this particular subset there was no significant difference in RFS between the treated and the control groups ($P = 0.26$).

A. Howell et al.

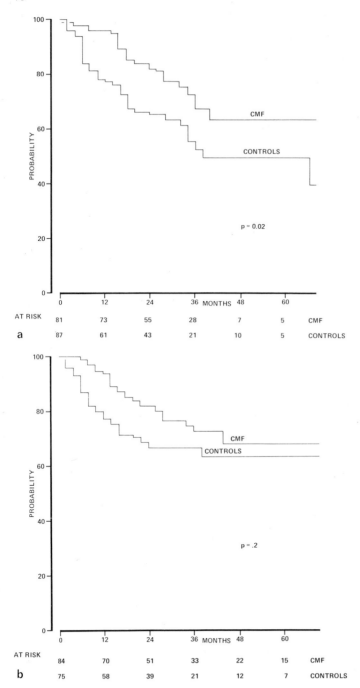

Fig. 2. a Postoperative RFS for premenopausal patients: CMF vs control. **b** Postoperative RFS for postmenopausal patients: CMF vs control

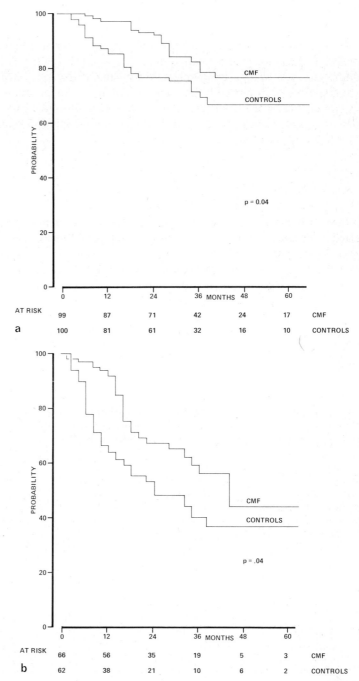

Fig. 3. a Postoperative RFS for patients with ≤ 3 axillary lymph nodes involved: CMF vs control.
b Postoperative RFS for patients with ≥ 4 axillary lymph nodes involved: CMF vs control

CMF Study

A comparison of the treatment and control groups is shown in Fig. 1b. Patients treated with CMF had a longer RFS than controls ($P = 0.005$); at the 3rd year of follow-up this difference was 17.4%. Premenopausal women treated with CMF also had a significantly longer RFS ($P = 0.02$; Fig. 2a) but the difference for postmenopausal women was not significant ($P = 0.13$; Fig. 2b). The groups of CMF-treated patients with 1−3 and $\geqslant 4$ involved axillary nodes had a significantly greater RFS than did controls ($P = 0.04$ and 0.02 respectively; Figs. 3a and 3b).

Site of Relapse

There was a close similarity in the distribution of recurrence sites, both of first recurrence and of all recurrences (Table 2), in the control and melphalan-treatment groups. These results do not support the suggestion that melphalan has specific action against any particular site of recurrence. However, for first recurrences, there was a significant reduction in locoregional relapses in the CMF-treated group ($P = 0.007$; 21% control vs 9% CMF-treated) but no difference in the proportion of patients with distant relapse (17% control vs 16% CMF-treated). When all sites of relapse were considered (i.e., not only first relapse) there were significantly more skin and lymphatic relapses in the controls than in the CMF-treated group ($P = 0.02$ and 0.04, respectively) but no differences in distant sites such as bone, lung, and liver (Table 2).

Table 2. Sites of first recurrence and of all recurrences (first + subsequent)

	Numbers of patients (%)			
	Controls $n = 162$	CMF $n = 165$	Controls $n = 183$	Melphalan $n = 187$
Sites of first relapse				
Locoregional	34 (21)	15 (9)	49 (27)	33 (18)
Distant	27 (17)	26 (16)	41 (22)	42 (22)
Locoregional + distant	1 (1)	0 (0)	4 (2)	5 (3)
Total	62 (38)	41 (25)	94 (51)	80 (43)
Sites of all relapses				
Contralateral breast	9 (6)	5 (3)	21 (11)	15 (8)
Skin	27 (16)	12 (7)	28 (15)	26 (14)
Lymphatics	19 (12)	8 (5)	34 (19)	15 (8)
Bone	25 (15)	23 (14)	36 (20)	26 (14)
Lung/pleura	15 (9)	14 (8)	21 (11)	24 (13)
Liver	6 (4)	8 (5)	27 (15)	19 (10)
Brain	5 (3)	1 (1)	11 (6)	5 (3)
Other	4 (2)[a]	3 (2)[a]	16 (9)[b]	8 (4)[b]

[a] Includes meninges (3), pericardium (1), eye (1), appendix (1), pancreas (1)
[b] Includes ascites (15), dura (2), mesentery (2), ovary (1), kidney (1), adrenal (1), gall bladder (1)

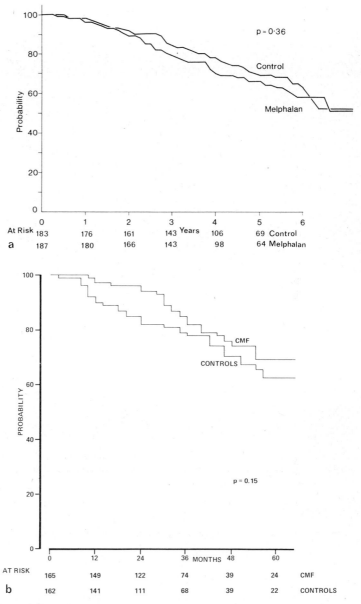

Fig. 4. a Survival of all patients: melphalan vs control. **b** Survival of all patients: CMF vs control

Survival

Adjuvant melphalan had no appreciable effect on survival (Fig. 4a); indeed, the trend was for better survival in the control group as after 5 years 34% of the treated and 31% of the control patients had died. Adjuvant CMF also had no appreciable effect on survival (Fig. 4b); after 3 years, 16% of the treated and 21% of the control patients had died. There was no survival advantage in any subgroup when these were analysed separately.

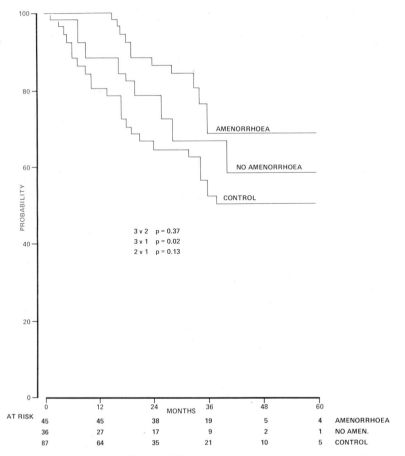

Fig. 5. Postoperative RFS for CMF-treated premenopausal patients with amenorrhoea (*1*) and without amenorrhoea (*2*) compared with premenopausal controls (*3*)

Amenorrhoea

The occurrence of amenorrhoea was studied, since an effect of chemotherapy on ovarian function may influence the prognosis in breast cancer. Twenty-four of 78 (31%) premenopausal patients treated with melphalan and 45 of 87 (52%) premenopausal patients treated with CMF developed amenorrhoea. In the melphalan study there was a trend in favour of a longer RFS in the group that developed amenorrhoea, but this did not reach statistical significance ($P = 0.17$). Similarly, in the CMF-treated premenopausal patients, those with amenorrhoea had a longer DFS (disease-free survival) than treated patients without amenorrhoea ($P = 0.13$): when the amenorrhoeic treated group were compared with untreated premenopausal controls there was a significant difference in DFI (disease-free interval) ($P = 0.02$; Fig. 5).

Receptor Status

The RFS was analysed for CMF and controls according to oestrogen and progesterone status of the primary tumour. Patients with progesterone receptor-positive tumours treated

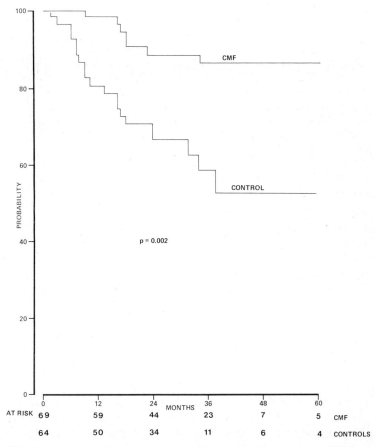

Fig. 6. Postoperative RFS in patients with progesterone receptor-positive tumours: CMF vs control

with CMF had a significantly longer RFS than controls; seven of 69 CMF-treated patients recurred, whereas 22 of 64 controls recurred ($P = 0.002$; Fig. 6). There were no significant differences in RFS between treated patients and controls in the groups with oestrogen receptor-positive, oestrogen receptor-negative, or progesterone receptor-negative tumours. The RFS in favour of CMF progesterone receptor-positive patients was significant for the premenopausal patients ($P = 0.02$), but although there was a trend in favor of CMF-treated postmenopausal patients this was not significant ($P = 0.14$). There were no differences in survival between treated and control patients for any receptor subgroup.

Toxicity

The subjective and haematological toxicity of melphalan and CMF are outlined in Table 3. Subjective toxicity from melphalan was almost exclusively nausea and vomiting and developed on one or more occasions in 25% of treated patients. Predictably CMF was more

Table 3. Toxicity attributable to CMF and melphalan

		CMF	Melphalan
		Number of patients (%)[a]	
		(n = 165)	(n = 187)
Nausea/vomiting		136 (82)	47 (25)
Alopecia		107 (65)	4 (2)
Conjunctivitis		51 (31)	0
Stomatitis		53 (32)	0
Diarrhoea		37 (22)	0
Cystitis		10 (6)	0
WBC ($\times 10^9$)/l)			
Manchester	Guy's		
< 3.5	< 4	103 (62)	41 (22)
< 2.5	< 2	13 (8)	33 (17)
Platelets ($\times 10^9$/l)			
< 125	< 100	11 (7)	25 (13)
< 100	< 70	6 (4)	7 (4)

[a] In whom the toxic effect was observed on one or more occasions

toxic, with 82% nausea and vomiting and 65% partial alopecia. Other side effects were less common but troublesome in a significant minority of patients.

Depression of the WBC count below $3.5-4 \times 10^9$/l was seen more often in CMF-treated patients, but there were proportionately more melphalan patients with counts below 2×10^9/l. Melphalan was more likely to cause thrombocytopenia. In order to estimate the long-term effect of adjuvant chemotherapy upon the bone marrow, 14 patients (2 melphalan and 12 CMF) consented to bone marrow examination 5−36 months after completion of chemotherapy. Cells were grown in vitro to detect the number of granulocyte-macrophage colony-forming cells and these were compared to the number of fibroblast colony forming units from patients and controls undergoing thoracotomy or orthopaedic operations. Although the fibroblast colony-forming unit numbers did not differ between adjuvant treated and control marrows (Fig. 7), the number of granulocyte-macrophage colony-forming cells was reduced below normal in 11 of 14 patients who had had adjuvant chemotherapy (Fig. 7).

The psychological morbidity of melphalan and CMF was estimated in a subgroup of 59 patients. Trained interviewers conducted the present-state examination shortly after surgery and 3, 12, and 18 months later. Of the 26 patients treated with CMF, 20 experienced an anxiety state, compared with 4 of the 15 given melphalan and 9 of the 18 control subjects. Depressive illness occurred more often in the CMF group (20 patients) than in the melphalan group (5 patients) or control group (9 patients; Table 4).

Dose

In the melphalan study 45 (24%) patients received $\geqslant$ 90% of the planned dose and 142 (76%) received < 90% of the planned dose. There was a trend towards a longer DFI in patients who received lower doses ($P = 0.07$).

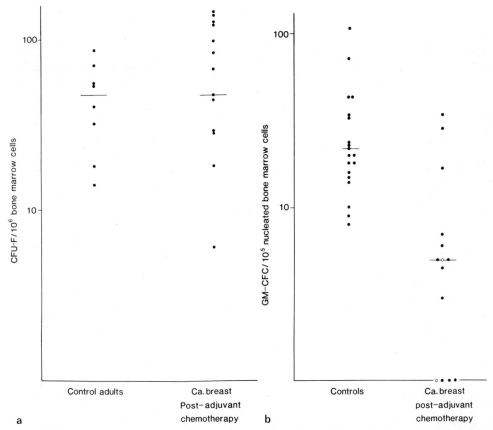

Fig. 7. a Bone-marrow fibroblast colony-forming units (*CFU-F*) in controls compared with patients after adjuvant chemotherapy. **b** Bone marrow granulocyte-macrophage colony-forming cells (GM-CFC) in controls compared with patients after adjuvant chemotherapy (○ post-melphalan; ● post-CMF)

In the CMF study, 37 (24%) patients received $\geq$ 85% of the planned dose, 47 (31%) received 65%−84% and 69 (45%) received < 65%. There was a trend in favour of a longer RFS for patients, who received the highest doses, but this was not statistically significant ($P = 0.19$; Fig. 8). The median number of cycles of CMF given per patient was 11.6 and the mean was 9.4.

Second Malignancies

In the melphalan study second malignancies other than breast cancer were observed in three patients in the control group (one carcinoma of appendix, one lung cancer, one ovarian cancer) and in two patients receiving melphalan (one rectal carcinoma, one pancreatic carcinoma). In the CMF study second malignancies were observed in two patients in the control group (one melanoma, one ovary) and in three patients receiving CMF (one acute myeloid leukaemia, two ovary).

Table 4. Presence or absence of psychiatric morbidity judged to require treatment in patients with breast cancer

Treatment group	Anxiety[a]		Depression[b]		Sexual problems[c]		Overall morbidity[d]	
	+ (%)	−	+ (%)	−	+ (%)	−	+ (%)	−
Mastectomy alone	9 (50)	9	9 (32)	19	5 (50)	5	9 (50)	9
Mastectomy and melphalan	4 (27)	11	5 (33)	10	3 (38)	5	5 (33)	10
Mastectomy and CMF	20 (77)	6	20 (77)	6	14 (70)	6	21 (81)	5

Significance of difference between numbers of patients showing morbidity and numbers of patients not showing morbidity at:
[a] $\chi^2 = 10.1$, $df = 2$, $P < 0.01$
[b] $\chi^2 = 8.0$, $df = 2$, $P < 0.02$
[c] $\chi^2 = 4.4$, $df = 2$, NS
[d] $\chi^2 = 9.9$, $df = 2$, $P < 0.01$

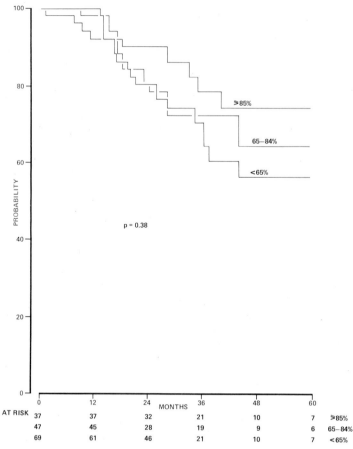

Fig. 8. Post operative RFS and dose of CMF

Discussion

The preliminary results of the NSABP trial in the USA suggested a significant prolongation of postoperative RFS with the use of adjuvant melphalan therapy in premenopausal patients and those with 1−3 involved axillary lymph nodes [1]. Although our trial reaffirms a trend towards a lower number of recurrences and longer postoperative RFS in all subgroups, particularly premenopausal patients and those with 1−3 nodes involved, in no case was this significant.

Our failure to confirm any of the original results of Fisher et al. [1] to find significant differences in any of the retrospective subgroup analyses raises a fundamental point as far as trials of adjuvant chemotherapy are concerned. With currently available treatments for breast cancer, large beneficial effects would not be expected but, in a common disease such as this, even a modest effect from a readily practicable treatment which reduces the mortality from this cause would be of substantial medical importance. Such an effect would, however, be extremely difficult to detect reliably in trials on only a few hundred patients, such as our own and previous studies, particularly when subset analyses are done. Consequently, one would expect that different trials of the same treatments might yield apparently different answers. Joint examination of our results and those of the NSABP does not necessarily indicate that melphalan works better in their hands than in ours, but rather that the overall evidence from the two studies suggests a slight difference in RFS but little difference in overall survival.

The preliminary results of the Milan trial demonstrated a significant improvement in RFS for patients treated with CMF compared with controls [2]. The improvement was seen initially in premenopausal and postmenopausal patients and in those with 1−3 and also 4+ nodes involved. The advantage in the postmenopausal group later disappeared, but after 8 years there remains an overall advantage in RFS for CMF-treated patients confined to premenopausal patients and those with 1−3 nodes involved [8]. Our results evolved in a similar manner to those from Milan. At an early stage there was a highly significant advantage in RFS for CMF-treated patients overall and for all subgroups [9]. Subsequently, although there is an overall treatment advantage it is no longer significant in the postmenopausal group of patients. The median follow-up period in our study is 33 months. It remains to be seen whether differences in RFS continue to be significant after a longer period of follow-up. At present it appears that CMF significantly delays relapse.

Both melphalan and CMF tended to reduce the number of first relapses in locoregional sites but had no effect upon distant relapses. A similar trend was seen when the sites of first and subsequent relapses were assessed. This contrasts with the Milan experience where a reduction in distant relapses was also found.

There was no difference in overall survival between the control group patients receiving adjuvant melphalan or adjuvant CMF. This is true for the pre- and postmenopausal groups of patients. In the Milan study there was no difference in overall survival for the whole group though premenopausal patients treated with CMF have consistently had a significantly improved survival compared with controls [2, 8]. Although RFS may give a preliminary indication of the results of adjuvant chemotherapy, the true efficacy of such treatment must ultimately be measured in terms of survival. It is possible that adjuvant chemotherapy compromises the effective use of chemotherapy for subsequent advanced disease, since the advantage of an increased RFS is lost when we look at survival. This study, therefore, fails to confirm the survival adavantage for premenopausal CMF-treated patients seen in the Milan trial.

In this study, CMF delays relapse in premenopausal women only. It is possible that this effect is produced by a chemical castration, since patients who developed CMF-induced amenorrhoea had a significantly longer RFS compared with controls, whereas RFS in those without amenorrhoea did not differ significantly from the controls. A trend towards longer DFS in patients with CMF-induced amenorrhoea was also seen in the Milan trial. In addition, when the relationship of RFS to receptor status was considered, CMF was found to delay relapse in the subgroup of premenopausal patients whose primary tumour contained measurable progesterone receptors: a group that would be expected to have a high probability of response to hormone therapy if they developed recurrent disease. However, the number of patients in each subgroup according to receptor status is small, and these findings must be treated with caution.

The protocol dose of CMF was reduced to 80% of the Milan dose because this was approximately what was administered in later cycles in that study [2]. However, despite this initial reduction, further reductions were necessary, mainly because of haematological toxicity. In contradistinction to the Milan study, improvement in RFS was not related to the dose of CMF administered [10]. In the melphalan study, reported here, there was a trend for patients who had dosage reduction to have longer RFS. It is of interest that a significant dose-response effect was not seen when the Milan group used 6 cycles of CMF [11]. A positive dose-response effect, if found, must be treated with caution in retrospective analyses, since compliant patients may be the ones able to tolerate high doses and may have longer DFS for reasons other than response to chemotherapy. It is known that patients on full-dose placebo live longer than those who require placebo dosage reduction.

The psychological, physical, and haematological toxicity of CMF was considerable [7]. More than half the patients had marked anxiety or depression, virtually all had some degree of physical toxicity and mild bone marrow depression was common. The development of acute myeloid leukaemia in a CMF-treated patient so early in the follow-up period (3 years) may have been purely coincidental, but it is of interest that the majority of patients tested had evidence of subclinical bone marrow depression as judged by normal or near-normal peripheral blood counts in association with reduced bone marrow colony-forming units 5–36 months after the completion of CMF treatment [12]. Long-term follow-up of all patients in adjuvant trials is mandatory.

The benefit of CMF to a limited proportion of treated patients must be weighed against the harm and inconvenience to those who would otherwise have been cured by operation alone and also to those whose tumours were not actually affected by the drugs used. If adjuvant chemotherapy results in a pronounced increase in the cure rate of breast cancer, then this toxicity is justifiable. However, our early results indicate a need for caution before advocating the widespread use of CMF as an adjuvant treatment for breast cancer.

Acknowledgements. We thank Dr R. R. Millis (Pathology), Miss C. L. Joyce, Miss N. M. H. Byrant, Mrs M. Hamer, Mr M. A. Halder, Miss M. Dias, Mr P. Lennard-Jones (data handling), Dr R. J. B. King (steroid receptor analyses), all of the Imperial Cancer Research Fund Breast Unit, and Dr M. Harris (Pathology), Miss G. Wood, Miss J. Redford (data managers), Dr D. M. Barnes (steroid receptor analyses), and Mrs Eileen Morgan (for typing the manuscript).

References

1. Fisher BF, Carbone P, Economou SG et al. (1975) L-phenylalanine mustard (L-PAM) in the management of primary breast cancer: a report of early findings. N Engl J Med 292: 117–122
2. Bonadonna G, Brusamolino E, Valagussa P et al. (1976) Combination chemotherapy as an adjuvant treatment in operable breast cancer. N Engl J Med 294: 405–410
3. Hayward JL, Meakin JW, Stewart HJ (1978) Assessment of response and recurrence in breast cancer. Semin Oncol 5: 445–449
4. Peto R, Pike MC, Armitage P et al. (1977) Design and analysis of randomised clinical trials requiring prolonged observations of each patient. II. Analysis and examples. Br J Cancer 35: 1–39
5. King RJB, Redgrave S, Hayward JL, Millis RR, Rubens RD (1979) The measurement of receptors for oestrogen and progesteron in human breast tumours. In: King RJB (ed) Steroid receptor assays in human breast tumours. Methodological and clinical aspects. Alpha Omega, Cardiff
6. Barnes DM, Ribeiro GG, Skinner LG (1979) Simultaneous estimation of oestrogen and progestin receptor activity in human breast tumours and correlation with response to treatment. In: King RJB (ed) Steroid receptor assay in human breast tumours. Methodological and clinical aspects. Alpha Omega, Cardiff, pp 16–31
7. Maguire GP, Howat JMT, Sellwood RA, Tait A, Bush H (1980) The psychological morbidity associated with adjuvant chemotherapy following mastectomy in patients with breast cancer. Br Med J 281: 1179–1180
8. Bonadonna G, Rossi A, Tancini G, Valagussa P (1983) Adjuvant chemotherapy in breast cancer. Lancet 1: 1157
9. Howat JMT, Hughes R, Durning P, George WD, Sellwood RA, Bush H, Phadke K, Grafton C, Crowther D (1981) A controlled clinical trial of adjuvant chemotherapy in operable cancer of the breast. In: Salmon SE, Jones SE (eds) Adjuvant therapy of cancer III. Grune and Stratton, New York, p 71
10. Bonadonna G, Valagussa P (1981) Dose-response effect of adjuvant chemotherapy in breast cancer. N Engl J Med 304: 10–15
11. Tancini G, Bonadonna G, Valagussa P, Marchini S, Veronisi U (1983) Adjuvant CMF in breast cancer: comparative 5 year results of 12 versus 6 cycles. J Clin Oncol 1/1: 2–10
12. Haworth C, Howell A, Testa NG (to be published) Long term bone marrow damage in patients treated with adjuvant chemotherapy

Adjuvant Chemoimmunotherapy with LMF + BCG in Node-Negative and Node-Positive Breast Cancer: 8 Year Results

H. J. Senn, W. F. Jungi, R. Amgwerd, E. Hochuli, J. Ammann,
G. Engelhart, C. Heinz, A. Wick, F. Enderlin, G. Creux,
B. Simeon, R. Lanz, R. Bigler, and S. Seiler*

Medizinische Klinik C, Kantonsspital, St. Gallen, Switzerland

Introduction

Since medium- to long-term survival expectancy, and thus mortality, for patients with operable breast cancer have remained essentially unchanged during the past 40−50 years in most countries, increasing numbers of clinical adjuvant studies have emerged during the past decade (reviewed in [3, 16]), prompted particularly by early optimistic reports from the NSABP and Milan groups [1, 5]. Most such investigations included only node-positive (N+) patients. We, however, felt the need to also incorporate (on a stratified basis) histologically node-negative (N−) women for the following three reasons: (1) our observation of a lower regional relapse-free survival (RFS) and overall survival (OAS) in N− patients [14] than is usually cited in the literature; (2) our assumption that N− patients with truly "minimal postoperative tumor cell burden" would constitute an ideal and completely curable population to test the present concept of adjuvant systemic chemotherapy, since to date at least 25%−30% of N− patients present recurrent, mostly incurable disease within 8−10 years of mastectomy; (3) our choice of a well-tolerated adjuvant regimen without the potential of hair-loss or significant gastrointestinal upset. Immunostimulation with bacillus Calmette-Guérin (BCG) was added to the chemotherapy (leukeran, methotrexate, fluorouracil − CMF) based on earlier claims that this treatment would "counter-balance" immunodepressive effects of cytotoxic treatment and potentially prolong RFS and/or OAS.

The present paper reports 8-year results (median duration of follow-up) of our study, OSAKO 06/74, which accepted its first patients exactly 10 years ago.

Patients and Study Design

Between 1974 and 1977, a total of 254 patients with stages T_{1-3a}, N_{0-1}, M_0 operable breast cancer have been randomized to either surgery alone (modified radical mastectomy without adjuvant radiotherapy) or the same type of surgery + 6 cycles of *oral* LMF, followed by monthly skin scarifications with Glaxo-strain BCG up to relapse or 2 years. The details of study design, patient selection, and follow-up program have been reported

---

* Ostschweizerische Arbeitsgruppe für Klinische Onkologie (OSAKO)

Table 1. Distribution of prognostic factors of 240 evaluable patients in adjuvant study OSAKO 06/74 (only general nodal status [N−, N+] was stratified prior to randomization in both treatments)

(Sub)group	All patients	Surgical controls	Surgery and LMF/BCG
N− and N+ (all)	240	123	117
N−	122	65	57
N+	118	58	60
N+ (1−3)	80	38	42
N+ ($\geq$ 4)	38	20	18
T_{1-2a}	218	112	106
T3a	22	11	11
Pre- and perimenopausal	126	63	63
Postmenopausal	114	60	54
Median age at surgery (years)	55.3	56.7	53.0

several times before [12−15]. No hormone receptor data were available during the years of patient accrual.

At the time of the 8-year analysis in January 1984, 240 of 254 randomized patients (= 94%) were fully evaluable. The two treatment groups were well balanced, regarding known risk factors (excluding hormone receptors) as shown in Table 1.

Results at 8 Years Median Follow-up

Eight-year results will be presented graphically for RFS and OAS in the whole patient population (N− and N+) as well as in the most important menopausal and nodal subgroups (N−, N+). Note that in contrast to the basic nodal status (N−, N+), menopausal status and nodal substatus were *not* stratified prior to randomization for surgery alone or surgery + LMF/BCG, thus limiting statistical conclusions and cross-study comparisons in these patient subgroups.

Figure 1a, b demonstrates a clear-cut distinction in RFS as well as OAS between our N− and N+ global study-patient population (both treatment regimens combined). This statistically highly evident difference is not seen by comparing pre- and postmenopausal women in our combined N+/N− study population (Fig. 2a, b). In this respect "premenopausal" patients included also perimenopausal women (up to 5 years after last menses or 55 years of age).

Figure 3a shows a prolonged and still significant increase of RFS for patients treated with LMF/BCG. This advantage no longer transforms into a significantly elevated OAS at 8 years (Fig. 3b), while it did up to the 7th year [14, 15].

This trend may however change significance again as follow-up goes on, since to date only half of the patients have reached the 8-year follow-up.

Figure 4a, b discloses significantly better RFS and borderline significantly higher OAS of *post*menopausal patients, treated with LMF/BCG compared with the entire patient population. The gains of +14% in RFS and of +11% in OAS are remarkable.

Figure 5a shows the evolution of the difference in RFS in both treatment groups of N− patients. Following an impressive divergence of the curves in favor of LMF/BCG-treated patients during the first 4 years, this difference vanished at 5−6 years. The difference in

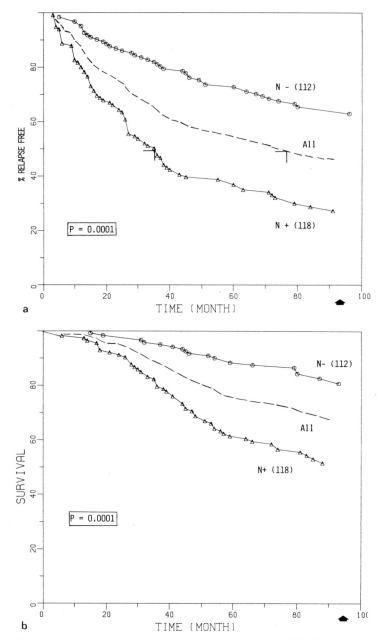

Fig. 1a, b. Prognostic influence of initial nodal status in OSAKO Study 06/74, all patients and both treatment arms combined. **a** Relapse-free survival; **b** overall survival

RFS for LMF/BCG (68.4%) and surgical controls (62.1%) is far from significant ($P = 0.28$). Interestingly enough, the OAS gain for N− patients with LMF/BCG continues, although there is a tendency towards merging of the curves at 8 years (84.2% vs 69.2%, $P = 0.07$). The median annual patient death rate of 3.2% in surgical controls has been reduced to 1.7% in LMF/BCG-treated patients.

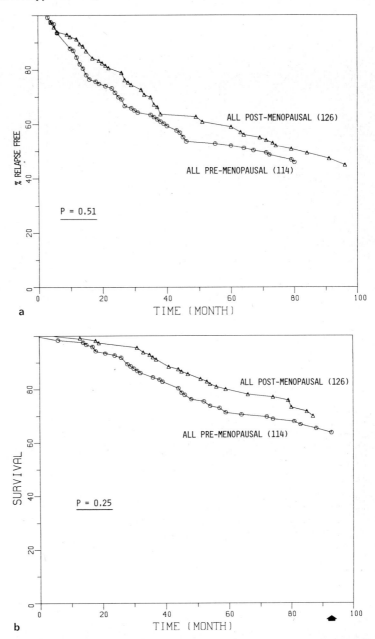

Fig. 2a, b. Missing prognostic influence of menopausal status at surgery in OSAKO-Study 06/74. **a** Relapse-free survival; **b** overall survival

In N+ patients, showing no benefit with LMF + BCG during the first 3 years, a persistent and rather increasing difference in RFS in favor of the LMF/BCG-treated women was emerging after the fourth year as demonstrated in Fig. 6a (40.0% vs 22.4%, $P = 0.05$). However, this late benefit in RFS at no time translated into increased OAS, with a median annual death rate of 6.3% in both treatments arms (Fig. 6b). All favorable effects of LMF

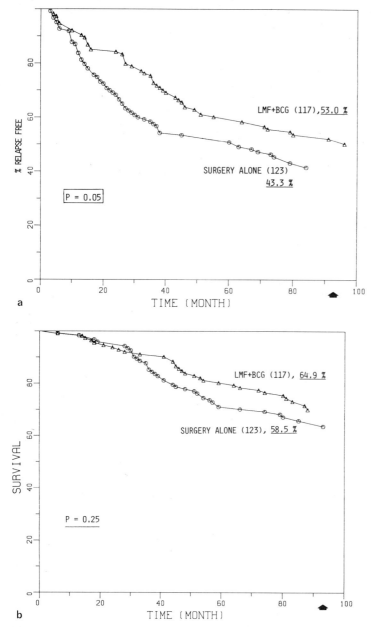

Fig. 3a, b. Results of LMF + BCG in OSAKO-Study 06/74, all patients. **a** Relapse-free survival;
b overall survival

+ BCG in node-positive patients were seen in women with 1−3 positive axillary nodes.
Virtually no differences between the two treatment regimens were observed for RFS and
OAS in highest-risk women with four or more positive nodes ($P = 0.94$ for RFS and 0.98
for OAS).

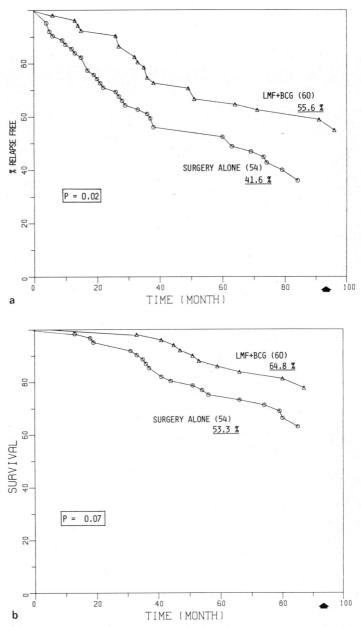

Fig. 4a, b. Results of LMF + BCG in OSAKO-Study 06/74, all postmenopausal patients.
a Relapse-free survival; **b** overall survival

There was a strong indication in N− (concerning OAS) as well as N+ patients (regarding RFS), that *post*menopausal benefited more than premenopausal women from LMF + BCG. But we resist presenting these data in detail, due to the small patient numbers in these nonstratified subgroups.

Figure 7 gives at least suggestive evidence that full total dose (greater than 90%) during the 6 cycles of LMF positively affected OAS (74% vs 60%, P = 0.08). However, the two

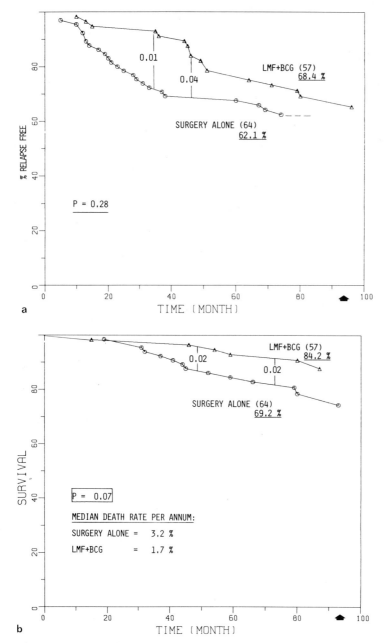

Fig. 5a, b. Results of LMF + BCG in OSAKO-Study 06/74, all node-negative patients. **a** Relapse-free survival; **b** overall survival

groups of treatment intensity are very imbalanced numerically, with 75% of patients completing 6 cycles of oral LMF with total drug doses of ≥ 90% (due to excellent drug tolerance) [14].

Immediate toxicity due to LMF + BCG was low, compared with other adjuvant regimens such as CMF, CMFVP, or adriamycin-containing combinations. There was usually mild GI

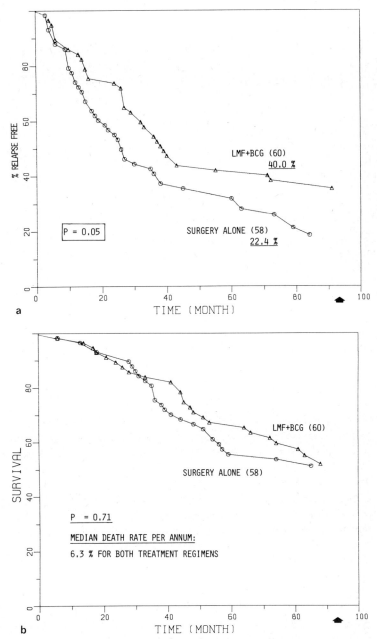

Fig. 6a, b. Results of LMF + BCG in OSAKO-Study 06/74, all node-positive patients. **a** Relapse-free survival; **b** overall survival

upset (in 28% of patients), but no hair-loss [12, 14]. No indication of late toxicity was observed up to 8 years, especially no increase of second tumors [8]. Two cases of acute leukemia (one combined with a colorectal carcinoma) were observed in the surgical control arm, but none in patients treated with LMF + BCG.

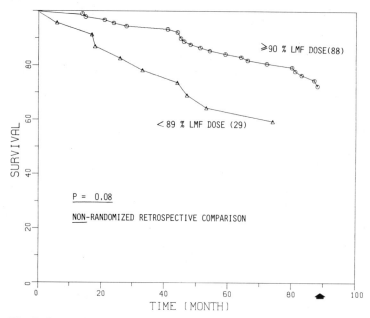

Fig. 7. Correlation of total dose of LMF (≥ 90% vs ≤ 89%) on overall survival of all LMF patients (N− and N+)

Discussion

As observed since the third year, patients treated with (oral) LMF + BCG continue to exhibit a marginal gain in RFS up to 8 years postmastectomy (medium follow-up). Due to a series of (partly nonneoplastic) late deaths in the LMF + BCG arm during the last year of observation, this RFS difference no longer expresses itself in an OAS gain, as observed up to the seventh year of follow-up. However, this might statistically change again in the future, since only half of the patients are presently at risk at 8 years and the survival curve of LMF + BCG-treated women has been constantly superior to the surgical controls since the fourth observation year. It should be kept in mind (also by some zealous critiques [11]), that the sequential statistical analysis of a clinical study is a dynamic process and not a final, irreversible verdict − at least as long as relapse or survival curves continue to separate and do not start to "criss-cross," as is the case for example, for OAS in our N+ patient subgroup (Fig. 6b).

The nominal gain of +10% RFS and of +7% OAS for LMF/BCG in the whole patient population at 8 years is not impressive. It is, however, a constant feature of our trial, that preferentially *post*menopausal women seem to profit from adjuvant LMF + BCG. This is in contradiction to two studies with L-PAM and CMF [2, 6], but is not at all unique. At least five current breast cancer trials show postmenopausal women benefiting from adjuvant chemo(hormono)therapy either to the same extent or even more than younger patients [3, 13, 16]. The discordance of therapeutic effect when making a cross-study comparison between the results reported for the Milan CMF trial and our LMF/BCG-OSAKO program does not constitute a scientific basis for drawing final conclusions about "inefficiency" of CMF in postmenopausal women and of (oral) LMF in premenopausal women [2, 15]. This can be ascertained only by making direct randomized comparisons of therapeutic effect and toxicity of CMF vs LMF in both menopausal patient subgroups, as is currently being done for N+(1−3) women (SAKK-Study 27/82).

Node-negative patients, treated with LMF + BCG experienced an impressive RFS increase during the first 4 years of observation. However, at 5 years of median follow-up, there was a strange accumulation of late relapses among LMF + BCG patients and a partial merging of the hitherto clearly separating curves. Whether this late drop in RFS features a biologic lesson on the limitations of our present concept of adjuvant chemotherapy, remains an open question. Regarding the moderate, nominal percentage gain in RFS (and OAS) through use of present adjuvant systemic therapy, the concept of late, repeated adjuvant consolidation treatments should be scientifically explored in advanced disease, as proposed by Plotkin and Wangh [10].

Interestingly enough, there has remained an OAS advantage for LMF/BCG-treated N− patients since the third study year (Fig. 4b), possibly now disappearing at 8 years. Since there are equal and few death due to causes other than breast cancer, one must conclude, that relapsing N− women with LMF + BCG pretreatment fare better and finally live longer than relapsing N− surgical-control patients. A detailed analysis of subsequent treatments and course of disease in all relapsing patients is presently in progress. No significant difference as to the distribution in site of first relapse was detected between N− patients with or without LMF + BCG adjuvant therapy.

Node-positive LMF + BCG patients continue to demonstrate a moderate, but still significant RFS gain, as reported since the fifth year of observation [14]. If analyzed in menopausal subgroups, this gain is nearly exclusively expressed in *post*menopausal N+ women. Due to small patient numbers and nonstratification of menopausal status prior to randomization, we hesitate to attach too much importance to this menopausal subgroup discordance, as pointed out earlier. Despite the marginal gain in RFS, no OAS benefit was observed for N+ women, treated with LMF + BCG (Fig. 6b), indicating that the course of relapsing disease in N+ patients is not altered by prior LMF + BCG as seems to be the case in N− women. As seen in other CMF and L-PAM-type studies [3, 12] all favorable effects of LMF + BCG in N+ patients were obtained in those with 1−3 positive axillary nodes, with virtually no effect on RFS and OAS in highest-risk women with N+ ≥ 4.

There is strong disagreement among various groups and investigators as to the correlation of adjuvant drug doses received and prognosis. While Bonadonna et al. repeatedly demonstrated a statistically significant influence of ≥ 85% CMF on RFS and OAS after 5 and now 9 years of follow-up [2], Fisher and NSABP investigators using various analytical methods [6] are not able to find such a correlation. In our OSAKO 06/74 study there is at least suggestive evidence that full dose (≤ 90%) of LMF for 6 cycles positively affected OAS at 8 years. Again, one must caution against overinterpretation of data, since these comparisons are retrospective and have never been answered in a prospective study. However, dose remains a critical factor in cancer chemotherapy [7].

It is extremly difficult to assess the potential impact of the nonspecific influence of prolonged BCG skin scarifications in our adjuvant regime, since we lack randomized comparisons with either LMF p.o. or BCG alone. However, in a subsequent Swiss national study (SAKK 27/78), comparing 6 vs 18 cycles of LMF p.o. without BCG, RFS and OAS of both regimens were slightly, but not statistically, worse than those of LMF + BCG-treated women in our OSAKO-study [9, 14]. This renders either a "positive" or "negative" influence of BCG rather unlikely. The same conclusion is reached by the Houston group, using adjuvant FAC + BCG [4].

There was no indication of any adverse long-term toxicity of LMF + BCG in our study population after a median follow-up of 8 years, especially no increase of second neoplasia and of acute leukemia. This is in agreement with many other studies and will be dealt with elsewhere this book. It emphasizes that increased late toxicity data from other diseases and treatment schedules (such as, e.g., chemoradiotherapy of Hodgkin's disease) cannot simply be extended to intermittent adjuvant chemotherapy of other types of neoplasia.

Conclusion

On the basis of our present 8-year study data on 240 patients, we tentatively conclude: (1) LMF + BCG as given in our trial significantly increases RFS in the whole patient population as well as in N+ women, especially those who are postmenopausal. (2) LMF + BCG marginally increases OAS in all postmenopausal patients and in N− women, possibly also in all those receiving ⩾ 90% of LMF. (3) The benefit for postmenopausal patients is a constant feature of this trial and cannot be explained by drug-dose calculations. (4) The moderate RFS gain for N+ patients does not transform into increased OAS, while the opposite seems to be the case for N− women. The differential behavior of relapsing N− and N+ patients is as yet unexplained. It looks, however, as if OAS gain for N− patients could be fading after 7 years. (5) The nominal percentage gain of most-benefited subgroups (+18% RFS in N+ women, +15% OAS in N− patients) compares well with other "positive" adjuvant studies, although overall clinical gain is moderate and less than expected. (6) Subjective and objective toxicity of LMF × 6 p.o. (+BCG) was well acceptable, and even at 8 years there is no evidence of an increase in second tumors in the adjuvant therapy arm.

Acknowledgements. We greatly acknowledge the skilful coordinating assistance of Miss Agnes Glaus, R.N, Head Nurse, Dept. of Medicine C, Kantonsspital St. Gallen and the statistical evaluation of our data by Dr. W. Berchtold, Aargauisches Technikum, Buchs, Switzerland.

References

1. Bonadonna G, Brusamolino E, Valagussa P et al. (1976) Combination chemotherapy as an adjuvant treatment in operable breast cancer. N Engl J Med 194: 405
2. Bonadonna G, Valagussa P (1981) Dose response effect of adjuvant chemotherapy in breast cancer. N Engl J Med 304: 10
3. Bonadonna G, Valagussa P (1982) Adjuvant therapy of primary breast cancer. In: Carter SK, Glatstein E, Livingstone RB (eds) Principles of cancer treatment. McGraw-Hill, New York, p 315
4. Buzdar AU, Blumenschein GR, Hortobagyi GN et al. (1980) 5-year follow up of FAC + BCG adjuvant therapy of stage II + III breast cancer. Cancer Chemother Pharm 5: 8
5. Fisher B, Wolmark N (1975) New concepts in the management of primary breast cancer. Cancer [Suppl 2] 36: 627
6. Fisher B (1980) Laboratory and clinical research in breast cancer − a personal adventure. Cancer Res 40: 3863
7. Frei E III (1980) Dose a critical factor in cancer chemotherapy. Am J Med 69: 585
8. Holdener EE, Osterwalder J, Senn HJ (1982) Zweitmalignome bei operiertem Mammakarzinom: Vergleich retro- und prospektiver Erfahrungen. Schweiz Med Wochenschr 112: 1800
9. Jungi WF, Alberto P, Brunner KW et al. (1981) Short- or long-term adjuvant chemotherapy of breast cancer? In: Salmon SE, Jones SE (eds) Adjuvant therapy of cancer III. Grune & Stratton, New York, p 395

10. Plotkin D, Wangh WJ (1983) Hypothesis: Discontinous chemotherapy for advanced breast cancer. Am J Clin Oncol 6: 375
11. Sauter C (1983) Hat die heutige adjuvante zytostatische Chemotherapie bei radikal operiertem Mammakarzinompatientinnen versagt? Schweiz Med Wochenschr 113: 414
12. Senn HJ, Mayr AC (1979) Adjuvant therapy in breast cancer − Swiss cooperative studies. Cancer Treat Rev [Suppl] 6: 79
13. Senn HJ (1982) Current status and indications for adjuvant chemotherapy in breast cancer. Cancer Chemother Pharmacol 8: 139
14. Senn HJ, Amgwerd R, Jungi WF et al. (1982) Adjuvant Chemoimmunotherapy with LMF + BCG in N− and N+ breast cancer patient − intermediate report at 4 years. In: Mathé G, Bonadonna G, Salmon E (eds) Adjuvant therapies of cancer. Springer, Berlin Heidelberg New York, p 177 (Recnet results in cancer research 80)
15. Senn HJ, Jungi WF, Amgwerd R et al (1983) 7-year results of adjuvant chemo(immuno)therapy with LMF/BCG in operable N− and N+ breast cancer (OSAKO-study 06/74). Second Europ Conf Clin Oncol, Amsterdam, Abstract 03-28
16. Senn HJ (1984) Adjuvante Chemotherapie beim operablen Mammakarzinom. Dtsch Med Wochenschr (in press)
17. Tancini G, Bonadonna G, Valagussa P et al. (1983) Adjuvant CMF in breast cancer: comparative 5-year results of 12 cycles vs 6 cycles. J Clin Oncol 1: 2

Ludwig Breast Cancer Trial LBCS III: Chemo- and Endocrine Adjuvant Treatment in Postmenopausal Patients

R. D. Gelber*

Ludwig Institut für Krebsforschung, Inselspital, 3010 Bern, Switzerland

Introduction

In 1978 the Ludwig Breast Cancer Study (LBCS) Group initiated four complementary randomized controlled clinical trials to evaluate adjuvant therapy in both pre- and postmenopausal patients with operable breast cancer and axillary lymph node involvement. The trial in postmenopausal patients 65 years old or younger (LBCS III), in which the combination of endocrine therapy with multiple cytotoxic chemotherapy was compared with endocrine therapy alone and with no adjuvant treatment after mastectomy, is the subject of this report (Fig. 1).

Materials and Methods

Postmenopausal women, defined by menstrual history or by endocrine testing, who were 65 years of age or less and who had histologically confirmed, noninflammatory, unilateral breast carcinoma with axillary lymph node metastases, were considered for eligibility in the

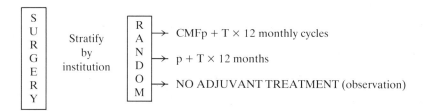

C :	cyclophosphamide	100 mg/m^2	p.o. days 1–14
M:	methotrexate	40 mg/m^2	i.v. days 1 and 8
F :	5-fluorouracil	600 mg/m^2	i.v. days 1 and 8
p :	prednisone	7.7 mg/day	p.o. (5 mg a.m., 2.5 mg p.m.) continuously
T :	tamoxifen	20 mg/day	p.o. continuously

Fig. 1. Study design

---

* Ludwig Breast Cancer Study Groups, see p. 108, 109

study. Treatment of the primary tumor was by total mastectomy and axillary clearance for disease staged according to the International TNM Classification as T_{1A} or T_{1B}, T_{2A} or T_{2B}, T_{3A}, N_0 or N_1 (but with histologically proven axillary node metastasis); M_0. A chest radiograph and bone scan (with X-rays of "hot spots," if applicable) were required for exclusion of detectable metastatic disease. A peripheral WBC count of $\geq$ 4,000/mm^3, a platelet count of $\geq$ 100,000/mm^3, creatinine of $<$ 130 µmol/l, bilirubin $<$ 20 µmol/l, and SGOT of $<$ 60 IU were also required.

The combination of chemotherapy and endocrine therapy [cyclophosphamide, metho-trexate, 5-fluorouracil, prednisone, and tamoxifen; CMFp + T (the use of the abbreviation p-rather than P-highlights the use of *low-dose* prednisone)] was compared with treatment by endocrine therapy (prednisone and tamoxifen; p + T), and with no adjuvant treatment, in 463 patients.

From July 1, 1978 to August 31, 1981, stratification by participating clinic (see Appendix A), and randomization of patients were done centrally by the Study Coordination Center.

Treatment was started within 6 weeks of surgery and continued through twelve 28-day cycles of chemoendocrine therapy or 12 months of endocrine therapy alone. Dosage was modified as follows: a full dose of CMF was administered to patients with WBC $\geq$ 4,000/mm^3 and platelet count $\geq$ 100,000/mm^3. Fifty percent dose was given to those with WBC 2,500−3,999/mm^3 and and/or platelet count $\geq$ 50,000/mm^3 but below 100,000/mm^3. CMF was not administered if blood counts were below these levels. Criteria were also established for prospective dosage modification due to extreme hematological toxicity, mucositis, and cystitis.

The participating laboratories adopted standardized methods for estrogen receptor (ER) and progesterone receptor assays of primary tumor following individual laboratory assessment of standards provided by the coordinating laboratory. ER results of $\geq$ 10 fmol/mg cytosol protein were considered positive and values below this as negative. ER results were available for 51% of the patients.

Clinical, hematological, and biochemical assessment of each patient was required every 3 months for 2 years and thereafter every 6 months until death. Chest X-rays and bone scans were required every 6 months. After 2 years a bone scan was required once yearly. All

Table 1. Patient entry and characteristics

	CMFp + T	p + T	Observation	Total
No. randomized patients	171	164	168	503
No. evaluable patients (% of total	154 (90%)	153 (93%)	156 (93%)	463 (92%)
Median age (range)	60 (45−65)	59 (45−65)	59 (40−65)	59 (40−65)
Nodal status				
N+ 1−3	58%	54%	56%	56%
N+ 4	42%	46%	44%	44%
ER status				
ER+	38%	29%	34%	33%
ER−	12%	20%	21%	18%
ER unknown	50%	51%	45%	49%

study records (on-study, treatment, toxicity, and recurrence) were reviewed centrally by the study coordinator. In addition, there was central data management review of all records during the course of the study. The time of relapse was defined as the time when recurrent disease was confirmed or was suspected and later confirmed. A total of 503 patients were randomized and 463 (92%) were evaluable for this report. Reasons for ineligibility and inevaluability were: refusal of treatment and follow-up ($n = 5$), primary stage T_{3A}, ($n = 5$), randomization to the wrong study based on menopausal status or age ($n = 8$), previous or concurrent malignancy other than basal cell carcinoma of the skin or cervical carcinoma in situ ($n = 5$), inadequate surgery ($n = 2$), node-negative ($n = 2$), and inadequate renal function ($n = 3$). Ten additional patients entered from a noncompliant clinic were excluded from analysis on a decision made in November 1981.

Table 1 summarizes the distribution of relevant patient characteristics for each therapy. The treatment groups were also well balanced for type of surgical procedure, tumor size, histological tumor type, and grade as determined by a central pathology review in 96% of evaluable cases.

Statistical Methods

This analysis utilized data available on all eligible patients as of October 1, 1983, with a median follow-up of 36 months. For the analysis of disease-free survival (DFS), failure was defined as any recurrence, appearance of a second primary malignancy, or death, whichever occurred first.

The Kaplan-Meier method [1] was used to estimate survival distributions for DFS and overall survival. The log-rank procedure [2] was utilized to assess the statistical significance of treatment differences between these survival distributions. Times were measured from the date of randomization. Tests of significance for treatment effects were carried out adjusting for prognostic factors (nodal status and ER status), using the Cox proportional hazard regression model [3].

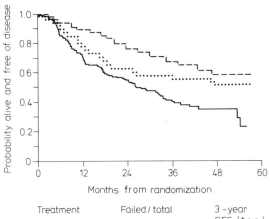

Treatment	Failed / total	3-year DFS ($\pm$ s.e.)
–– CMFp+T	48 / 154	67% ($\pm$ 4%)
····· p+T	66 / 153	56% ($\pm$ 4%)
—— OBS	93 / 156	39% ($\pm$ 4%)

Fig. 2. Disease-free survival by treatment. Patients who relapsed, developed second malignancies, or died without recurrence were considered as failures. Log-rank tests yielded $P = 0.0001$ for the three treatment comparisions, $P = 0.0001$ for CMFp + T vs observation, $P = 0.008$ for p + T vs observation, and $P = 0.02$ for CMFp + T vs p + T

Results

DFS was significantly increased for women who received CMFp + T as compared with those who received endocrine therapy ($P = 0.02$) or no adjuvant treatment (observation) after mastectomy ($P < 0.0001$). The estimated DFS curves are presented in Fig. 2. As shown in Table 2, DFS was longer for patients with ER+ tumors who received CMFp + T ($P = 0.01$) *or* p + T ($P = 0.03$) than for the observation group. There was virtually no difference in DFS between patients with ER+ tumors who received CMFp + T and those who received p + T ($P = 0.86$).

Table 2. Three-year DFS and overall survival

	CMFp + T	p + T	Observation	P
DFS				
All Patients	67 ± 4	56 ± 4	39 ± 4	0.0001
Nodal status				
N+ 1–3	76 ± 5	68 ± 5	49 ± 6	0.0008
N+ 4	56 ± 7	43 ± 6	27 ± 6	0.0014
ER status				
ER+[a]	70 ± 6	68 ± 7	43 ± 7	0.02
ER−[b]	58 ± 15	35 ± 9	35 ± 9	0.12
ER unknown	66 ± 6	58 ± 6	39 ± 6	0.0002
Overall survival	75 ± 4	71 ± 4	79 ± 4	0.76

Values derived using Kaplan-Meier method. For DFS, failure is defined as recurrence, second primary, or death, whichever occurred first
[a] ER+: CMFp + T vs obs., $P = 0.01$; CMFp + T vs p + T, $P = 0.86$; p + T vs obs., $P = 0.03$
[b] ER−: CMFp + T vs obs., $P = 0.11$; CMFp + T vs p + T, $P = 0.03$; p + T vs obs., $P = 0.54$

Table 3. Site of first failure by treatment regimen

	CMFp + T	p + T	Observation
Total patients	154	153	156
Total failures	48 (33)	66 (38)	93 (36)
First evidence of failure			
Mastectomy scar alone[a]	4 (2)	14 (7)	23 (4)
Contralateral breast alone	1	1	1
Other regional or local/regional without distant	6 (1)	10 (6)	18 (3)
Distant or distant + other sites	27 (20)	37 (21)	48 (27)
Second primary (not breast)	2 (2)	1 (1)	2 (1)
Death without recurrence	8	3	1

Figures in parentheses are deaths
[a] Twenty of these patients (two CMFp + T, p + T, nine obs.) subsequently developed systemic failure

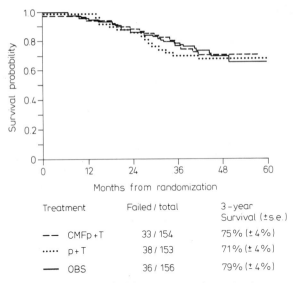

Fig. 3. Overall survival by treatment ($P = 0.76$)

Table 4. Incidence of toxicity by treatment regimen (%)

Side effect	CMFp + T		p + T	
	Mild/mod	Severe	Mild/mod	Severe
Leukopenia[a]	76	4	6	−
Thrombocytopenia[a]	40	7	3	−
Nausea, vomiting, xerostomia, anorexia, epigastric pain	77	9	10	1
Diarrhea	19	0.7	1	−
Stomatitis, mucositis	28	4	−	−
Conjunctivitis, keratitis	13	1	0.7	−
Skin toxicity (rash)	3	0.7	5	−
Alopecia (complete/incomplete)	26/43	−	−	−
Hepatotoxicity	1	−	−	−
Cystitis	18	0.7	−	−
Thrombosis, thrombophlebitis, embolism	6	4	3	0.7
Cushingoid, weight gain, edema	21	0.7	17	0.7
Hot flashes, vaginal bleeding	9	0.7	9	−
Hyperglycemia	−	−	4	−
Neurological, depression, euphoria, etc.	10	3	5	−
Infection	15	0.7	3	−
Hemorrhage	3	−	−	0.7
Reported worst degree	70	22	43	3

[a] Mild/moderate: WBC $3,999-1,000/mm^3$; platelets $99,999-50,000/mm^3$
   Severe: WBC $< 1,000/mm^3$; plateles $< 50,000/mm^3$

Analysis of sites of first failure showed a reduced number of all types of relapse (local, regional, and distant) in the CMFp + T group as compared with the p + T and mastectomy alone groups (Table 3).

There are no significant differences in overall survival between treatment groups at this point in the study (Table 2, Fig. 3).

Toxic Effects

The frequency of severe hematological and nonhematological toxic effects (excluding alopecia) in patients who received CMFp + T (22%) was higher than the same grade of complications observed in patients who had p + T alone (4%; $P < 0.0001$) (Table 4). No fatalities were definitely attributable to treatment. Twelve patients died without recurrence, six of them within the first year.

Discussion

With a median follow-up of 36 months, our randomized controlled study showed a significant increase in DFS using a combination of chemoendocrine therapy given after mastectomy in postmenopausal patients aged ≤ 65 years with histologically proven axillary lymph node metastases. This treatment advantage was noted for CMFp + T when compared with p + T or with mastectomy alone (Fig. 2, Table 2). Estimated failure rates at 3 years were 33%, 44% ($P = 0.02$), and 61% ($P < 0.0001$), respectively.

The advantage of CMFp + T compared with mastectomy alone was consistently apparent within all major prognostic subgroups including those relating to ER status (Table 2). While CMFp + T may be superior to p + T for patients with ER– tumors, the outcome for these two treatments was virtually identical for patients with ER+ tumors. The chemoendocrine regimen continued to show significant superiority in an analysis controlling for prognostic factors.

The marked reduction in the number of relapses following adjuvant treatment might have been expected to reduce the mortality rate in the treated population. However, to date, no difference in survival has been observed. This notable absence of survival advantage might be due either to insufficient duration of follow-up or to the different patterns of relapse after adjuvant therapy compared with relapses in patients without adjuvant therapy.

In the Milan study [4], in which CMF was compared with mastectomy alone, the estimated 3-year relapse-free survival (RFS) rates for postmenopausal patients did not differ significantly (64% with CMF and 60% with mastectomy alone). In our study DFS rather than RFS was used as a measure of treatment outcome to avoid unduly optimistic interpretation of early results. For purposes of comparability, the 3-year RFS probabilities in our study were as follows: 72% CMFp + T, 59% p + T, 40% observation. The marked difference in the natural histories of patients in the control groups in the Ludwig and Milan trials emphasizes the value of including a concurrent randomized control group in clinical trials designed to compare adjuvant treatments for breast cancer. This will continue to be true as long as the magnitude of expected treatment differences remains in the 10%–20% range observed to date.

Although no overall survival benefit has been demonstrated, the advantage of the CMFp + T regimen must be measured in terms of control of disease in local and regional as well as distant sites.

Ludwig Breast Cancer Study Group: LBCS (Toxicity Report. Pilot and First Series)

Institution	
Ludwig Institute for Cancer Research, Inselspital, Bern, Switzerland	A. Goldhirsch (*Study Coordinator*), W. Hartmann, B. Davis, D. Zava, M. de Marval
Frontier Science and Technology Research Foundation, Boston, USA	R. Gelber (*Study Statistician*), M. Isley, L. Szymoniak, M. Zelen
Auckland Breast Cancer Study Group, Auckland, New Zealand	R. G. Kay, J. Probert, B. Mason, H. Wood, E. G. Gifford, J. F. Carter, J. C. Gillmann, J, Anderson, L. Yee, I. M. Holdaway, G. C. Hitchcock, M. Jagusch
Groote Schuur Hospital, Cape Town, Rep. of South Africa	A. Hacking, D. M. Dent, J. Terblanche, A. Tiltman, A. Gudgeon, E. Dowdle, R. Sealy, P. Palmer
University of Essen, West German Tumor Center, Essen, Germany	C. G. Schmidt, F. Schüning, K. Höffken, L. D. Leder, H. Ludwig, R. Callies, P. Faber, H. Bender, H. Bojar
Swedish Western Breast Cancer Study Group, Göteborg, Sweden	C.-M. Rudenstam, E. Cahlin, H. Salander, I. Branehög, G. Jäderström, R. Hultborn, U. Wannholt, S. Nilsson, J. Fornander, J. Säve-Söderbergh, Ch. Johnsén, O. Ruusvik, G. Ostberg, L. Mattsson, C. G. Bäckström, S. Bergegardh, U. Ljungqvist, I. Dahl, Y. Hessman, S. Holmberg, S. Dahlin, G. Wallin
The Institute of Oncology, Ljubljana, Yugoslavia	J. Lindtner, J. Novak, J. Cervek, O. Cerar, P. Mavec, R. Golouh, J. Lamovec, J. Jancar, S. Sebek
Madrid Breast Cancer Group, Madrid, Spain	H. Cortés-Funes, F. Martinez-Tello, F. Cruz Caro, M. L. Marcos, M. A. Figueras, F. Calero, A. Suarez, F. Pastrana, R. Huertas
Anti-Cancer Council of Victoria, Melbourne, Australia	J. Collins, I. Russell, M. A. Schwarz, J. F. Forbes, P. R. B. Kitchen, L. Sisely, R. Reed, E. Guli, R. C. Bennett, J. W. Funder, L. Harrison, G. Brodie, W. I. Burns, R. D. Snyder, P. Jeal, J. H. Colebatch
Sir Charles Gairdner Hospital Nedlands, Western Australia	M. Byrne, P. M. Reynolds, H. J. Sheiner, S. Levitt, D. Kermode, K. B. Shilkin, R. Hähnel
SAKK (Swiss Group for Clin. Cancer Res.) − Basel, Kantonsspital	J. P. Obrecht, F. Harder, A. C. Almendral, U. Eppenberger, J. Torhorst
− Bern, Inselspital	K. Brunner, P. Aeberhard, H. Cottier, K. Burki, A. Zimermann, E. Dreher, G. Locher, M. Berger, M. Walther, R. Joss, A. Gervasi, P. Herrmann
− Geneva, Hopital Cantonal Universitaire	P. Alberto, F. Krauer, R. Egeli, R. Mégevand, M. Forni, P. Schäfer, E. Jacot des Combes, A. M. Schindler, F. Leski
− Neuchatel, Hôpital des Cadolles	P. Siegenthaler, V. Barrelet, R. P. Baumann
− St. Gallen, Kantonsspital	W. F. Jungi, H. J. Senn, A. Mutzner, U. Schmid, Th. Hardmeier, E. Hochuli, O. Schildknecht

Institution	
– Bellinzona, Ospedale San Giovanni	F. Cavalli, M. Varini, P. Luscieti, E. S. Passega, G. Losa
– Zurich, Universitätsspital	G. Martz, T. Muller, R. Maurer, E. S. Siebenmann, W. E. Schreiner, V. Engeler, C. Genton, H. J. Schmid
Ludwig Institute for Cancer Research, and Royal Prince Alfred Hospital, Sydney, Australia	M. H. N. Tattersall, R. Fox, A. Coates, D. Raghavan, F. Niesche, R. West, S. Renwick, D. Green, J. Donovan, P. Duval, A. Ng, T. Foo, D. Glenn, T. J. Nash, R. A. North, J. Beith, G. O'Connor
Wellington Hospital, Wellington, New Zealand	J. S. Simpson, L. Hollaway, C. Unsworth

References

1. Kaplan EL, Meier P (1958) Nonparametric estimation from incomplete observation. J Am Statist Assoc 53: 457–481
2. Peto R, Pike MC, Armitage P, Breslow NE et al. (1977) Design and analysis of randomized clinical trials requiring prolonged observation of each patient. Br J Cancer 35: 1–39
3. Cox DR (1972) Regression models and life tables (with discussion). J Roy Statist Soc B (Methodol) 34: 187–220
4. Bonadonna G, Rossi A, Valagussa P, Banfi A, Veronesi U (1977) The CMF programm for operable breast cancer with positive axillary nodes. Cancer 39: 2904–2915

Postmenopausal Node-Positive Comparison of Observation with CMFP and CMPF + Tamoxifen Adjuvant Therapy: An Eastern Cooperative Oncology Group Trial

D. C. Tormey, S. G. Taylor, IV, R. Gray, and J. E. Olson*

Department of Human Oncology, K4/666 Clinical Science Center,
600 Highland Avenue, Madison, WI, 53792, USA

Introduction

Adjuvant chemotherapy of postmenopausal axillary node-positive women with breast carcinoma in 1977 suggested a disease-free survival benefit but no overall survival benefit with cyclophosphamide, methotrexate, and 5-fluorouracil (CMF) [1]. In advanced disease the subsequently reported results with CMF + prednisone (CMFP) were superior to CMF [2] and the addition of tamoxifen to a chemotherapy regimen appeared to enhance effectiveness [3]. Accordingly, in 1977 the Eastern Cooperative Oncology Group (ECOG) designed an adjuvant trial for axillary node-positive postmenopausal patients to compare observation with 1 year of postoperative therapy with CMFP of CMFP + tamoxifen (CMFPT). The current results from this trial are presented.

Methods

Women < 66 years of age and with a histopathologic diagnosis of breast carcinoma confined to the breast and ipsilateral axillary nodes were considered for study. Eligibility details were similar to those of a previous trial [4] except that an estrogen receptor (ER) analysis and a negative bone scan were required. Randomization was performed and treatment initiated within 10 weeks of radical or modified radical mastectomy. No additional systemic antitumor therapy or radiotherapy was allowed. Postmenopausal status was defined as no menses within the 12 months prior to diagnosis or age ≥ 52 years in the case of prior hysterectomy. Absence of systemic disease was demonstrated by normal liver and renal function tests and chest X-ray, history, and physical examination in addition to the bone scan. Surgically free margins − as judged by the original pathologist and by a central pathology review − were required.

Randomization was by permuted blocks within strata designed by a central office for North American patients. Patients were stratified by axillary nodal status, 1−3 and ≥ 4 nodes involved, and ER status, negative or positive (≥ 10 fm/mg cytosol protein was defined as positive).

Treatment assignments were (1) no adjuvant therapy, (2) CMFP, and (3) CMFPT.

---

* For the Eastern Cooperative Oncology Group

Recent Results in Cancer Research. Vol. 96
© Springer-Verlag Berlin · Heidelberg 1984

Chemotherapy was repeated every 28 days for a total of 12 cycles beginning 2−10 weeks postoperatively. The drug schedules for each cycle were cyclophosphamide 100 mg/m^2 orally days 1 through 14, methotrexate 40 mg/m^2 i.v. days 1 and 8, 5-fluorouracil 600 mg/m^2 i.v. days 1 and 8, prednisone 40 mg/m^2 orally days 1 through 14, and tamoxifen 10 mg orally twice daily throughout each treatment cycle. The lesser of the ideal and actual body weights was used for dosage calculations. Standard toxicity-related dosage modifications were used. Hematologic toxicity led to a CMF reduction of 50% for WBC 2,500−4,000/mm^3 or platelets 75,000−100,000/mm^3. A delay of day 1 therapy for up to 2 weeks was allowed to enable full dosage administration. If the WBC was < 2,500/mm^3 or the platelets were < 75,000/mm^3 on day 1, therapy was delayed; if on day 8, CMF was omitted. The protocol allowed a 25% reduction in CMF dosage in subsequent cycles if WBC count fell to < 2,000/mm^3 or the platelet count to < 75,000/mm^3.

Follow-up consisted of history, physical examination, and blood chemistry values every 3 months, chest X-rays every 6 months, bone scans at 6 and 12 months and then yearly, and mammograms yearly. Toxicity was assessed using standard ECOG criteria [5]. Relapse was based upon "acceptable evidence" as defined elsewhere [6].

The method of Kaplan and Meier [7] was used to estimate time to relapse and survival from the date of randomization. The crude relationships of treatment or other patient characteristics with time to relapse or survival were analyzed using the log-rank test [8]. A proportional hazards model [9] was used to analyze these relationships while adjusting simultaneously for other patient characteristics. Associations of endpoints having ordered categories with treatment were evaluated using an exact test [10]. The associations of relpase sites with treatment were evaluated using Fisher's exact test [11]. All P values are based on two-sided alternatives and are considered "significant" if ≤ 0.05.

Results

There were 265 patients randomized between March 1978 and July 1981. There were insufficient data for evaluation of nine cases, and 32 cases were ineligible. The major analysis was performed upon the remaining 224 cases although the results of separate analyses including all randomized cases were similar. Table 1 lists selected patient characteristics. The regimens were well balanced with respect to these and other variables. Minor imbalances were controlled for in the analyses. The median follow-up is 44 months, with 48% having relapsed and 22% having died.

The overall comparisons of time to relapse (TTR) revealed a significant advantage for systemic therapy in year 1 ($P < 0.001$), but this had diminished by years 3 and 4 ($P = 0.09$) (Fig. 1). A similar benefit from systemic therapy was observed in all subgroups during the first year. Survival was not different for any treatment approach (Fig. 2). TTR was significantly better for patients with 1−3 nodes involved compared with > 3 nodes involved ($P = 0.04$), tumor size < 3 cm compared with ≥ 3 cm ($P = 0.003$) and for ER+ compared with ER− patients ($P = 0.04$). This latter difference was significant only for the observation group ($P = 0.001$). There was a significant ER and treatment interaction, demonstrating no treatment difference among ER+ patients but a significant advantage for treatment in ER− patients ($P = 0.006$) (Table 2, Fig. 3). Within these subgroups only the TTR advantage of 1−3 node-positive and ER+ disease extended to survival ($P = 0.02$ and 0.004, respectively).

There were no difference between the regimens with respect to sites of first recurrence (Table 3). The majority of the first recurrences were distant metastases.

Table 1. Patient characteristics

Characteristic	Observation	CMFP	CMFPT	Total
Nodes examined[a]	14	14	18	15
Nodes positive[a]	3	4	3	3
Tumor size (cm)[a]	2.8	3.0	2.5	2.8
Age (years)[a]	57	58	57	57
Days surgery to Rx[a]	–	35	34	35
% ER+	61	63	65	63

[a] Median

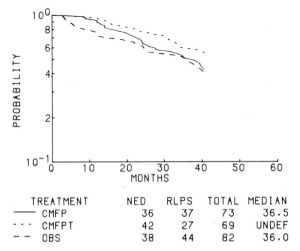

TREATMENT	NED	RLPS	TOTAL	MEDIAN
—— CMFP	36	37	73	36.5
· · · CMFPT	42	27	69	UNDEF
– – OBS	38	44	82	36.0

Fig. 1. Time to relapse for all evaluable patients on each regimen; $P = 0.09$

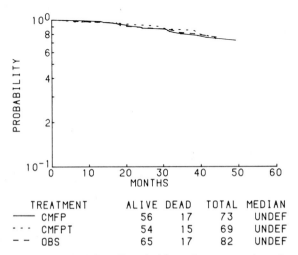

TREATMENT	ALIVE	DEAD	TOTAL	MEDIAN
—— CMFP	56	17	73	UNDEF
· · · CMFPT	54	15	69	UNDEF
– – OBS	65	17	82	UNDEF

Fig. 2. Survival for all evaluable patients on each regimen

Table 2. ER and treatment interaction

ER status	Disease free at 4 years (%)		
	Observation	CMFP	CMFPT
Negative	16	41	53
Positive	54	45	55

Table 3. Sites of first recurrence by treatment regimen

	Observation	CMFP	CMFPT	Total
Local only	12	10	7	10
Regional only	6	4	4	5
Local + regional	1	1	–	1
Distant only	29	30	26	29
Local + distant	5	4	1	4
Regional + distant	–	1	–	0.4
Local + regional + distant	–	–	–	–
Local ± regional only	20	15	12	16
Distant ± local/regional	34	36	28	32

Local refers to the area bounded by the sternal midline, clavicle, posterior lateral edge of the latissimus dorsi and costal margin; regional includes the internal mammary, supraclavicular, and axillary area; all other sites are considered distant. Included are 44 relapses on observation, 37 on CMFP, and 27 on CMFPT. Values are percentages of evaluable patients

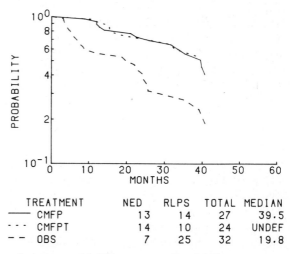

TREATMENT	NED	RLPS	TOTAL	MEDIAN
—— CMFP	13	14	27	39.5
- - - CMFPT	14	10	24	UNDEF
– – OBS	7	25	32	19.8

Fig. 3. Time to relapse for patients on each regimen with ER− tumors; $P = 0.006$

Table 4. Major side effects with CMFP and CMFPT (%)

Events	CMFP	CMFPT
Nausea and emesis requiring support	4	6
Clinical/documented sepsis	5/1	4/1
Neurologic → Rx modification	6	7
WBC < 2,000/< 1,000/mm^3	22/7	19/6
Platelets < 50,000/mm^3	7	7
Thrombophlebitis peripheral/deep vein	1/4	6/13[a]
Peripheral edema	26	25
Cushingoid changes	22	12
Musculoskeletal pain	18	23
Weight gain > 20%	12	9
Hot flashes	12	18

[a] Overall, $P = 0.01$; deep vein only, $P = 0.07$

The side effects associated with the two systemic therapy regimens were compared. Table 4 shows that the incidence of clinically significant events was similar for both regimens except that thrombotic events were significantly greater with the addition of tamoxifen.

Discussion

The present trial is similar to the Milan CMF vs observation trial in demonstrating a significant advantage of systemic chemotherapy only during the first 1−2 years [1]. As with the previous trial there is no survival advantage. However, the availability of ER analyses in the current trial enabled an evaluation of the impact of this variable upon and results. The observation group supports previous data [12, 13] demonstrating an advantage for patients with ER+ tumors. The introduction of systemic therapy to patients with ER− disease converted their TTR prognosis to that of ER+ untreated patients resulting in a significant advantage at the present time. Further follow-up will be required to assess whether or not this advantage will extend to survival.

The reason for this selective advantage in ER− patients is not known. It can be hypothesized that holding the ER+ cohorts in G_1 by the hormonal agents results in a higher porportion of ER− cells entering the proliferative pool and being reduced by chemotherapy, resulting in a more prolonged TTR. This explanation would be consonant with the proposed lower proliferative activity of ER+ cells [14] and the G_1 block produced by hormonal agents [15, 16]. Further follow-up and attention to cell population changes will be needed to verify or refute this hypothesis.

The present study supports other trials in showing the prognostic impact of nodal status [1, 4, 17], tumor size [1, 4, 17], and ER status [17, 18] upon TTR, and nodal status [17] and ER status [17, 18] upon survival.

Side effects with CMFP and CMFPT were similar to those from previous studies of advanced disease, with the exception that the addition of tamoxifen to CMFP in these postmenopausal patients resulted in a higher incidence of thrombotic events. This has not been observed in premenopausal patients. Although thrombotic events must be considered when using the drug, it is possible that it was an artifact of multiple statistical analyses.

In summary, the present trial suggests an early advantage to systemic therapy in node-positive postmenopausal patients. The failure to sustain this advantage to survival suggests that the cell kill achieved is insufficient, although long-term survival differences could yet emerge. The apparant greater advantage of systemic therapy in ER− patients compared with ER+ patients raises hypothetical possibilities that need to be addressed in future studies.

Acknowledgements. This trial was conducted by the Eastern Oncology Group and supported by PHS grants from the National Cancer Institute, National Institutes of Health and DHHS.

References

1. Bonadonna G, Brusamolino E, Valagussa P, Rossi A, Brugnatelli L, Brambilla C, DeLena M, Tancini G, Bajetta E, Musumeci R, Veronesi U (1976) Combination chemotherapy as an adjuvant treatment in operable breast cancer. N Engl J Med 294: 405−410
2. Tormey DC, Gelman R, Band PR, Sears M, Rosenthal SN, DeWys W, Perlia C, Rice MA (1982) Comparison of induction chemotherapies for metastatic breast cancer: an Eastern Cooperative Oncology Group Trial. Cancer 50: 1235−1244
3. Tormey DC, Falkson G, Crowley J, Falkson HC, Voelkel J, Davis TE (1982) Dibromodulcitol and adriamycin ± tamoxifen in advanced breast cancer. Cancer Clin Trials 5: 33−39
4. Tormey DC, Weinberg VE, Holland JF, Weiss RB, Glidewell OJ, Perloff M, Falkson G, Falkson HC, Henry PH, Leone LA, Rafla S, Ginsberg SJ, Silver RT, Blom J, Carey RW, Schein PS, Lesnick GJ (1983) A randomized trial of five and three drug chemotherapy and chemoimmunotherapy in women with operable node positive breast cancer − a cancer and leukemia group B study. J Clin Oncol 1: 138−145
5. Oken MM, Creech RH, Tormey DC, Horton J, Davis TE, McFadden ET, Carbone PP (1982) Toxicity and response criteria of the Eastern Cooperative Oncology Group. Am J Clin Oncol 5: 649−655
6. Tormey D, Fisher B, Bonadonna G, Carter S, Davis H, Glidewell O, Hahn RG, Payne S, Zelen M, Sears ME (1977) Proposed guidelines. In: Carbone PP, Sears ME (eds) Report from the Combined Modality Trials Working Group in Breast Cancer: suggested protocol guidelines for combination chemotherapy trials and for combined modality trials. DHEW, Washington (DHEW publication no. [NIH] 77-1192, pp 20−35)
7. Kaplan EL, Meier P (1958) Nonparametric estimation from incomplete observations. J Am Stat Assoc 53: 457−481
8. Peto R, Peto J (1972) Asymptotically efficient rank invariant test procedures. J R Stat Soc [A] 135: 185−198
9. Cox DR (1972) Regression models and life tables (with discussion). J R Stat Soc [B] 34: 187−220
10. Lehman EL (1975) Nonparametrics: Statistical methods based on ranks. Holden Day, San Francisco
11. Fisher RA (1934) Statistical methods for research workers. University Press, Edinburgh
12. Knight WA, Livingston RB, Gregory EJ, McGuire WL (1977) Estrogen receptor as an independent prognostic factor for early recurrence in breast cancer. Cancer Res 37: 4669−4671
13. Hähnel R, Woodings T, Vivian AB (1979) Prognostic value of estrogen receptors in primary breast cancer. Cancer 44: 671−675
14. Bertuzzi A, Daidone MG, DiFronzo G, Silvestrini R (1981) Relationship among estrogen receptors, proliferative activity and menopausal status in breast cancer. Breast Cancer Res Treat 1: 253−261

15. Ernst P, Killmann S-A (1970) Perturbation of generation cycle of human leukemic blast cells by cytostatic therapy in vivo: effect of corticosteroids. Blood 36: 689–696

16. Osborne CK, Blodt DH, Clark GM, Trent JM (1983) Effects of tamoxifen on human breast cancer cell cycle kinetics: accumulation of cells in early G_1 phase. Cancer Res 43: 3583–3585

17. Fisher B, Redmond C, Brown A, Wickerham DL, Wolmark N, Allegra J, Escher G, Lippman M, Savlov E, Wittliff J, Fisher ER (1983) Influence of tumor estrogen and progesterone receptor levels on the response to tamoxifen and chemotherapy in primary breast cancer. J Clin Oncol 1: 227–241

18. Hubay CA, Pearson OH, Marshall JS, Stellato TA, Rhodses RS, DeBanne SM, Rosenblatt J, Mansour EG, Hermann RE, Jones JC, Flynn WJ, Eckert C, McGuire WL (1981) Adjuvant therapy of stage II breast cancer. Breast Cancer Res Treat 1: 77–82

Adjuvant Systemic Therapy in High-Risk Breast Cancer: The Danish Breast Cancer Cooperative Group's Trials of Cyclophosphamide or CMF in Premenopausal and Tamoxifen in Postmenopausal Patients

H. T. Mouridsen, C. Rose, H. Brincker, S. M. Thorpe, F. Rank, K. Fischerman, and K. W. Andersen

Department of Oncology I, Finsen Institute,
49 Strandboulevarden, 2100 Copenhagen Ø, Denmark

Introduction

At the annual meeting of the Danish Surgical Society in December 1975, a task force was set up to nationally coordinate the new principles of systemic therapy of breast cancer. Over the following 2 years the structure of the Danish Breast Cancer Cooperative Group (DBCG) was organized and in 1977 the first clinical program, DBCG-77, was activated [1, 8]. This paper will briefly review the present status of this program.

Clinical Study Design

Surgery

The primary surgical treatment is total mastectomy and partial axillary dissection [5]. Detailed surgical instructions are distributed to all 80 participating surgical departments.

Pathology

The examination of the pathological specimen has been standardized at the 28 participating departments of pathology. The microscopic examination includes evaluation of degree of anaplasia and tumor classification according to WHO [15], and evaluation of several other pathological factors.

Receptor Studies

Estrogen (ER) and progesterone (PgR) receptors are measured in a single laboratory according to the methods recommended by the EORTC [7]. Continuous quality-control studies of steroid receptor assay methods are performed in collaboration with other European laboratories in the EORTC [9].

Recent Results in Cancer Research. Vol. 96
© Springer-Verlag Berlin · Heidelberg 1984

Patient Allocation

Patients are allocated one of two groups: Group I includes patients with tumors peroperatively estimated to be ≤ 5 cm in diameter and without histologically demonstrable invasion of skin or deep resection line and without demonstrable spread to axillary lymph nodes. Group II includes patients with tumors > 5 cm or with invasion of skin or deep resection line or with positive axillary lymph nodes.

Postoperative Radiotherapy

Patients in group I are not given postoperative radiotherapy.
All group II patients receive postoperative radiotherapy to the supraclavicular and axillary lymph nodes and to the mastectomy area at a dose equivalent to 1,335 rets. The radiotherapy is administered by the five radium centers or by the eight radiological departments of major county hospitals. With the available capacity for various radiation qualities, about 80% of the patients receive high voltage treatment, while the remainder receive orthovoltage radiotherapy. The radiotherapy is standardized according to a protocol with description of field positions, field sizes, absorbed dose to target areas, and fractionation.

Adjuvant Systemic Treatment

Patients in group I (Table 1) are observed after operative treatment (protocol DBCG-77-1a). The follow-up of these patients is undertaken by 5 radium centers, 38 surgical departments, and by 5 medical departments.
Group II (Table 1) is divided into two subgroups, with premenopausal and perimenopausal patients in one and postmenopausal patients in the other. A woman is defined as being postmenopausal when menostasia has persisted for at least 5 years. In the former subgroup the effect of adjuvant treatment for 1 year with levamisole or cyclophosphamide (C) alone or cyclophosphamide, methotrexate, and 5-fluorouracil (CMF) is evaluated and compared with no adjuvant therapy (protocol DBCG-77-1b). In the postmenopausal subgroup the

Table 1. DBCG-77 program: protocols

Menopausal			Adjuvant treatment
Risk group	Group	Protocol	
I Low risk	Pre + post	DBCG 77-1a	None
II High risk	Pre	DBCG 77-1b	⌈ RT ⊢ RT + L ⊢ RT + C ⌊ RT + CMF
II High risk	Post	DCCG 77-1c	⌈ RT ⊢ RT + L ⌊ RT + T

effect of a 1-year treatment with levamisole or tamoxifen is compared with no adjuvant therapy (protocol DBCG-77-1c).

The dose of levamisole was 2.5 mg per kg body weight given for 2 consecutive days and repeated weekly. Each cycle of C consisted of 130 mg/m^2 p.o. days 1–14, every 4 weeks for 12 cycles. Each cycle of CMF consisted of C 80 mg/m^2 p.o. days 1–14, M 30 mg/m^2 i.v. days 1 and 8, and F 500 mg/m^2 i.v. days 1 and 8, every 4 weeks for 12 cycles. Tamoxifen was administered continuously at a daily dose of 10 mg × 3.

The systemic treatment and follow-up of these group II patients has also been carried out at the five radium centers in collaboration with eight radiological departments and 14 medical departments in major county hospitals.

Program of Clinical Examinations

Physical examinations, laboratory tests, chest X-rays, and bone scintigraphy or bone X-rays were done before entry to the study and at regular intervals thereafter as described in detail elsewhere [1].

A patient may enter a protocol only if these examinations reveal no indications of disseminated disease. The diagnosis of recurrence is based on clinical and/or roentgenological criteria and, if possible, is histologically verified. An abnormal bone scintigraphy must be verified roentgenologically to be diagnosed as bone metastases. The diagnosis of liver metastases requires palpable enlargement of the liver or a diagnosis by CT scanning or ultrasound scanning.

Data Management

All relevant data are registered in the DBCG secretariat, where they are checked, stored, processed, and analyzed by computer.

In the present studies patient entry has been from August 1977 to November 1982. The results in the present report were evaluated as of November 1983. Life-table analysis has been performed on all data. The rates of recurrence given all derived from these analyses. The log-rank test was used to evaluate recurrence rates. Levels of significance are represented by P values for a two-tailed test.

Results

Quantitative Aspects

Since 1978, the annual number of patients registered in DBCG has been close to 2,000. Two small counties did not participate. From the other counties this patient entry represents 99% of all new breast cancer cases.

A total of 9,844 patients have been registered in the DBCG-77 program. Thirty-seven percent of the patients did not enter the protocols and, as can be seen in Table 2, this is due to accepted criteria of exclusion in 92% of cases. A detailed analysis of this subject will be given elsewhere in connection with presentation of the specific protocols.

Table 2. Criteria of exclusion in the DBCG-77 protocols (%)

According to protocol	
Incorrect operation	25
Medical contraindication	29
Previous breast cancer	11
Metastases	10
Other malignant disease	7
Bilateral breast cancer	6
Patient refusal	4
Total	92
Other (errors)	8

Protocol DBCG-77-1a

Protocol DBCG-77-1a has been entered by 3,125 patients. At 5 years, 31% of the patients have experienced recurrent disease and 16% have died. Details of this protocol will be presented elsewhere.

Protocol DBCG-77-1b

Adjuvant levamisole treatment increased the early rate of recurrence compared with the control group, and for this reason entry to the levamisole arm was stopped in December 1979 [3]. These results have been confirmed by later follow-up [6].

In the following only the two chemotherapy arms and the control group will be considered.

The groups consisted of: 155 patients randomized to the radiotherapy (RT) arm, 421 to the RT + C arm, and 422 to the RT + CMF arm. The number of patients in the control arm is smaller than in the two chemotherapy arms because accrual to the control arm was stopped in January 1981 when it became evident that the chemotherapy patients had a significantly better prognosis. The median time of observation is 39 months in the RT arm and 27 months for the other two arms. It appears from Fig. 1 that RFS is significantly superior in the two groups receiving chemotherapy but that there is no RFS difference between the C and CMF groups. Seventy-six recurrences were observed in the RT arm, of which 6 were local. In the RT + C arm and the RT + CMF arm, 59 and 76 recurrences respectively were observed, of which 14 and 4 were local. To date, no significant difference is observed in survival (RT vs RT + C, $P = 0.52$ and RT vs RT + CMF, $P = 0.09$).

The RFS data have also been analyzed in relation to the number of positive lymph nodes and tumor size. As shown in Table 3, the effectiveness of chemotherapy at 4 years is significant in all groups except for the patients with more than four positive lymph nodes treated with C. The efficacy of chemotherapy was most pronounced in tumors between 3 and 5 cm in diameter (Table 4).

Physician compliance with the protocol was excellent, with close agreement between intended doses, with or without dose reduction due to toxicity, and doses given. As described in detail elsewhere [4], hematological toxicity was more severe with C than with CMF. The average given doses were 59% for C and 61% for CMF. Only 47% of CMF patients received more than 75% of the scheduled dose in all 12 cycles, compared with 38%

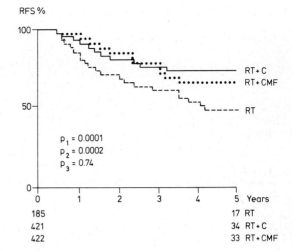

Fig. 1. DBCG-77-1b: overall RFS.
p_1, RT vs RT + C; p_2, RT vs RT +
CMF; p_3, RT + C vs RT + CMF

Table 3. DBCG-77-1b: RFS in relation to number of positive nodes

Treatment	Number of nodes					
	0–3			≥ 4		
	RT	RT + C	RT + CMF	RT	RT + C	RT + CMF
n	138	309	290	47	106	123
RFS%	58	80	73	35	45	45
P values						
RT vs RT + C		0.0001			0.08	
RT vs RT + CMF		0.0010			0.01	

n, number of patients at entry; RFS%, 4-year life-table analysis

Table 4. DBCG-77-1b: RFS in relation to tumor size

Treatment	Tumor size								
	< 3 cm			3–5 cm			> 5 cm		
	RT	RT + C	RT + CMF	RT	RT + C	RT + CMF	RT	RT + C	CT + CMF
n	41	100	103	103	223	223	38	89	85
RFS%	73	84	82	41	73	63	40	52	55
P values									
RT vs RT + C		0.09			0.0001			0.56	
RT vs RT + CMF		0.19			0.0010			0.11	

n, number of patients at entry; RFS%, 4-year life-table analysis

Table 5. DBCG-77-1b: RFS in relation to drug dose

Drug dose	Treatment			
	C		CMF	
	< 75%	> 75%	< 75%	> 75%
n	264	91	247	103
RFS%	77	78	72	68
P		0.52		0.62

n, number of patients having completed 12 courses of chemotherapy; RFS%, 4-year life-table analysis

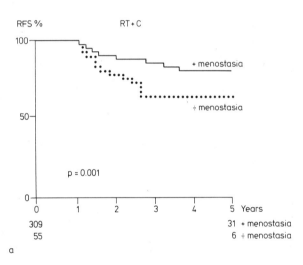

a

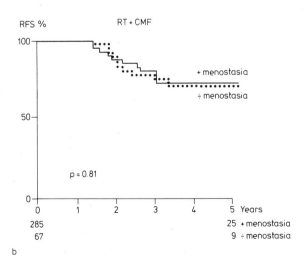

b

Fig. 2a, b. DBCG-77-1b: RFS in relation to occurrence of menostatia in patients having completed 12 cycles of chemotherapy: **a** RT + C; **b** RT + CMF

of C patients. Using 75% of the scheduled dose as limit, no significant relationship was observed between RFS and dose level, neither with C nor with CMF (Table 5).

The frequency of nausea and vomiting was greater with CMF than with C, whereas alopecia occurred more often with C [4].

The incidence of amenorrhea rose steadily during the adjuvant therapy until at 12 months it occurred in 85% of patients treated with C and 81% of those treated with CMF. When RFS was analyzed in relationship to occurrence of menostasia, it appeared that RFS was significantly higher in patients with this symptom treated with C, while no such relation was observed in patients treated with CMF (Fig. 2).

Protocol DBCG-77-1c

Clinical Data

After mastectomy and postoperative radiotherapy, 827 patients were randomized to treatment with tamoxifen (T) for 1 year (RT + T) and 820 were randomized to no further therapy (RT). Overall RFS is shown in Fig. 3. Only 70 patients have been at risk for 5 years, and the median time of observation is 25 months. The RFS after 5 years of life-table analysis is 48% in the RT + T group and 40% in the control group. This difference is significant ($P = 0.013$). The numbers of both local and distant metastases are reduced by systemic treatment with tamoxifen. In the RT group 235 recurrences were observed, of which 21 were local. The corresponding figures in the RT + T arm were 172 and 15, respectively. For the overall survival analysis a total of 107 patients have been observed for 5 years. Survival is 58% in the RT group and 62% in the RT + T group ($P = 0.65$).

The RFS has also been analyzed in relation to age. The greatest difference in RFS according to decade of age was observed in the youngest group of postmenopausal patients, aged 50−59 years (Table 6). The trend in favor of the tamoxifen-treated group is less apparent in the groups of patients 60−69 and 70−79 years of age and does not reach significance in either of these two groups.

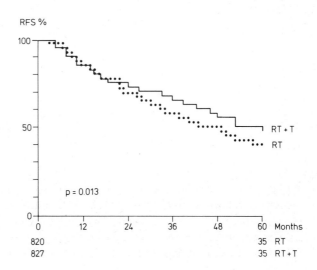

Fig. 3. DBCG-77-1c: overall RFS in patients aged 50−79 years

Table 6. DBCG-77-1c: RFS in relation to age

Treatment	Age (years)					
	50–59		60–69		70–79	
	RT	RT + T	RT	RT + T	RT	RT + T
n	179	190	383	387	258	250
RFS%	45	58	54	57	45	51
P		0.05		0.06		0.65

n, number of patients at entry; RFS%, 4-year life-table analysis

Table 7. DBCG-77-1c: RFS in relation to anaplasia grade

Treatment	Anaplasia grade					
	I		II		III	
	RT	RT + T	RT	RT + T	RT	RT + T
n	211	199	383	386	119	127
RFS%	59	72	46	53	39	36
P		0.0004		0.12		0.2

n, number of patients at entry; RFS%, 4-year life-table analysis

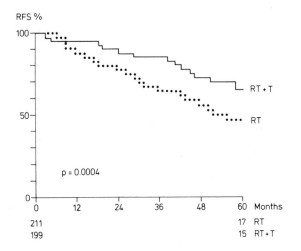

Fig. 4. DBCG-77-1c: RFS in relation to anaplasia degree I

The RFS in relation to degree of anaplasia is shown in Fig. 4 and Table 7. The rate of recurrence is lower in grade I and II tumors for patients treated with tamoxifen, although the difference is significant only for patients with grade I tumors ($P = 0.0004$). Approximately 96% of the 410 patients with grade I tumors are ER+, and the difference in rate of recurrence in this group of patients is 13% at 4 years.

Table 8. DBCG-77-1c: RFS in relation to number of positive nodes

Treatment	Number of nodes			
	0–3		≥ 4	
	RT	RT + T	RT	RT + T
n	584	602	236	224
RFS%	60	62	23	39
P		0.37		0.002

n, number of patients at entry; RFS%, 4-year life-table analysis

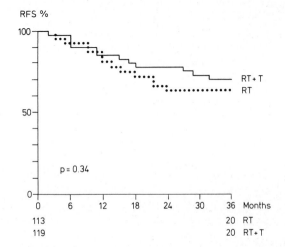

Fig. 5. DBCG-77-1c: RFS in ER+ (≥ 10 fmol/mg protein) tumors

A trend towards lower recurrence rates in patients treated with tamoxifen is seen in those with tumors < 5 cm. Approximately 50% of the patients have tumors between 3 and 5 cm, and the difference in RFS at 5 years is 11% in favor of the tamoxifen-treated patients ($P = 0.06$).

There is no difference in rate of recurrence between the two treatment groups for patients with 0–3 positive lymph nodes (Table 8), but in the group of patients with 4 or more positive nodes the difference in RFS is highly significant.

ER Data

A subset of approximately 17% of the patients in this study had ER determinations performed between September 1, 1979 and November 1, 1983. The median time of observation is 16 and 21 months in ER− and ER+ patients, respectively. Regardless of treatment the RFS in the ER+ group is 73% compared with 35% in the ER− group after 2 years of life-table analysis ($P = 0.0001$). Fig. 5 compares the RFS for the ER+ patients only in the two treatment groups. There is a trend for a higher RFS in the

Table 9. DBCG-77-1c: RFS in relation to ER content

Treatment	ER content (fmol/mg protein)					
	< 10		10–100		> 100	
	RT	RT + T	RT	RT + T	RT	RT + T
n	33	27	43	43	70	76
RFS%	32	40	72	61	65	87
P		0.62		0.17		0.007

n, number of patients at entry; RFS%, 4-year life-table analysis

tamoxifen-treated patients, but the difference is not significant after 3 years of analysis. The RFS data have also been analyzed in relation to the concentration of ER protein in the primary tumors (Table 9). It appears, that while the prognosis is significantly better for patients with ER concentrations above 10 fmol/mg cytosol protein, a beneficial effect of tamoxifen treatment can only be demonstrated in patients with an ER content of more than 100 fmol/mg cytosol protein, whereas patients with levels between 10 and 100 fmol/mg have the same rate of recurrence irrespective of treatment.

Discussion

The present study has confirmed the ability of CMF to increase RFS in premenopausal, high-risk, primary breast cancer patients. A similar effectiveness was demonstrated with single-agent therapy with intermittent cyclophosphamide. A number of other studies have compared multiple-drug therapy with single-agent therapy using L-PAM. All of these studies (for review see [10]) demonstrated the superiority of the multiple-drug regimes. However, the only published major trial with adjuvant cyclophosphamide treatment, the Scandinavian trial [11], also demonstrated that cyclophosphamide is active, although duration of treatment was very short.

Conflicting studies have been reported concerning drug dose and drug-induced toxicity related to RFS [10]. In agreement with the majority of these studies, no relation was observed in this study between drug dose and RFS. These retrospective analyses, however, may be invalidated by factors unrelated to the dose level as such, and prospective trials are needed for conclusive evidence concerning this relation.

It has been argued that some of the effects of adjuvant therapy given to premenopausal patients might be attributed to drug-induced ovarian suppression [10]. In the present study a significant relation between occurrence of menostasia was observed in patients treated with C but not in those treated with CMF. So far, this observation cannot be explained, and it should be emphasized that the number of patients who did not experience menostasia, was small.

The main objective of the DBCG-77-1c trial was to define the value of adjuvant antiestrogen treatment in postmenopausal patients with high-risk primary breast cancer. In agreement with our previous findings [14], this update confirms that systemic treatment with tamoxifen significantly increases the RFS. Furthermore, there is a tendency toward an increased overall survival and there appears to be an equal reduction in the number of both local and distant metastases. The increase in RFS is significant in women less than 70 years of age, in patients with four or more positive lymph nodes, and in patients with grade-I tumors.

ER+ patients have a significantly better prognosis regardless of treatment when a cut-off limit of 10 fmol/mg cytosol protein is used. In the present study, this cut-off limit seems of little value in predicting the effect of antiestrogen treatment. However, a cut-off level of 100 fmol/mg cytosol protein identifies a subgroup of patients in whom tamoxifen treatment has a substantial impact on the RFS.

Other adjuvant trials have evaluated the therapeutic effect of adjuvant tamoxifen treatment in postmenopausal patients [2, 12, 13, 16]. The mean follow-up time in most of these studies is short, but the results generally indicate that tamoxifen treatment delays recurrence in certain subgroups of patients. However, longer observation periods and more thorough analysis of the relationship between ER status and the outcome of tamoxifen treatment are needed.

The present studies have demonstrated that adjuvant systemic therapy in high-risk breast cancer patients is active in increasing the recurrence-free survival. However, this applies only to some subgroups of patients. Furthermore, the period of observation is still too short to evaluate the effect of adjuvant therapy on survival. For these reasons the ultimate role of adjuvant systemic therapy is still poorly defined.

The experience with DBCG, so far, has demonstrated the feasibility of conducting nationwide trials of adjuvant therapy in primary breast cancer. Such studies in nonselected patient populations in close cooperation with basic research programs can hopefully improve our knowledge of the natural history and biology of the disease and thus improve the rationale for selection of patients for the various therapies possible.

References

1. Andersen KW, Mouridsen HT, Castberg T, Fischerman K, Andersen J, Hou-Jensen K, Brincker H, Johansen H, Henriksen E, Rørth M, Rossing N, DBCG (1981) Organization of the Danish Adjuvant Trials in Breast Cancer. Dan Med Bull 28: 102–106
2. Baum N, other members of the Nolvadex Adjuvant Trial Organization (1983) Control trial of Tamoxifen as adjuvant agent in management of early breast cancer. Lancet 1: 257–261
3. Brincker H, Mouridsen HT, Andersen KW, Andersen J, Castberg T, Fischerman K, Henriksen E, Hou-Jensen K, Johansen H, Rossing N, Rørth M, DBCG (1980) Increased breast-cancer recurrence rate after adjuvant therapy with levamisole. Lancet 2: 824–827
4. Brincker H, Mouridsen HT, Andersen KW (1983) Adjuvant chemotherapy with cyclophosphamide or CMF in pre-menopausal women with stage II breast cancer. Breast Cancer Res Treat 3: 91–95
5. Cady B (1973) Total mastectomy and partial axillary dissection. Surg Clin North Am 53: 313–317
6. Danish Breast Cancer Cooperative Group (1983) Informationsblad no 11
7. EORTC Breast Cancer Cooperative Group (1980) Revision of standards for the assessment of hormone receptor in human breast cancer. Report of the second EORTC workshop. Eur J Cancer 16: 1513–1515
8. Fischerman K, Mouridsen HT (1977) Danish Breast Cancer Cooperative Group – DBCG. Ugeskr Læger 139: 2493–2494
9. Koenders A, Thorpe SM (1983) Standardization of steroid receptor-assays in human breast cancer – I: Reproducibility of estradiol- and progesterone-receptorassays. Eur J Cancer Clin Oncol 19: 1221–1229

10. Mouridsen HT, Palshof T (1983) Adjuvant systemic therapy in breast cancer. A review. Eur J Cancer Clin Oncol 19: 1753–1770
11. Nissen-Meyer R, Kjellgren K, Månsson B (1982) Adjuvant chemotherapy in breast cancer. In: Mathé G, Bonadonna G, Salmon S (eds) Adjuvant therapies of cancer. Springer, Berlin Heidelberg New York (Recent results in cancer research, vol 80)
12. Palshof T, Mouridsen HT, Daehnfeldt JL (1980) Adjuvant endocrinotherapy of primary operable breast cancer. Report on the Copenhagen Breast Cancer Trials. Eur J Cancer [Suppl] 1: 183–189
13. Ribeiro G, Palmer MK (1983) Adjuvant tamoxifen for operable carcinoma of breast: report of clinical trial by Christie Hospital and Holt Radium Institute. Br Med J 286: 827–830
14. Rose C, Thorpe SM, Mouridsen HT, Andersen JA, Brincker H, Andersen KW (1983) Antiestrogen treatment of postmenopausal women with primary high risk breast cancer. Breast Cancer Res Treat 3: 77–84
15. Scharf RW, Tarloni H (1968) Histological typing of breast tumors. World Health Organization, Geneva
16. Wallgren A, Ideström K, Glas U, Kaigas M, Theve NO, Wilking N, Nordenskjöld B, Karnström L, Silverswärd C (to be published) Adjuvant tamoxifen treatment in operable breast cancer. N Engl J Med

Clinical Results II: Experience of Non-Randomized Trials with Historical or Mached Surgical Controls

FAC + BCG as Adjuvant Therapy in Breast Cancer: An 8-Year Update

G. R. Blumenschein, A. U. Buzdar, and G. N. Hortobagyi

University of Texas System Cancer Center, M.D. Anderson Hospital and Tumor Institute, Department of Medical Oncology, Medical Breast Service, 6723 Bertner Avenue, Houston, TX 77030, USA

Introduction

In January 1974, the Medical Breast Service at M.D. Anderson Hospital began investigation of a combination of fluorouracil, doxorubicin (adriamycin), and cyclophosphamide (FAC) as adjuvant therapy for stage II and III breast cancer. Earlier results of these studies have been published [1−3]. Here the results of the initial study are presented, with the median follow-up of FAC-treated patients being 85 months. As this is the first adjuvant program utilizing FAC with such long-term follow-up, it seemed important to review the results of stage II and III patients so treated.

Materials and Methods

Between January 1974 and April 1927, 222 patients with stage II, III, and IV (according to UICC classification criteria; IV included T_4 or N_3 patients) breast cancer were treated with FAC chemotherapy. In this trial all patients also received nonspecific immunotherapy with bacillus Calmette-Guerin (BCG). The details of the chemotherapy program have been

Table 1. Pretreatment characteristics of FAC and control group

Characteristics	FAC (%)	Control (%)	P
Total no. of patients	222	186	−
Stage			
II	153 (69)	117 (63)	0.24
III, IV	69 (31)	69 (37)	
No. of involved nodes			
1− 3	73 (33)	71 (38)	
4−10	93 (42)	63 (34)	0.25
> 10	56 (25)	52 (28)	
Age (years)			
< 50	111 (50)	63 (34)	< 0.01
≥ 50	111 (50)	123 (66)	

previously reported [1]. All patients had received prior surgery and most also had irradiation before starting FAC chemotherapy. In terms of disease-free interval and survival, the FAC-treated patients were compared with a historical control group which included 186 patients with stage II or III breast cancer treated at M.D. Anderson Hospital between 1971 and 1973. The control patients were treated with surgery and irradiation but did not receive systemic therapy following primary treatment of breast cancer. The pretreatment characteristics of the FAC and control patients are shown in Table 1. These two groups were comparable for number of involved nodes and stage of disease; there was a significantly higher proportion of patients in the control group who were postmenopausal. When calculating hazard ratio according to known prognostic factors, however, there was a similarity between the control and the FAC-treated groups. The detailed description of the hazard ratio has been previously published [1]. The calculation is based on a regression model which incorporates three factors determined to be the most predictive of disease-free interval at the time of entry into study in 1974−1977: number of involved nodes, stage, and menopausal status. Statistical methods used for analysis of this study have been previously published [1].

Results

Ninety-four patients in the FAC group have developed recurrent disease at the median follow-up of 85 months. The estimated fraction of patients free of disease at 85 months was approximately 55% for the entire FAC-treated group as compared with 35% for the control group (Table 2). The difference in the overall distribution was highly statistically significant ($P < 0.01$). Only four patients have relapsed between 60 and 85 months. The fraction of stage II patients free of disease was 66% for the FAC-treated group and 38% for

Table 2. Disease-free survival

Characteristics stage	Estimated at 7 years (%)		P (two-tailed)
	FAC	Control	
All patients	55	35	< 0.01
II	66	38	< 0.01
III, IV	38	25	0.02
Stage II Age (years)			
< 50	69	28	< 0.01
≥ 50	61	41	0.02
Nodes			
1−3	70	43	0.01
4−10	68	40	< 0.01
> 10	48	22	0.17
Stage III and IV Age (years)			
< 50	33	18	0.02
≥ 50	40	25	0.09

Table 3. Survival

Characteristics stage	Estimated at 7 years (%)		P (two-tailed)
	FAC	Control	
All patients	66	48	< 0.01
II	75	54	< 0.01
III, IV	47	37	0.08
Age (years)			
< 50	72	51	< 0.01
≥ 50	72	55	0.02

the historical control group. Stage III and IV patients had similar disease-free survival intervals, but superior to those for the control patients ($P = 0.02$). There was no difference between the disease-free survival intervals of the FAC-treated stage III and IV patients by menopausal status (Table 2).

Thirty-three percent of FAC-treated patients < 50 years of age remained disease-free as compared with 18% of controls; for patients ≥ 50 years of age these figures were 40% and 25%, respectively.

Upon examination of prognostic factors for stage II disease, significant disease-free survival has been observed for both those FAC-treated patients ≥ 50 years and those < 50 Table 2). Sixty-nine percent of stage II patients < 50 years of age treated with chemotherapy remained disease-free at 7 years, as opposed to 28% of control patients. This difference was highly significant ($P < 0.01$). Of patients ≥ 50 years, 61% treated with FAC remained free of disease, as compared with 41% of the control population ($P = 0.02$). Examination for number of lymph nodes involved revealed differences amongst patients, especially between those having 1–10 nodes and those with > 10 nodes involved with metastatic disease. Of those patients with 1–3 nodes and 4–10 nodes involved, 70% and 68%, respectively, enjoyed disease-free survival at 7 years, as opposed to 43% and 40% of the control patients; the difference between the FAC-treated patients and the control group was significant in both categories. When > 10 nodes were involved with stage II disease, the estimated proportion of patients remaining disease-free at 7 years fell to 48%, while the control population showed only 22% disease-free; because the numbers were small this difference was not significant in the two-tailed T-test.

Seventy-five percent of stage II FAC-treated patients remained alive at 7 years as opposed to 54% of stage II control patients, while 47% of stage III and IV patients remained alive as compared with 37% of their controls (Table 3). It was interesting to note that 72% of patients in both age-groups (≥ 50 years and < 50 years) in the stage II FAC-treated patient category remained alive after 7 years, compared with 51% and 55%, respectively, in the stage II control category (Table 3).

Discussion

The results of this study after long follow-up have demonstrated that doxorubicin combination therapy is associated with significant improvement in the disease-free survival and overall survival of high-risk patients with breast cancer. The effectiveness of the chemotherapy is independent of menopausal status. There was no difference in the disease-free survival between patients with 1−3 metastatic nodes and 4−10 nodes. However, when stage II patients had > 10+ nodes, the disease-free survival interval decreased − when compared with the stage II control population with > 10+ nodes, these patients do not enjoy a significant disease-free survival advantage. Subsequent studies have failed to show any therapeutic advantage from the addition of irradiation and/or BCG therapy [4].

References

1. Buzdar AU, Gutterman JU, Blumenschein GR et al. (1978) Intensive postoperative chemoimmunotherapy for patients with stage II and stage III breast cancer. Cancer 41: 1064−1075
2. Buzdar AU, Blumenschein GR, Gutterman JU et al. (1979) Postoperative adjuvant chemotherapy with fluorouracil, doxorubicin, cyclophosphamide, and BCG vaccine: A follow-up report. JAMA 242: 1509−1513
3. Buzdar AU, Smith T, Blumenschein GR et al. (1981) Adjuvant chemotherapy with fluorouracil, doxorubicin, and cyclophosphamide (FAC) for stage II or III breast cancer: 5-year results. In: Salmon SE, Jones SE (eds) Adjuvant therapy of cancer III. Grune and Stratton, New York, p 419
4. Buzdar AU, Blumenschein GR, Smith T et al. (1984) Adjuvant chemotherapy with fluorouracil, doxorubicin, and cyclophosphamide, with or without Bacillus Calmette-Guerin and with or without irradiation in operable breast cancer. Cancer 53: 384−389

Current Results of the University of Arizona Adjuvant Breast Cancer Trials (1974–1984)

S. E. Jones, R. J. Brooks, B. J. Takasugi, H. S. Garewal, G. F. Giordano, S. J. Ketchel, R. Jackson, R. S. Heusinkveld, S. R. Kemmer, T. E. Moon, and S. E. Salmon

Departments of Medicine and Radiology, Cancer Center, University of Arizona, College of Medicine, Tucson, AZ 85724, USA

Introduction

In this paper we update the results of a series of clinical trials of chemotherapy and radiotherapy for patients with early stage breast cancer seen and treated at the University of Arizona Cancer Center between 1974 and 1984. Preliminary results have been presented at earlier conferences on the adjuvant therapy of cancer [1−7]. The basic chemotherapy employed in these adjuvant trials consisted of the two-drug combination of doxorubicin (adriamycin) and cyclophosphamide (AC) administered at 3-week intervals. These agents were picked for study because of their efficacy in treating patients with advanced breast cancer, the subsequent evidence of drug synergism from animal tumor systems, and for their ease of administration in an outpatient setting. This report includes data based on an analysis made in October, 1983.

Patients and Methods

The temporal sequence of the adjuvant trials carried out at the University of Arizona between 1974 and 1984 is shown in Table 1. Detailed information on methodology may be found elsewhere [1−7]. However, a brief description of patient eligibility is necessary to understand these trials. Patients were eligible for these studies if they had undergone radical or modified radical mastectomy and did not have a history of prior breast cancer or

Table 1. Temporal sequence of Arizona early breast cancer trials

Time	Stage II (node-positive)	Stage I (node-negative)
1974	Pilot study: AC × 8	−
1975	AC ± XRT	AC × 3
1977	AC ± XRT	AC × 3 T_1N_0
		AC × 8 T_2N_0
1979	AC ± XRT	AC × 3
1981−1984	1−3 + Nodes: AC/XRT/AC	AC × 3
	3 + Nodes: alternating regimens	

heart disease which would exclude them from treatment with doxorubicin. Treatment could be initiated within 4 months of mastectomy though with the majority of patients it was begun within 6 weeks of surgery. Staging included pretreatment chest radiographs, bone scans (with correlative radiographs of abnormal sites on scan), and routine laboratory work. Staging classification was based on pathologic assessment of tumor size and nodal status according to the TNM classification [8]. Patients with tumors greater than 5.0 cm (T_3) were considered to have stage III breast cancer and were treated on other protocols not reported here. A brief description of each of these studies follow.

Stage II (Node-Positive)

Beginning in 1974 a pilot study was carried out employing eight courses of chemotherapy with AC administered at 3-week intervals. The dose of doxorubicin was 30 mg/m^2 administered intravenously on the first day followed by cyclophosphamide 150 mg/m^2 administered orally on days 3−6 (4 days total) for each course of therapy. As previously reported, 85% of patients were able to tolerate 85% or more of the planned drug dosages in this program [6]. In 1975, this trial was modified to examine the question of chemotherapy alone (AC) vs chemotherapy + radiotherapy (AC + RT). Radiotherapy was administered in a split course between the second and third courses of chemotherapy. In general, patients received comprehensive regional lymph node and chest wall irradiation to a dose of 5,000 rads. The majority of patients were randomized, but there were a group of patients who could not be randomized as they were unable to stay in Tucson for 5 weeks for radiotherapy. Randomized and nonrandomized patients are considered together in this analysis. In 1981, at the Third International Conference on Adjuvant Therapy of Cancer, we reported that there was a significant difference in relapse-free survival (RFS) for the patients receiving AC + RT compared with AC alone in the 1−3 node-positive group [6]. For that reason the study was modified in 1981 so that additional patients with stage II breast cancer and 1−3 positive nodes received combined therapy (AC + RT). This study design continues to the present time.

Stage II (> 3 + Nodes)

Between 1975 and 1981 patients with stage II breast cancer with more than three positive nodes were treated with AC or AC + RT as described above. Based upon the analysis presented in 1981 [6], the trial was modified to evaluate short-course, high-dose, intravenous alternating chemotherapy regimens as adjuvant therapy for this group of patients at high risk of recurrence. This program was based on animal data which suggested that early intensive treatment with potentially non-cross-resistant or alternating combinations of drugs might be more effective than one combination of drugs given repeatedly in an effort to avoid the rapid acquisition of drug resistance which would occur in patients with a high residual occult tumor burden [9]. In addition, it was our belief that this type of chemotherapy program might be effective even if given over a short period of time [10, 11]. Accordingly, we picked three drug regimens with the intention of giving each combination once. The three regimens were VAC (vincristine 1.0 mg/m^2 i.v. day 1, doxorubicin 40 mg/m^2 i.v. day 1, and cyclophosphamide 750 mg/m^2 i.v. day 1), CMF (cyclophosphamide 600 mg/m^2 i.v. day 22, methotrexate 40 mg/m^2 i.v. day 22, and 5-fluorouracil 600 mg/m^2 i.v. day 22 − these are the doses currently used by the Milan group [12]), and mitomycin-vinblastine (mitomycin C 10 mg/m^2 i.v. day 43 and vinblastine 5 mg/m^2 i.v. day 43 − this program was piloted in patients with advanced disease [13]). All drugs were given intravenously at 3-week intervals. Chemotherapy was completed in 6 weeks. Patients with node-positive stage III breast cancer (T3 > 5.0 cm) received the same chemotherapy followed by comprehensive regional lymph node and chest wall irradiation as previously described. This pilot program which was begun in September 1981, continues to the present time for patients with high-risk stage II breast cancer as well as those with stage III breast cancer. These results are preliminary and will not be discussed.

Stage I (Node-Negative)

Beginning in 1975, a pilot program was initiated for patients with pathologically negative axillary lymph nodes. Our initial plan was to administer three courses of chemotherapy with AC at 3-week intervals. Based upon an analysis in 1977, we modified the protocol so that patients with T_1N_0 breast cancer continued to receive three courses of AC, whereas patients with T_2N_0 breast cancer (primary tumor size 2.1 cm−5.0 cm) received eight courses of AC. In 1979, based upon another analysis [4], we decided to administer only three courses of AC to patients with both T_1 and T_2N_0 breast cancer. That policy continues to the present time.

General Procedures

Subsequent careful follow-up of all patients after therapy was carried out every 3 months for the first year and every 4−6 months thereafter. Relapse was confirmed radiographically or histologically whenever possible. RFS and overall survival have been calculated by standard techniques and comparisons using several statistical tests have been employed.

Results

All clinical trials have been updated through October 1983. The results are summarized in Table 2.

Table 2. Results of Arizona adjuvant trials, 1974−1984

Stage	No. eligible	No. evaluable[a]	No. relapses	Median follow-up (months)
I (T_1N_0)	49	47	1	51
II (T_2N_0)	78	74	9	40
II (1−3 + nodes)	166	144	25	60
II (> 3 + nodes)	99	88	48	60

[a] Evaluable = completed planned therapy

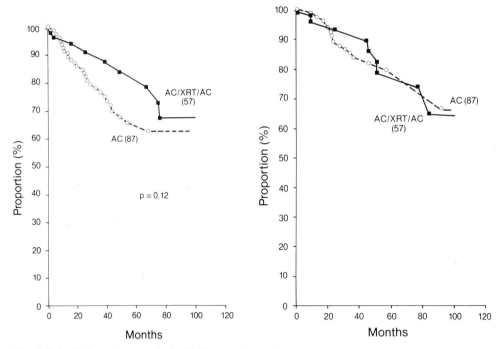

Fig. 1 *(left).* Relapse-free survival of 144 evaluable patients with stage II breast cancer (1−3 positive nodes) according to treatment

Fig. 2 *(right).* Survival of patients with stage II breast cancer (1−3 positive nodes) according to treatment

Stage II (Node-Positive)

Between 1974 and 1984, 265 eligible patients with stage II (node-positive) breast cancer were entered on these trials and 232 are presently fully evaluable (e.g., have completed all therapy). The median time of follow-up is 60 months. The primary comparison was between results with AC vs AC + RT. Of 144 evaluable patients with 1−3 positive nodes, 87 received AC and 57 received AC + RT. RFS was compared for the two treatments as shown in Fig. 1. Although the difference favors AC + RT, this differences is of marginal statistical significance ($P = 0.12$). Moreover, overall survival of the two treatments is identical (Fig. 2).

For patients with more than three positive lymph nodes, 48 relapses have occurred among 88 evaluable patients at median time of follow-up of 60 months. Thirty-nine patients have received AC and 49 have received AC + RT. RFS for these patients is shown in Fig. 3. There is no difference in RFS or in overall survival according to treatment.

Effect of Treatment Delay

In March 1983, we performed an analysis to assess the impact of delay in the initation of adjuvant chemotherapy in stage II breast cancer [14]. According to our original protocol,

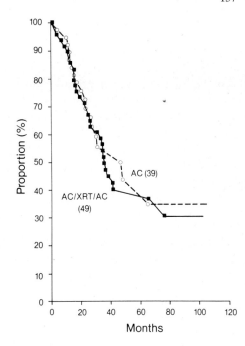

Fig. 3. Relapse-free survival of 88 evaluable patients with stage II breast cancer (> 3 positive nodes) according to treatment

Table 3. Effect of delay on outcome in stage II breast cancer[a]

| | 1–3 positive nodes | | > 3 positive nodes | |
	≤ 4 weeks	> 4 weeks	≤ 4 weeks	> 4 weeks
No. at risk	48	37	46	38
% Free of disease at 48 months	85%	59%	46%	61%
	$P = 0.02$		$P = 0.6$	

[a] Based on an analysis done in March 1983 (the numbers of patients differ slightly from those in Table 1)

patients were eligible for this study if chemotherapy had been initiated within 4 months of surgery. For the majority of patients treatment was initiated within 6 weeks. For the purposes of this analysis we included patients who received AC alone if they had 1–3 positive axillary nodes and either AC or AC + RT if they had more than three positive axillary lymph nodes. RFS curves were generated for groups of patients according to the week after surgery when chemotherapy with AC was initiated. The only clear-cut difference in RFS noted (for patients with 1–3 positive nodes) was between those treated within 4 weeks and those treated more than 4 weeks after surgery (Table 3). Of those women with 1–3 positive lymph nodes who had a delay of more than 4 weeks, only 59% were free of disease at 4 years, compared with 85% of those women who began treatment within 4 weeks ($P = 0.02$). For patients with more than three positive nodes there was no significant effect of delay and the overall recurrence rates were substantially higher than for women with 1–3 positive nodes irrespective of treatment or delay (see Fig. 2).

Stage I and II (Node-Negative)

One hundred and twenty-seven eligible patients have been entered on this trial and presently 121 are evaluable; ten relapses have occurred (Table 2). Among patients with T_1N_0 breast cancer only a single relapse has occurred in 47 evaluable patients with median follow-up of 51 months. Among patients with T_2N_0 breast cancer, nine relapses have occurred in 74 patients with a median follow-up time of 40 months.

Discussion

In this paper we have updated our results of treatment of early breast cancer from prior reports [1–7]. The last published update was from the Third International Conference on Adjuvant Therapy of Cancer held in Tucson in 1981 and included data on node-positive as well as node-negative breast cancer [6, 7]. Our conclusions remain essentially unchanged from prior reports. AC is a well-tolerated and effective adjuvant chemotherapy program for women with operable breast cancer irrespective of menopausal status [6, 7]. We have consistently been able to administer full doses of chemotherapy (85% of planned doses) in over 80% of women, in contrast to the use of cyclophosphamide, methotrexate, and 5-fluorouracil (CMF) which could be given in full doses in only 20%–40% of women [6, 7, 12, 15]. Other investigators have reported that dose of chemotherapy is a significant prognostic factor affecting outcome with the best results observed in women who received full doses [15].

As we reported previously, the number of axillary lymph nodes involved by breast cancer is the single most important prognostic factor in affecting outcome with AC (Table 2) [6]. Among women with 1–3 involved lymph nodes, two additional factors appear to be important: treatment (AC or AC + RT) and delay in initiating chemotherapy. In 1981, we reported that RFS was significantly better for the 24 women with 1–3 positive nodes who received AC + RT than for the 63 patients who received AC alone ($P < 0.05$) [6]. However, the number of evaluable patients was small. At the present time 144 women are evaluable and the median follow-up is now 60 months. Although RFS is somewhat better for AC + RT than for AC (Fig. 1), the difference is of marginal significance ($P = 0.12$) and there is no difference in overall survival (Fig. 2).

One of our initial objectives was to evaluate the effect of timing of chemotherapy after surgery. With the recent analysis (Table 3) it appears that beginning chemotherapy with AC within 4 weeks of surgery produces superior results compared with a delay of more than 4 weeks in women with limited axillary node involvement (1–3 positive) [14]. Although this was a retrospective analysis, timing of chemotherapy as well as the dose of chemotherapy appear to be important determinants of outcome in adjuvant therapy.

Among women with more than three positive lymph nodes, results with AC were no different than with AC + RT (Fig. 3) [6]. We would conclude that there is no demonstrable advantage to adding postoperative RT to adjuvant chemotherapy with AC. The major problem facing women with multiple involved axillary lymph nodes is a high relapse rate despite the use of adjuvant chemotherapy which has proven effective in women with less extensive node involvement (AC, CMF, etc.) [6, 12]. In our trial 48 (55%) of 88 women with more than three positive nodes have already relapsed (Table 2). Better treatments are needed for this group of women. Our current protocol evaluates the use of three potentially non-cross-resistant regimens (VAC, CMF, and mitomycin-vinblastine) as one test of the Goldie-Coldman hypothesis [9]. Our results are still too preliminary to assess. Various new approaches (e.g., intensive perioperative chemotherapy) may prove necessary to improve the prognosis of women with advanced stage II breast cancer with extensive nodal involvement.

In 1981, we reported on our pilot trial of AC in node-negative breast cancer [7]. Two relapses had occurred in 80 evaluable patients at a median follow-up of 37 months. At the present time 121 women are evaluable, with a median follow-up of 50 months for those with T_1N_0 and 40 months for those with T_2N_0 breast cancer (Table 2). Only a single relapse has occurred in 47 women with T_1N_0 and nine relapses have occurred in 74 women with T_2N_0 cancer (which is considered stage II by the TNM criteria [8]). While there is no surgery-alone control group in our series, the data still suggest benefit, particularly in women with T_1 primary tumors. Similar observations have been made in several randomized trials involving node-negative cancer [10, 11, 16], and additional controlled randomized trials are now underway [17].

Acknowledgements. These studies were supported by grant CA 17094 from the National Cancer Institute, DDHS, Washington, DC, USA.

References

1. Hammond N, Jones SE, Salmon SE, Giordano G, Jackson R, Miller R, Heusinkveld R (1977) Adjuvant treatment of breast cancer with adriamycin-cyclophosphamide with or without radiation therapy. In: Salmon SE, Jones SE (eds) Adjuvant therapy of cancer. North-Holland, New York, pp 153−160
2. Salmon SE, Jones SE (1979) Studies of the combination of adriamycin and cyclophosphamide (alone or with other agents) for the treatment of breast cancer. Oncology 36: 40−47
3. Salmon SE, Wendt A, Jones SE, Jackson R, Giordano G, Miller R, Heusinkveld R, Moon TE (1979) Treatment of early breast cancer with adriamycin-cyclophosphamide with or without radiation therapy: initial results of a brief and effective adjuvant program. In: Bonadonna G, Mathe G, Salmon SE (eds) Adjuvant therapies and markers of post-surgical minimal residual disease I. Springer, Berlin Heidelberg New York, pp 98−104
4. Wendt AG, Jones SE, Salmon SE, Giordano GF, Jackson RA, Miller RS, Heusinkveld RS, Moon TE (1979) Adjuvant chemotherapy of breast cancer with adriamycin-cyclophosphamide with or without radiation therapy. In: Jones SE, Salmon SE (eds) Adjuvant therapy of cancer II. Grune and Stratton, New York, pp 285−293
5. Jones SE, Salmon SE, Allen H, Giordano GF, Davis S, Chase E, Moon TE, Heusinkveld RS (1982) Adjuvant treatment of node-positive breast cancer with adriamycin-cyclophosphamide with or without radiation therapy: Interim results of an ongoing clinical trial. In: Mathé G, Bonadonna G, Salmon S (eds) Adjuvant therapies of cancer. Springer, Berlin Heidelberg New York, pp 162−169 (Recent results in cancer research, vol 80)
6. Allen H, Brooks R, Jones SE, Chase E, Heusinkveld RS, Giordano GF, Ketchel SJ, Jackson RA, Davis S, Moon TE, Salmon SE (1981) Adriamycin-cyclophosphamide (AC) + radiotherapy (XRT). In: Salmon SE, Jones SE (eds) Adjuvant therapy of cancer III. Grune and Stratton, New York, pp 453−462
7. Brooks R, Allen H, Salmon SE, Jones SE, Chase E, Moon TE, Giordano GF (1981) Adjuvant use of adriamycin and cyclophosphamide in node-negative carcinoma of the breast. In: Salmon SE, Jones SE (eds) Adjuvant therapy of cancer III. Grune and Stratton, New York, pp 463−470
8. American Joint Committee for Cancer Staging and End Results Reporting (1983) Manual for staging of cancer, 2nd ed. Chicago, pp 127−130
9. Goldie JH, Coldman AJ, Gudauskas GA (1982) Rationale for the use of alternating non-cross-resistant chemotherapy. Cancer Treat Rep 66: 439−449

10. Nissen-Meyer R, Kjellgren K Malmio K et al. (1978) Surgical adjuvant chemotherapy: results with one short course with cyclophosphamide after mastectomy for breast cancer. Cancer 41: 2088–2098

11. Nissen-Meyer R (1979) One short chemotherapy course in primary breast cancer: 12-Year follow-up in series 1 of the Scandinavian adjuvant chemotherapy study group. In: Jones SE, Salmon SE (eds) Adjuvant therapy of cancer II. Grune and Stratton, New York, pp 207–213

12. Bonadonna G, Valagussa P, Rossi A, Tancini G, Brambilla C, Marchini S, Veronesi U (1981) Multimodal therapy with CMF in resectable breast cancer with positive axillary nodes: The Milan Institute experience. In: Salmon SE, Jones SE (eds) Adjuvant therapy of cancer III. Grune and Stratton, New York, pp 435–444

13. Garewal HS, Brooks RJ, Jones SE, Miller TP (1983) Treatment of advanced breast cancer with mitomycin c combined with vinblastine or vindesine. J Clin Oncol 1: 772–775

14. Takasugi B, Garewal H, Jones S et al. (to be published) Effect of delayed adjuvant chemotherapy in stage II breast cancer

15. Bonadonna G, Valagussa P (1981) Dose-response effect of adjuvant chemotherapy in breast cancer. N Engl J Med 304: 10–15

16. Senn H, Jungi WF, Amgwerd R (1981) Chemo (immuno) therapy with LMF + BCG in node-negative and node-positive breast cancer. In: Salmon SE, Jones SE (eds) Adjuvant therapy of cancer III. Grune and Stratton, New York, pp 385–393

17. Valagussa P, Di Fronzo G, Bignami P, Buzzoni R, Bonadonna G, Veronesi U (1981) Prognostic importance of estrogen receptors to select node negative patients for adjuvant chemotherapy. In: Salmon SE, Jones SE (eds) Adjuvant therapy of cancer III. Grune and Stratton, New York, pp 329–334

Significance of Drug Dose, Timing and Radiotherapy in Adjuvant Therapy of Breast Cancer

A. U. Buzdar, T. L. Smith, C. E. Marcus, G. N. Hortobagyi, and G. R. Blumenschein

University of Texas System Cancer Center, M.D. Anderson Hospital and Tumor Institute, Department of Medical Oncology, Medical Breast Service, 6723 Bertner Avenue, Houston, TX 77030, USA

Introduction

In the past decade, many adjuvant chemotherapy trials in operable breast cancer have been conducted. The results of these trials have answered a number of questions, but have also raised new issues. Among other issues, results have suggested that relapse-free survival was dependent on the dose of cytotoxic drugs and the timing of initiation of chemotherapy [1, 2]. Routine postoperative irradiation was shown to have a detrimental effect on the efficacy of adjuvant chemotherapy [2, 3]. At M.D. Anderson Hospital, since 1974, a combination of fluorouracil, doxorubicin (adriamycin), and cyclophosphamide (FAC) has been utilized following regional therapy in patients with operable breast cancer. In this paper the dose of cytotoxic drugs, timing of initiation of chemotherapy, and the role of routine postoperative irradiation are evaluated.

Material and Methods

Between January 1974 and April 1980, 460 patients with stage II or III breast cancer were treated with FAC adjuvant chemotherapy. The details of the chemotherapy regimens have been previously reported [4, 5]. The initial 222 patients also received nonspecific immunotherapy with bacillus Calmette-Guérin (BCG), and most had postoperative irradiation. The second protocol was initiated in 1977; this study included a randomization for BCG immunotherapy, and chemotherapy cycles were repeated at 3-week instead of 4-week intervals. A randomization for routine postoperative irradiation was also included in the latter part of the second study. The data for all patients were updated through October 1983; the median follow-up was 85 months for the first study and 51 months for the second study.

The FAC chemotherapy program consisted of 400 mg/m^2 fluorouracil i.v. on day 1 and day 8, 40 mg/m^2 doxorubicin i.v. on day 1, and 400 mg/m^2 cyclophosphamide i.v. on day 1 of each 21- to 28-day cycle. When a total dose of 300 mg/m^2 of doxorubicin was reached, a maintenance regimen which included fluorouracil, methotrexate, and cyclophosphamide was begun. The chemotherapy was continued for 2 years. For each patient the percent of protocol dose of FAC administered in cycles one, three, and six was tabulated and the length of disease-free survival (DFS) was compared according to drug dosage. DFS was also compared by degree of myelosuppression (as measured by nadir absolute granulocyte/mm^3) observed in these cycles of chemotherapy. One hundred and ninety-five patients were omitted from this analysis due to the lack of data regarding the myelosuppression.

DFS of patients treated on the initial protocol was compared with that of the patients treated on the second protocol. There were no significant DFS differences in comparable patient population between the two studies. Therefore, for analysis of the relationship between DFS and timing of chemotherapy initiation, patients from both studies were combined.

Patients were started on chemotherapy as soon as possible after being referred to our clinic. The effect of delay in the initiation of chemotherapy on DFS was evaluated between patients with similar characteristics. In addition, a regression model developed in a control group of patients and used in analyzing our initial FAC adjuvant therapy program was employed to determine comparable subgroups [6]. The model, which relates DFS to patients' characteristics, allowed simultaneous consideration of the three most important prognostic factors: number of involved nodes, stage of disease, and menopausal status. A hazard ratio indicating risk of recurrence was calculated for each patient, and patients with similar risk were compared.

Randomization for routine postoperative irradiation was included in the second study beginning in May, 1978. Patients who had postoperative irradiation prior to coming to the institution were included in the radiation therapy subgroup, but were randomized for BCG. Seventy-five patients did not receive radiation therapy. DFS was compared between patients treated with or without postoperative irradiation. DFS was compared using a generalized Wilcoxon test in the case of two groups [7], the Breslow test in the case of three or more groups [8].

Results

Dose of the Drugs

Characteristics of patients according to FAC therapy dosage are shown in Table 1. There were differences in distribution of patient characteristics between those receiving full dose and reduced dose in both studies. To adjust for these differences, patients were grouped according to hazard ratios and data were analyzed in each study by hazard ratios. Patients with hazard ratio < 2 and ≥ 2 in the first study tended to have lower DFS with reduced dose, but none of the differences were statistically significant (Table 2). In the second study, there was no suggestive evidence of shortened DFS with a reduced dose in any of the subgroups. DFS was also analyzed according to the degree of myelosuppression observed in these cycles of chemotherapy. The pretreatment characteristics were similar in all three categories of patients grouped according to myelosuppression (Table 3). There was no significant relationship between length of DFS and extent of myelosuppression (Table 4).

Timing of Initiation of Chemotherapy

The median length of delay was 13 weeks (range 1–54 weeks). Patients treated with routine postoperative radiation had longer delays of chemotherapy; of 361 patients in this subgroup only 13% (47 patients) had chemotherapy started within 10 weeks of surgery. Of

Table 1. Characteristics of patients with and without FAC dose reduction

Characteristics	First study		Second study	
	No reduction n %	Reduction n %	No reduction n %	Reduction n %
Total	178	22	179	42
Stage				
II	121 (68)	13 (59)	110 (62)	24 (57)
III, IV	57 (32)	9 (41)	69 (38)	18 (43)
No. of positive nodes				
1–3	62 (35)	5 (23)	51 (29)	15 (36)
4–10	77 (43)	8 (36)	70 (39)	19 (45)
> 10	39 (22)	9 (41)	58 (32)	8 (19)
Hazard ratio				
< 0.5	22 (12)	2 (9)	18 (10)	6 (14)
0.5–0.99	63 (35)	6 (27)	49 (27)	17 (40)
1–1.99	53 (30)	7 (32)	54 (30)	10 (24)
≥ 2	40 (22)	7 (32)	58 (32)	9 (21)

Table 2. Disease-free survival by FAC dose[a] (cycles 1, 3, and 6) and hazard ratio

	n	Estimated disease-free at 5 years (%)	P (two-tailed)
First study			
Hazard ratio < 2			
100	138	66	0.2
≤ 80	15	47	
Hazard ratio ≥ 2			
100	40	53	0.37
≤ 80	7	28	
Second study			
Hazard ratio < 2			
100	121	46	0.12
≤ 80	33	63	
Hazard ratio ≥ 2			
100	58	37	0.44
≤ 80	9	44	

[a] FAC doses given as percentages in left-hand column

the 99 patients not treated with postoperative radiation, 81% (80 patients) had chemotherapy initiated within 10 weeks of surgery. The distributions of major prognostic characteristics of patients treated within 10 weeks, at 10–13 weeks, at 14–17 weeks, and at ≥ 18 weeks were similar [9]. The DFS for four subgroups of patients according to length of delay is summarized in Table 5. There were no evident trends for earlier treatment being

Table 3. Patient characteristics according to myelosuppression. Low granulocyte count, cycles 1, 3, and 6

Characteristics	> 3,000 n %	1,000−3,000 n %	< 1,000 n %	P
Total granulocyte count	25	194	46	
Stage				
II	14 (56)	124 (64)	26 (57)	0.53
III, IV	11 (44)	70 (36)	20 (43)	
No. of nodes involved				
1−3	4 (16)	69 (36)	18 (39)	
4−10	11 (44)	72 (37)	19 (41)	0.22
> 10	10 (40)	53 (27)	9 (20)	

Table 4. Disease-free survival by myelosuppression in FAC-treated patients (cycles 1, 3, and 6)

Lowest granulocyte/mm^3	Both studies		
	n	Estimated disease-free at 5 years (%)	P
> 3,000	25	63	
1,000−3,000	194	55	0.92
< 1,000	46	57	
Unknown	195	49	

associated with longer DFS. DFS at 5 years from initiation of chemotherapy was similar in the various subgroups. The data were analyzed in similar prognostic subgroups and DFS was compared according to delay from surgery to initiation of chemotherapy. There were no statistically significant differences in DFS within any subgroup, though for patients with stage III there were somewhat earlier recurrences among patients who did not receive chemotherapy until or later than 14 weeks following surgery.

Another method employed classified patients into similar subgroups by estimating prognosis based on regression equation. Patients were then grouped according to prognosis and the relationship of delay of chemotherapy to the outcome was examined within these subgroups. These results are also summarized in Table 5. In three subgroups there was no evidence of significant differences in DFS according to the length of delays in the treatment. Among 124 patients with the worst prognosis (hazard ratio > 2) there were statistically significant differences in DFS according to the length of delay of chemotherapy. However, there was not a consistent trend for shorter DFS as the delay of treatment increased.

Irradiation

The pretreatment characteristics of patients treated with or without postoperative radiation were similar [5]. DFS for patients treated with or without routine postoperative radiation

Table 5. Disease-free survival according to timing of initiation of chemotherapy

Characteristics	Delay (weeks)	n	Recur-rences	Estimated disease-free at 5 years (%)	P (Wilcoxon two-tailed test)
Stage II					
1−3 nodes	< 10	25	5	77	
	10−13	38	13	64	
	14−17	32	9	67	0.37
	≥ 18	16	2	86	
> 3 nodes	< 10	50	19	59	
	10−13	49	16	58	
	14−17	51	25	47	0.35
	≥ 18	29	13	48	
Stage III, IV	< 10	52	31	36	
	10−13	46	20	50	
	14−17	47	31	34	0.13
	≥ 18	25	16	38	
All patients	< 10	127	55	52	
	10−13	133	49	59	
	14−17	130	65	48	0.22
	≥ 18	70	31	52	
Hazard ratio					
< 0.5	< 10	14	3	77	
	10−13	17	6	59	
	14−17	16	5	59	0.33
	≥ 18	8	0	100	
0.5−0.9	< 10	37	13	59	
	10−13	40	15	58	
	14−17	43	14	62	0.92
	≥ 18	22	6	67	
1−1.9	< 10	35	12	62	
	10−13	40	16	55	
	14−17	39	21	48	0.75
	≥ 18	23	13	35	
≥ 2.0	< 10	41	27	25	
	10−13	36	12	63	
	14−17	31	25	17	< 0.01
	≥ 18	17	12	35	

was similar for groups of patients with stage II and those with stage III and IV disease. Survival was also similar in both subgroups treated with or without radiation (Table 6). Table 7 summarizes the sites of first recurrence for patients treated with or without radiation. The incidences of local or regional failure in the two groups were not significantly different. The incidence of second primary breast cancer also was similar in the two groups.

Table 6. Disease-free and overall survival by irradiation status

Irradiation	n	Estimated disease-free at 5 years (%)	P (two-tailed)	Estimated alive at 5 years (%)	P (two-tailed)
All patients					
No	75	52	0.93	70	0.90
Yes	163	41		71	
Stage II					
No	49	61	0.74	72	0.70
Yes	94	44		77	
Stage III, IV					
No	26	38	0.65	62	0.84
Yes	69	35		61	

Table 7. Site of first recurrence and irradiation status

Site	Irradiation status	
	No	Yes
	n %	n %
Local/regional	10 (13)	11 (7)
Systemic	16 (21)	45 (28)
CNS	4 (5)	5 (3)
Opposite breast	1 (1)	3 (2)

Discussion

The first objective of this paper was to present our data on the effect of dose, timing, and irradiation on the length of DFS in patients treated with FAC chemotherapy. Too small a number of patients received chemotherapy at reduced dose in our study to draw any definite conclusions. In the first trial, where chemotherapy was administered at 4-week intervals, there was some suggestion that lower dose of drugs was associated with inferior DFS; in the second protocol, where chemotherapy was administered at 3-week intervals, there was no apparent trend for a lower dose of drugs administered to be associated with shorter DFS. It is possible that shorter DFS associated with lower dose observed in the first study could be related to the less frequent administration of drugs. However, the schedule of administration at 3 vs 4 weeks has not shown any substantial therapeutic benefit and DFS has been similar for the studies [10].

The second objective of this paper was to evaluate the timing of initiation of chemotherapy and its effect on DFS. In this analysis, as in our earlier analysis [9], there was not a clear correlation between the length of DFS and the length of delay in initiation of chemotherapy following surgery. This is in contrast to other studies which have suggested that longer delays markedly decrease the efficacy of adjuvant chemotherapy [1, 3].

DFS for patients treated with or without postoperative radiation was similar and use of routine postoperative irradiation did not decrease the effectiveness of chemotherapy as was reported by earlier observation [1, 3]. The incidence of local failures was not significantly different between the two subgroups.

Acknowledgement. We thank Vickie E. Richard for her help in the preparation of this paper.

References

1. Cooper RG, Holland JF, Glidewell O (1979) Adjuvant chemotherapy of breast cancer. Cancer 44: 793–798
2. Bonadonna G, Valagussa P (1981) Dose response effect of adjuvant chemotherapy in breast cancer. N Engl J Med 304: 10–15
3. Nissen-Meyer R, Kjellgren K Malmio K et al. (1978) Surgical adjuvant chemotherapy results with one short course with cyclophosphamide alter mastectomy for breast cancer. Cancer 41: 2008–2098
4. Buzdar A, Smith T, Blumenschein G, Hortobagyi G, Hersh E, Gehan E (1981) Adjuvant chemotherapy with fluorouracil, doxorubicin and cyclophosphamide (FAC) for stage II or III breast cancer: 5-year results. In: Salmon SE, Jones SE (eds) Adjuvant therapy of cancer III. Grune and Stratton, New York, pp 419–426
5. Buzdar A, Blumenschein G, Smith T et al. (1984) Adjuvant chemotherapy with fluorouracil, doxorubicin, and cylophosphamide, with our without Bacillus Calmette-Guerin and with or without irradiation in operable breast cancer. A prospective randomized trial. Cancer 53: 384–389
6. Buzdar A, Gutterman J, Blumenschein G et al. (1978) Intensive postoperative chemoimmunotherapy for patients with operable breast cancer. Cancer 41: 1064–1075
7. Gehan EA (1965) A generalized Wilcoxon test for comparing arbitrarily singly-censored samples. Biometrika 52: 203–225
8. Breslow N (1970) A generalized Kruskal-Wallis test for comparing K samples subject to unequal patterns of censorship. Biometrika 57: 579–594
9. Buzdar A, Smith T, Powell K et al. (1982) Effect of timing of initiation of adjuvant chemotherapy on disease-free survival in breast cancer. Cancer Res Treat 2: 163–169
10. Buzdar A, Smith T, Blumenschein G et al. (1984) Adjuvant therapy for stage II or III breast cancer M.D. Anderson Hospital experience. In: Blumenschein GR, Montague E (eds) Current controversy in breast cancer. Proceedings of the 26th annual clinical conference, New York, pp 171–184

The Use of a Natural History Data Base
to Compare Outcome Among Several Trials
of Adjuvant Chemotherapy for Stage II Breast Cancer

S. E. Jones and T. E. Moon

Cancer Center, University of Arizona, Health Sciences Center, Tucson, AZ 85724, USA

Introduction

Three international conferences on the adjuvant therapy of cancer have been held in Tucson since 1977. Reports on the results of adjuvant chemotherapy in operable breast cancer have been a major component of those meetings [1−3]. At the time of the second conference in 1979, a consensus among most investigators was that adjuvant chemotherapy reduced recurrence rates after surgery and probably also resulted in improved survival, although this was not consistent in all studies [2]. Because of the original reports of the NSABP and Milan trials [1−3], many second-generation adjuvant trials did not include a control group of patients who had undergone surgery alone, but instead compared different forms of adjuvant chemotherapy or chemotherapy + radiotherapy. Indeed, our own trial at the University of Arizona, initiated in 1974, looked at the question of chemotherapy alone or chemotherapy + radiotherapy as adjuvant treatments for patients with operable breast cancer [4]. Thus, by 1979, there were a large number of clinical trials which did not have an untreated control group for comparison. Many questions were raised: Does adjuvant treatment work in postmenopausal women? Are there differences in therapeutic efficacy between various treatment programs? These questions could not be answered directly because appropriate clinical trials did not exist or had just been established. Accordingly, we initiated a plan to acquire data on a large number of patients who had undergone primary surgery (± irradiation), which could be used to compare results of various adjuvant programs in matched populations of patients with known prognostic factors. This data set later became known as the "Natural History Data Base" or NHDB [5]. Moreover, modern statistical methodology would provide comparison of the results of treatment from different studies even if the initial important prognostic factors were not well balanced. The initial phase of this ambitious project was reported on in 1981 [5, 6]. Since that time, additional work has been accomplished and a considerably updated version of this was presented at the Fourth International Conference on Adjuvant Therapy of Cancer in Tucson in March 1984. This paper represents an interim report on the status of the NHDB and its comparison of various adjuvant trials.

Methods

A list of the five participating cancer centers or clinical oncology study groups and the cooperating investigators is shown in Table 1. We first agreed what clinical information on

Table 1. Participating institutions and investigators

Institution	Investigators
National Cancer Institute, Milan, Italy	G. Bonadonna
	U. Veronesi
	P. Valagussa
Royal Marsden Hospital, Sutton, Surrey, England	T. Powles
M.D. Anderson Hospital, Houston, Texas, USA	A. Buzdar
	E. Montague
University of Arizona, Tucson, Arizona, USA	S. Jones
	T. Moon
Southwest Oncology Group, San Antonio, Texas, USA	S. Rivkin

Table 2. Known potential prognostic factors in the natural history data base (NHDB) and in the adjuvant treated patients

NHDB
   Age
   Menopausal status
   Tumor location
   Size of tumor (pathologic assessment)
   Lymph node status (pathologic assessment)
   Type of surgery
   Postoperative radiotherapy
   Estrogen receptor status[a]
   Progesterone receptor status[a]

Adjuvant therapy groups
   Same factors as above plus:
      Type of chemotherapy
      Dose of chemotherapy
      Duration of treatment

[a] Not available for most cases

prognostic factors would most likely be available on all patients both in the NHDB and in the adjuvant-treated groups of patients. The prognostic factors and details about treatment collected on each patient are shown in Table 2. Estrogen receptor (ER) data were not available on most patients except for those treated recently. Data on additional node-negative cases with ER receptor status are also being added to the NHDB [7], as are data from M.D. Anderson [8]. A description of the methodology employed in constructing and analyzing the NHDB can be found elsewhere [5, 9].

Data on patients who received adjuvant chemotherapy (± radiotherapy) came from the following sources: (a) the Milan studies conducted from 1973–1978, which involved the postoperative administration of either 6 or 12 courses (months) of cyclophosphamide, methotrexate, and 5-fluorouracil (CMF) [10]; (b) the Southwest Oncology Group (SWOG) study, initiated in 1975 and closed to patient entry in 1978, which compared

2 years of melphalan (L-PAM) with the five drug program of cyclophosphamide, methotrexate, 5-fluorouracil, vincristine, and prednisone (CMFVP) given for 12 months after surgery [11]; (c) the Arizona study (1974–1984), which evaluated adriamycin and cyclophosphamide (AC) for 6 months (± radiotherapy) postoperatively [4]. More recently, investigators from M.D. Anderson Hospital have provided data from their trials of adjuvant chemotherapy with 5-fluorouracil, adriamycin, and cyclophosphamide (FAC) ± radiotherapy [8]. This data has not yet been fully analyzed. Outcomes for patients on the various series have been updated to 1983 for the Milan and Arizona studies, and to 1982 for the trial of the SWOG.

Statistical methods employed in these analyses have been discussed elsewhere [5, 9, 12–14]. Separate analyses of each treatment group as well as of all patients were carried out to identify important patient characteristics prognostic for relapse-free survival (RFS) and survival. RFS and survival comparisons between treatment groups simultaneously adjusted for multiple prognositc factors were carried out.

Results

Complete data on initial prognostic factors and subsequent clinical course are available on 3,712 patients as shown in Table 3. Not all of this information is currently assimilated into the NHBD or into treated groups for analysis, but it will be completed before the end of 1984. At present, full data in the NHDB consist of 835 patients with node-negative cancer and 1,014 patients with node-positive cancer with primary tumors ≤ 5.0 cm. The single

Table 3. Distribution of cases for NHDB and comparative analysis of clinical trials

NHDB	Node-negative (T_1 or T_2 N_0)	Node-positive (T_1 or T_2 N_+)
Milan NCI	324	524
Additional cases with ER (to be added in 1984)	413	–
Royal Marsden	98	272
M.D. Anderson (to be added in 1984)	–	218
Subtotals	835	1,014
Adjuvant-treated patients		
Milan NCI:	–	645
CMF (6 or 12 courses)		
Southwest Oncology Group		
L-PAM	–	141
CMFVP	–	314
University of Arizona		
AC ± XRT	121	232
M.D. Anderson		
FAC ± XRT ± BCG (to be added in 1984)	–	410
Subtotals	121	1,742

most important prognostic factor affecting outcome (e.g., RFS) was nodal status, as shown in Fig. 1, with tumor size being of secondary importance. We evaluated tumor size for patients with node-negative cancer and found three distinct patterns of RFS, all significantly different ($P = 0.05$) from each other (Fig. 1). Among 1,014 patients with stage II node-positive breast cancer, we evaluated the effect of nodal involvement by groups of two nodes (.i.e., 1 or 2 vs 3 or 4 vs 5 or 6 etc.). Three significantly different RFS curves were apparent (Fig. 1), with the curve for one or two positive nodes being considerably superior to those associated with more nodal involvement.

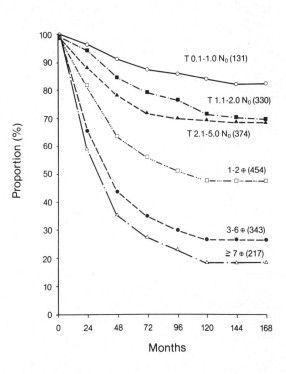

Fig. 1. Relapse-free survival of 835 patients with node-negative breast cancer according to primary tumor size and of 1,014 patients with node-positive breast cancer (primary size ≤ 5.0 cm) according to the number of involved axillary lymph nodes. Data are derived from the NHDB and include information from the Milan, Royal Marsden, and M.D. Anderson cancer centers

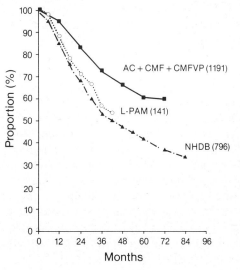

Fig. 2. Relapse-free survival of 1,191 patients with stage II breast cancer treated with combination chemotherapy compared with 141 treated with single agent chemotherapy (L-PAM) and 796 who received no adjuvant chemotherapy after surgery ($\pm$ irradiation). Data from M.D. Anderson Hospital are not included in this analysis but will be added later in 1984

In 1981 the NHDB consisted of data on 796 patients with stage II node-positive cancer [5]. The additional cases did not change the overall RFS of this group. The original 796 cases were used to compare the impact of adjuvant chemotherapy in groups of patients carefully adjusted for differences in important prognostic factors (e.g., number of involved lymph nodes). Data from FAC-treated patients have not yet been analyzed. As reported previously, the single agent L-PAM produced significantly less favorable RFS (and survival) than the five-drug CMFVP program [11]. Alll of the combination chemotherapy programs produced significant improvment in RFS compared with surgery (± radiotherapy) alone in the NHDB. In Fig. 2, RFS of the entire group of 1,191 patients who received combination chemotherapy (CMF, AC, or CMFVP) is compared with the RFS of patients treated with L-PAM or surgery (± radiotherapy) (NHDB).

Discussion

With the help of investigators around the world (Table 1), we have developed a NHDB involving a large number of patients who were well studied and followed at three major cancer centers (Milan, Royal Marsden, and M.D. Anderson). The most important pieces of prognostic information, with the exception of ER and PR status (Table 2) were available on all patients. Obviously, there are prognostic factors about which we have no information (e.g., histologic features such as vascular invasion, tumor necrosis, and biologic features such as labeling index). These have been reported individually as important factors [15, 16]. This type of specialized laboratory information is also not available in the vast majority of randomized clinical trials. Furthermore, the possibility that these laboratory-derived prognostic factors may highly correlate with prognosis and thus substitute for more commonly available factors (e.g., nodal status or tumor size) has yet to be evaluated and confirmed by prospective studies in large numbers of patients.

There has been considerable discussion about what prognostic factors should be used to select a group of patients with node-negative breast cancer for inclusion in trials of adjuvant chemotherapy [7, 17–19]. The most commonly mentioned factor is ER status [17] but this may not be available in all cases (e.g., small tumors). Our data in Fig. 1 suggest that a relatively simple factor (tumor size as measured by the pathologist) separates node-negative cancer into three distinct groups (all with significantly different RFS) and indeed very small primary cancers (< 1.0 cm) may not require adjuvant treatment. Whether additional information (e.g., ER data) in this particular subset of node-negative cancers would further separate prognostic groups remains to be determined.

The primary purpose of the NHDB was to assess the impact of adjuvant therapy from various series, most of which did not have surgery-alone control groups. With the availability of information on prognostic factors, we could make reasonable comparisons on groups of patients treated at different centers and statistically compensate for observed differences in the distribution of important prognostic factors between groups. This concept has been discussed at length elsewhere [9].

What has proven remarkable about this study is the similar outcome in patients who received effective adjuvant therapy (i.e., two or more drugs) compared with the minimal effect of L-PAM (which may not be absorbed well in some patients [20]) and in comparison with surgery alone (Fig. 2). In our previous report, we provided data on RFS of each of the adjuvant programs and all except L-PAM produced very similar results in most groups of patients [6].

Over the next several months we plan to fully incorporate additional data from M.D. Anderson [8]. The NHDB will provide a useful reference source for those investigators wishing to compare their adjuvant programs to surgery alone or to other adjuvant series (e.g., CMF, CMFVP, AC). The use of a NHDB does not supplant randomized clinical trials nor does it abolish the need for proper controls. However, it does provide a rational basis for making the kinds of comparisons most investigators now make with "eyeball" methods and it may provide clues for the design of new randomized clinical trials.

Acknowledgement. This work was supported in part by grants CA 23074 and CA 17094 from the National Cancer Institute, DHHS, Washington, D.C.

References

1. Salmon SE, Jones SE (eds) (1977) Adjuvant therapy of cancer. North-Holland, New York, p 646
2. Jones SE, Salmon SE (eds) (1979) Adjuvant therapy of cancer II. Grune and Stratton, New York, p 674
3. Salmon SE, Jones SE (eds) (1981) Adjuvant therapy of cancer III. Grune and Stratton, New York, p 603
4. Allen H, Brooks R, Jones SE et al (1981) Adriamycin-cyclophosphamide (AC) ± radiotherapy (XRT). In: Salmon SE, Jones SE (eds) Adjuvant therapy of cancer III. Grune and Stratton, New York, pp 453−462
5. Moon TE, Jones SE, Davis SL et al. (1981) Development of a natural history data base for breast cancer. In: Salmon SE, Jones SE (eds) Adjuvant therapy of cancer III. Grune and Stratton, New York, pp 471−482
6. Jones S, Moon T, Davis S et al. (1981) Comparative analysis of selected breast cancer adjuvant trials in relation to the natural history data base (NHDB). In: Salmon SE, Jones SE (eds) Adjuvant therapy of cancer III. Grune and Stratton, New York, pp 483−494
7. Valagussa P, Di Fronzo G, Bignami P et al. (1981) Prognostic importance of estrogen receptors to select node-negative patients for adjuvant chemotherapy. In: Salmon SE, Jones SE (eds) Adjuvant therapy of cancer III. Grune and Stratton, New York, pp 329−334
8. Buzdar A, Smith T, Blumenschein G et al. (1981) Adjuvant chemotherapy with fluorouracil, doxorubicin, and cyclophosphamide (FAC) for stage II or III breast cancer: Five-year results. In: Salmon SE, Jones SE (eds) Adjuvant therapy of cancer III. Grune and Stratton, New York, pp 419−426
9. Moon TE, Jones SE, Bonadonna G et al. (to be published) Using a data base of protocol studies to evaluate therapy: A breast cancer example. Statist Med
10. Bonadonna G, Valagussa P, Rossi A et al. (1981) Multimodal therapy with CMF in resectable breast cancer with positive axillary nodes: The Milan Institute experience. In: Salmon SE, Jones SE (eds) Adjuvant therapy of cancer III. Grune and Stratton, New York, pp 435−444
11. Rivkin SE, Glucksberg H, Rasmussen S (1981) Adjuvant chemotherapy for operable breast cancer with positive axillary nodes: a comparison of CMFVP versus L-PAM (Southwest Oncology Group Study). In: Salmon SE, Jones SE (eds) Adjuvant therapy of cancer III. Grune and Stratton, New York, pp 445−454
12. Peto R, Pike MC, Armitage P et al. (1976, 1977) Design and analysis of randomized clinical trials requiring prolonged observation of each patient. Br J Cancer 34: 585−612, 35: 1−39
13. Cox DR (1972) Regression models and life tables. J R Stat Soc [B] 34: 187−220
14. Kalbfleisch JD, Prentice RL (1980) The statistical analysis of failure time data. Wiley and Sons, New York, p 321

15. Fisher ER, Redmond C, Fisher B et al. (1983) Pathologic findings from the national surgical adjuvant breast project. Cancer 51: 181–191
16. Silvestrini R, Daidone MG, Gentili C (1981) Biologic characteristics of breast cancer and their clinical relevance. Commentaries on research in breast cancer. Liss, New York, pp 1–40
17. Clark GM, McGuire WL, Hubay CA et al. (1983) Progesterone receptors as a prognostic factor in stage II breast cancer. N Engl J Med 309: 1343–1347
18. Brooks R, Allen H, Salmon SE et al. (1981) Adjuvant use of adriamycin and cyclophosphamide in node-negative carcinoma of the breast. In: Salmon SE, Jones SE (eds) Adjuvant therapy of cancer III. Grune and Stratton, New York, pp 463–470
19. Senn HJ, Jungi WF, Amgwerd R (1981) Chemo (immuno) therapy with LMF + BCG in node-negative and node-positive breast cancer. In: Salmon SE, Jones SE (eds) Adjuvant therapy of cancer III. Grune and Stratton, New York, pp 385–393
20. Alberts DS, Chang SY, Chen GH-S et al. (1979) Oral melphalan kinetics. Clin Pharmacol Ther 26: 737–745

Clinical Results III:
Experience of Randomized Trials Without Surgical Controls

Adjuvant Systemic Therapy in Postoperative Node-Positive Patients with Breast Carcinoma: The CALGB Trial and the ECOG Premenopausal Trial

C. Tormey

Department of Human Oncology, K4/666 Clinical Science Center,
600 Highland Avenue, Madison, WI 53792, USA

Introduction

The initial results of the comparison of no systemic treatment to L-phenylalanine mustard (L-PAM) and cyclophosphamide, methotrexate, and 5-fluorouracil (CMF) suggested a benefit in treatment of both premenopausal and postmenopausal node-positive (N+) postoperative patients with breast carcinoma [1, 2]. Based on these results and the superiority of CMF over L-PAM in advanced disease [3] the Cancer and Leukemia Group B (CALGB) chose CMF as a control treatment for a trial initiated in 1975. Preliminary animal and human data [4, 5] led to the decision to administer the methanol extraction residue (MER) of bacillus Calmette-Guérin added to CMF (CMF + MER), in one arm of the trial. The early analyses of a previous trial (subsequently published [6]) determined the choice of as a second experimental regimen. The CMFVP (V = vincristine, P = prednisone) regimen was a continuing therapy, whereas the CMF regimen was intermittent with treatment being given for 2 out of each 4 weeks. An ongoing CALGB advanced-disease trial in 1975 suggested that a 6-week continuous induction therapy was well tolerated [7]. Accordingly, all patients were to receive a 6-week continuous induction of their assigned therapy followed by 10 intermittent cycles at 4-week intervals in the first year. In an attempt to eliminate slow-growing residual cells, all patients received six cycles of CMF at 8-week intervals in the second year. The initial results in patients with four or more axillary nodes involved were published in 1983 [8].

In 1977, the Eastern Cooperative Oncology Group (ECOG) developed a premenopausal trial in postoperative node-positive patients using a CMF control based on the initial results from Milan [2] and the advanced-disease results with CMF vs L-PAM [3]. Prednisone was added to CMF (CMFP) as the second regimen based upon the ECOG's results in advanced disease [9] demonstrating its superiority over CMF. Finally, early data from another advanced-disease trial [10] led to the addition of tamoxifen (T) to CMFP (CMFPT) as a third regimen. CMF and CMFP were given for 2 of each 4 weeks for a total of 12 cycles. The tamoxifen in CMFPT was administered continuously. The early results from this trial were presented in 1982 [11].

Methods

CALGB Trial

Postoperative women with a histopathologic diagnosis of carcinoma confined to the breast and ipsilateral axillary nodes were considered for study. The trial was initiated in May 1975 for patients with ≥ 4 nodes involved. Women with $1-3$ involved nodes were included in September 1975. Randomization to one of the regimens, CMF + MER, was discontinued in October 1978 and the trial was closed to further entry of patients with ≥ 4 nodes involved in June 1980 and to patients with $1-3$ nodes involved in October 1980. Details of the eligibility characteristics for this trial are detailed elsewhere [8] and are similar to those described previously in this volume [12].

Patients were stratified by clinical tumor size (< 3 or ≥ 3 cm) and age (< 50 or ≥ 50 years). They were then randomly assigned to receive CMF, CMFVP, or CMF + MER. Treatment was to start between 2 and 12 weeks postoperation.

All patients underwent a 6-week continuous drug exposure followed by a 2-week rest before starting intermittent therapy. In each regimen doses during the initial 6 weeks were: C 80 mg/m²/day p.o.; M 40 mg/m²/week i.v. (30 mg/m²/week if age ≥ 60); and F 500 mg/m²/week i.v. The CMFVP regimen also included: V 1.0 mg/m²/week (max. dose 1.5 mg/week) and P 40 mg/m²/day p.o. for 21 days, then tapering to zero by day 28. MER in CMF + MER was given intradermally as 200 µg in each of five sites at weeks 2, 3, and 5. Subsequent intermittent therapy consisted of ten 14-day courses of the randomized CMFVP, CMF, or CMF + MER therapy with 14-day recovery intervals followed by six 14-day courses of CMF with 42-day recovery intervals for all patients. The doses were the same as during the first 6 weeks except that C was raised to 100 mg/m²/day for days 1 through 14, M, F, and V were given on days 1 and 8 only, P was given days 1 through 14, and MER was administered on day 8. Drug doses were calculated using the lesser of patient's actual or ideal body weight.

Standard dosage modification criteria were employed as detailed elsewhere [8]. With respect to hematologic toxicity, CMF dose reductions of 50% were made for WBC counts of 2,500–3,999/cu mm or for platelet counts of 75,000–99,999/cu mm. CMF was omitted (during the first 6 weeks and on day 8 thereafter) or delayed along with VP and MER (on day 1 of intermittent courses) for WBC $< 2,500$/cu mm and CMFV doses were omitted (during the first 6 weeks and on day 8 thereafter) or delayed along with P and MER (day 1 of intermittent courses) for platelet counts $< 75,000$/cu mm.

In addition to specific drug monitoring parameters at frequent intervals during therapy, follow-up consisted of history taking, physical examination, blood studies, and chest X-rays at 3-month intervals, and skeletal examinations at 6-month intervals.

ECOG Trial

The entry criteria were identical to the ECOG postmenopausal node-positive trial detailed earlier in this volume [12] except for the requirement that patients be premenopausal. This was defined as at least one menses within 12 months prior to definitive surgery or, if a prior hysterectomy had been made age ≤ 52 years. As in the postmenopausal trial, an ER analysis was required along with a normal bone scan. Randomization was performed and treatment initiated within 10 weeks of receiving a radical or modified radical mastectomy. No additional systemic antitumor chemotherapy or radiotherapy was allowed. Other entry criteria and the stratification and randomization were as described earlier in this volume [12].

Treatment assignments were: (1) CMF, (2) CMFP, and (3) CMFPT. Chemotherapy was repeated every 28 days for a total of 12 cycles beginning 2−10 weeks postoperatively. The drug schedules for each cycle were: C 100 mg/m^2 p.o. days 1 through 14; M 40 mg/m^2 i.v. days 1 and 8; F 600 mg/m^2 i.v. days 1 and 8; P 40 mg/m^2 p.o. days 1 through 14; and, T 10 mg p.o. twice daily throughout each treatment cycle. The lesser of the ideal and actual body weight was used for dosage calculations. Standard toxicity guidelines were used for dosage modifications. Hematologic toxicity led to a CMF reduction of 50% for a WBC count of 2,500−4,000/cu mm or a platelet count of 75,000−100,000/cu mm. A delay of day 1 therapy for up to 2 weeks was allowed to enable full-drug administration: if the WBC count was < 2,500/cu mm or the platelets < 75,000/cu mm on day 1, therapy was delayed; if on day 8, CMF was omitted. A 25% CMF reduction was allowed in subsequent cycles if the nadir WBC count of < 2,000/cu mm or platelet count of < 75,000/cu mm was reached. Escalation of CMF by 25% was permitted if the nadir WBC count was > 3,500/cu mm and platelet count was > 125,000/cu mm.

In addition to specific drug-monitoring studies, follow-up consisted of history taking, physical examination, and blood chemistry values every 3 months, chest X-rays every 6 months, bone scans at 6 and 12 months and then yearly, and mammograms yearly.

Statistical Analyses

The date of disease recurrence was taken as the first date of suspicion of subsequently documented recurrence. Relapse was based upon "acceptable evidence" of disease as defined elsewhere [13]. Disease-free survival (DFS) was defined in the CALGB trial as the time from mastectomy plus axillary dissection to the date of disease recurrence or death without recurrence, and survival was measured from mastectomy until death. In the ECOG trial the starting date for analysis was the date of randomization. Time to relapse (TTR) was defined as the time to disease recurrence; deaths without recurrence were not counted as treatment failures, and survival was measured to the date of death from any cause.

The method of Kaplan and Meier [14] was used to estimate DFS, TTR, and survival. The crude relationships of treatment or other patient characteristics with DFS, TTR, or survival were analyzed using the log-rank test [15]. A proportional-hazards model [16] was used to analyze these relationships while adjusting simultaneously for other patient characteristics. Associations of endpoints having ordered categories with treatment were evaluated using an exact test [17]. The associations of relapse sites with treatment were evaluated using Fisher's exact test [18]. All *P*-values are based on two-sided alternatives and are considered "significant" if ≤ 0.05.

Results

CALGB Trial

There were 906 patients entered on study; of these 15 were improperly randomized or never treated, 68 were ineligible, 10 had major early protocol violations, and currently 63 records are either inadequate or too early. A further 76 cases have been deleted from the analysis because these patients received elective postoperative radiotherapy. The 674 remaining cases were analyzed as two series to evaluate CMFVP (258 cases) and CMF (270 cases) across the entire trial (total series) and to evaluate CMF + MER (146 cases), CMF (144 cases), and CMFVP (134 cases) during the concurrent randomization with CMF + MER (concurrent series). Selected patient characteristics are listed in Table 1. The regimens were well balanced with respect to these characteristics. The incidence of an ER unknown status decreased after October 1978 as reflected in the change from the concurrent to total series. Among the cases concurrently randomized with CMF + MER the median DFS follow-up is 44.5 months. The median DFS follow-up in the total series comparison of CMFVP and CMF is 29.7 months.

Figure 1 shows the DFS for patients treated with either CMFVP, CMF, or CMF + MER. Although the DFS with CMF + MER appears to be inferior, length of survival is not significantly different with the three regimens (Fig. 2).

The comparison of CMFVP to CMF reveals no overall difference in either DFS or survival (Figs. 3, 4). Separate analyses demonstrated that a worse DFS prognosis was associated with increasing nodal involvement (1−3, 4−9, ≥ 10 nodes involved, $P < 0.00001$), increasing tumor size (< 2, 2−5, ≥ 5 cm, $P < 0.00001$), and a postmenopausal state ($P = 0.001$).

Table 1. Selected patient characteristics in CALGB trial

Characteristic	Total series		Concurrent series		
	CMF	CMFVP	CMF	CMF + MER	CMFVP
No. positive nodes[a]	4	4	4	4	4
Tumor size (cm)[a]	3.0	3.0	3.0	3.0	3.0
Age (years)[a]	51	51	50	50	52
Days from mastectomy to Rx[a]	25	26	27	26	25
Premenopausal	47	46	47	47	45
% ER+	23	29	15	14	5
% ER unknown	53	52	73	68	83

[a] Median

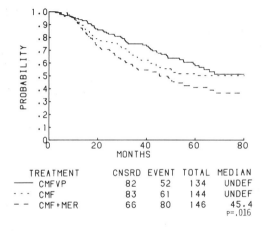

TREATMENT	CNSRD	EVENT	TOTAL	MEDIAN
—— CMFVP	82	52	134	UNDEF
· · · CMF	83	61	144	UNDEF
− − CMF+MER	66	80	146	45.4
				p=.016

Fig. 1. Disease-free survival for the concurrent series of patients treated with CMF, CMF + MER, or CMFVP; $P = 0.016$

Among the nodal involvement, tumor size, and menopausal subsets, the DFS with CMFVP is superior to CMF only in those patients with ≥ 4 nodes involved (Fig. 5). This difference was not observed among patients with 4−9 nodes involved but was still observed in patients with ≥ 10 nodes involved ($P = 0.025$). Within the ≥ 4 nodes involved subgroups patients receiving CMFVP tend to do better, whether premenopausal ($P = 0.12$) or postmeno-

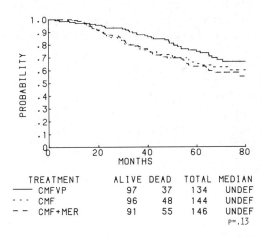

TREATMENT	ALIVE	DEAD	TOTAL	MEDIAN
—— CMFVP	97	37	134	UNDEF
- - - CMF	96	48	144	UNDEF
– – CMF+MER	91	55	146	UNDEF
				p=.13

Fig. 2. Survival for the concurrent series of patients treated with CMF, CMF + MER, or CMFVP; $P = 0.13$

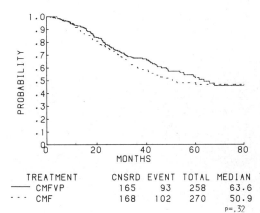

TREATMENT	CNSRD	EVENT	TOTAL	MEDIAN
—— CMFVP	165	93	258	63.6
- - - CMF	168	102	270	50.9
				p=.32

Fig. 3. Disease-free survival for the total series of patients treated with CMF or CMFVP; $P = 0.32$

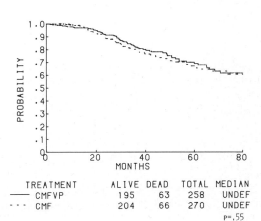

TREATMENT	ALIVE	DEAD	TOTAL	MEDIAN
—— CMFVP	195	63	258	UNDEF
- - - CMF	204	66	270	UNDEF
				p=.55

Fig. 4. Survival for the total series of patients treated with CMF or CMFVP; $P = 0.55$

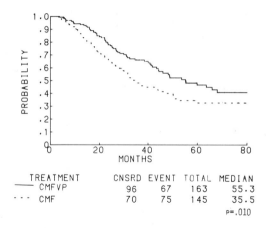

TREATMENT	CNSRD	EVENT	TOTAL	MEDIAN
—— CMFVP	96	67	163	55.3
- - - CMF	70	75	145	35.5

P=.010

Fig. 5. Disease-free survival for the total series of patients with ≥ 4 nodes involved treated with CMF or CMFVP; $P = 0.01$

Table 2. Sites of first recurrence in CALGB trial[a]

	CMF	CMFVP	Total
Local/regional only	7	4	6
Distant only	26	25	26
Both	3	4	4
Unknown	0.4	1	1

[a] Included are 101 relapses on CMF and 87 on CMFVP. Relapses are given as % of analyzed cases

Table 3. Patient characteristics in ECOG trial

Characteristic	CMF	CMFP	CMFPT	Total
No. nodes examined[a]	15	15	15	15
No. nodes positive[a]	3	3	4	3
Tumor size (cm)[a]	3.5	3.0	3.0	3.0
Age (years)[a]	44	43	43	43
Days from surgery to Rx[a]	32	29	28	29
% ER+	53	51	51	52

[a] Median

pausal ($P = 0.04$). None of these DFS differences were associated with a significant impact on survival. The majority of first recurrences were at distant sites with both CMF and CMFVP (Table 2). The toxicities associated with these regimens have been previously reported [8].

ECOG Trial

There were 662 patients randomized between March 1978 and March 1982. There is insufficient data on 22 patients, one patient refused therapy, and 83 were found ineligible.

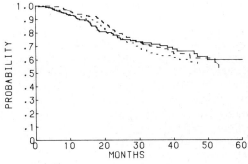

Fig. 6. Time to relapse for patients treated with CMF, CMFP, or CMFPT; $P = 0.53$

TREATMENT	NED	RLPS	TOTAL	75%-ILE
CMF	132	55	187	24.6
CMFP	124	62	186	25.4
CMFPT	128	55	183	27.9

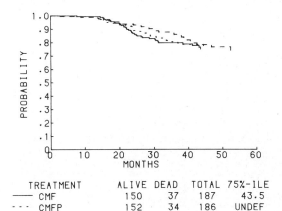

Fig. 7. Survival for patients treated with CMF, CMFP, or CMFPT; $P = 0.53$

TREATMENT	ALIVE	DEAD	TOTAL	75%-ILE
CMF	150	37	187	43.5
CMFP	152	34	186	UNDEF
CMFPT	153	30	183	52.4

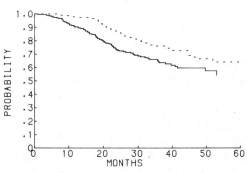

Fig. 8. Time to relapse related to the presence or absence of the development of amenorrhea; $P = 0.006$

AMENORRHEA	NED	RLPS	TOTAL	75%-ILE
NO	185	89	274	23.0
YES	175	57	232	38.2

Table 4. Sites of first recurrence in ECOG trial[a]

	CMF	CMFP	CMFPT	Total
Local only	5	6	4	5
Regional only	5	5	3	4
Local + regional	0.5	0.5	–	0.4
Distant only	14	19	20	18
Local + distant	3	2	–	2
Regional + distant	0.5	1	3	1
Local + regional + distant	–	0.5	1	0.5
Unknown	0.5	–	–	0.2
Local ± regional only	11	11	6	10
Distant ± local/regional	18	22	23	21

[a] Local refers to the area bounded by the sternal midline, clavicle, posterior lateral edge of the latissimus dorsi and costal margin; regional includes the internal mammary, supraclavicular and axillary area; all other sites are considered distant. Included are 55 relapses on CMF, 62 on CMFP, and 55 on CMFPT. Relapses are given as % of evaluable patients

The major analysis was performed upon the remaining 556 cases although separate analyses including all randomized cases gave similar results. Selected patient characteristics are shown in Table 3. Although there is good balance between regimens, minor imbalances were controlled for in the analyses. The median follow-up is 39 months with 31% having relapsed and 18% having died.

The overall comparisons of TTR (Fig. 6) and survival (Fig. 7) show no differences between the regimens. At the present time there are also no treatment regimen-associated TTR or survival differences across nodal involvement and ER subgroups.

Favorable prognostic features for TTR included 1–3 nodes involved ($P = 0.0000003$), ER+ status ($P = 0.0004$), and tumor size < 3 cm ($P = 0.05$). Tumor size is not presently a significant variable for survival although a progesterone receptor (PgR) positive status was favorable ($P = 0.05$). An analysis of amenorrhea revealed that those patients developing amenorrhea had a significantly greater TTR (Fig. 8, $P = 0.006$) and survival ($P = 0.001$, stratified Mantel-Byar tests). The development of hot flashes did not have this same prognostic impact, although they were reported more frequently with CMFPT (71%) than with CMFP (58%) ($P = 0.009$) or CMF (57%). Amenorrhea was reported more frequently with CMFP (46%) than with CMF (40%) ($P = 0.06$), and with CMFPT (51%) than with CMFP ($P > 0.10$). Preliminary analyses suggest that the TTR of ER+ amenorrheic patients is significantly better than of ER+ menorrheic and ER− amenorrheic patients, and that of ER− amenorrheic patients is significantly better than of ER− menorrheic patients.

The majority of first recurrences occurred at distant sites (Table 4). There is a suggestion of decreasing local-regional recurrences with CMFPT compared to CMFP and CMF. Table 5 shows the significantly increased incidence of side effects occurring with the addition of prednisone to CMF and with the addition of tamoxifen to CMFP. Unlike the postmenopausal trial [12] the addition of tamoxifen did not increase the incidence of thrombotic events but did increase the incidence of hot flashes and peripheral edema.

Table 5. Comparative side effects related to the addition of prednisone to CMF and tamoxifen to CMFP in the ECOG trial

CMF[a]	CMFP[b]	CMFPT[c]
Nausea/emesis	Other gastrointestinal	Peripheral edema
Thrombocytopenia	Infection	Hot flashes
	Neurologic	
	Leukopenia	
	Peripheral edema	
	Cushingoid changes	
	Musculoskeletal pains	
	Weight gain	
	Hypertension	

[a] Side effects occurring with a significantly greater incidence than is the case with CMFP treatment

[b] Side effects occurring with a significantly greater incidence than is the case with CMF treatment

[c] Side effects occurring with a significantly greater incidence than is the case with CMFP treatment

Discussion

These two trials represent successive generations of studies despite being designed from the initial Milan experience. The eligibility criteria for the CALGB trial were nearly identical to the initial L-PAM placebo [1] and CMF-observation [2] studies. Two years later the ECOG trial added requirements for bone scans and ER status and developed separate trials based on menopausal status. Although the CALGB and ECOG utilized separate experimental arms they both based their controls upon the Milan experience. The use of CMF by that group continues to provide a survival advantage in premenopausal patients but only an early TTR advantage in postmenopausal patients [2, 19].

The results of the CALGB and ECOG trials do not currently demonstrate an overall DFS, TTR, or survival advantage for adding either prednisone ± tamoxifen or vincristine + prednisone to CMF. Unlike the Milan trial [20], the ECOG study found that the development of amenorrhea was prognostically favorable for both TTR ($P = 0.006$) and survival ($P = 0.001$). Patients developing amenorrhea did significantly better within both ER+ and ER− subgroups. Although not formally tested, it appeared that ER− amenorrheic patients did about as well as ER+ patients not developing amenorrhea. These preliminary results suggest that ovarian ablation may be a beneficial procedure to test prospectively in both ER+ and ER− patients. The added benefit of amenorrhea in ER− patients also supports the hypothesis that the tumors are heterogeneous with respect to ER-containing cell populations.

Other factors found to be associated with an improved TTR in the ECOG premenopausal trial included fewer nodes involved, smaller tumor size, and an ER+ tumor. These same parameters were prognostic in the ECOG postmenopausal trial, although the ER+ advantage was limited to the untreated patients [12]. In both ECOG studies survival was improved for those with fewer nodes involved and ER+ tumors. The premenopausal trial also found PgR+ tumors were associated with an improved survival. At present there are no TTR or survival differences between the regimens in these various subgroups of premenopausal patients.

The CALGB trial also demonstrated an improved prognosis for DFS in patients with fewer nodes involved and smaller tumor sizes. This trial also demonstrated a DFS advantage avoring premenopausal patients over postmenopausal patients. The CALGB trial demonstrated a significant DFS advantage with CMFVP in the ≥ 4 nodes-involved subgroup. Although this advantage was limited to postmenopausal patients, there was a similar trend for premenopausal patients with ≥ 4 nodes involved. Increased dissociation of the nodal involvement revealed that the CMFVP advantage is restricted further to patients with ≥ 10 nodes involved. Additional follow-up will be needed to ascertain whether this advantage for CMFVP will continue.

It is of interest that a continuous-exposure CMFVP regimen has been found superior to L-PAM with respect to TTR and survival in both premenopausal and postmenopausal patients [21]. This result is particularly interesting in view of results from advanced-disease trials. CALGB previously found a continuous CMFVP regimen tended to be superior to an intermittent regimen [7]. The ECOG found CMF to be distinctly better than L-PAM [2] but only slightly less effective than CMFP [9]. Taken in concert with the current trials, it would appear that minor differences observed in advanced disease will not translate into readily apparent adjuvant-therapy differences, e.g., CMFP vs CMF. However, major advanced-disease differences will translate into adjuvant therapy differences, e.g., L-PAM vs CMF (VP). Thus, if small differences exist in advanced disease it will be necessary to provide large numbers of adjuvant patients to detect those differences if they exist in the postoperative setting.

As with other trials [1, 2, 21], the major sites of relapses continue to be distant in both studies. Whether or not this would be reduced by the use of postoperative or postsystemic therapy radiation therapy is not yet known. At present the results would suggest that the cell kill achieved with the current systemic therapy regimens is insufficient to eliminate disease in the majority of patients.

The overall toxicity with CMF is clearly less than with CMFVP [8] or with CMFPT or CMFP. Considering this parameter in concert with the results to date, it is not possible to routinely recommend these more toxic regimens − as used in the CALGB and ECOG trials − outside of research settings.

Acknowledgements. The author thanks all those investigators contributing to these trials. Special thanks go to James F. Holland, M.D. and Paul P. Carbone, M.D. The statistical analyses for the present paper were performed by Robert Gray, Ph.D. (ECOG) and Ann Korzun, M.S. (CALGB).

References

1. Fisher B, Carbone P, Economou SG, Frelick R, Glass A, Lerner H, Redmond G, Zelen M, Band P, Katrych DL, Wolmark N, Fisher ER (1975) L-Phenylalanine mustard (L-PAM) in the management of primary breast cancer − a report of early findings. N Engl J Med 292: 117−122
2. Bonadonna G, Brusamolino E, Valagussa P, Rossi A, Brugnatelli L, Brambilla C, DeLena M, Tancini G, Bajetta E, Musumeci R, Veronesi U (1976) Combination chemotherapy as an adjuvant treatment in operable breast cancer. N Engl J Med 294: 405−410
3. Canellos GP, Pocock SJ, Taylor SG III, Sears ME, Klaasen DJ, Band PR (1976) Combination chemotherapy for metastatic breast carcinoma. Prospective comparison of multiple drug therapy with L-phenylalanine mustard. Cancer 38: 1882−1886

4. Weiss DW (1976) MER and other mycobacterial fractions in the immunotherapy of cancer. Med Clin North Am 60: 473–497

5. Perloff M, Holland JF, Lumb GJ, Bekesi JG (1977) Effects of methanol extraction residue of Bacillus Calmette-Guérin in humans. Cancer Res 37: 1191–1196

6. Cooper RG, Holland JF, Glidewell O (1979) Adjuvant chemotherapy of breast cancer. Cancer 44: 793–798

7. Tormey DC, Weinberg VE, Leone LA, Glidewell OJ, Perloff M, Kennedy BJ, Cortes E, Silver RT, Weiss RB, Aisner J, Holland JF (to be published) A comparison of intermittent vs continuous and of adriamycin vs methotrexate 5-drug chemotherapy for advanced breast cancer – a cancer and leukemia group B study. Am J Clin Oncol

8. Tormey DC, Weinberg VE, Holland JF, Weiss RB, Glidewell OJ, Perloff M, Falkson G, Falkson HC, Henry PH, Leone LA, Rafla S, Ginsberg SJ, Silver RT, Blom J, Carey RW, Schein PS, Lesnick GJ (1983) A randomized trial of five and three drug chemotherapy and chemoimmunotherapy in women with operable node-positive breast cancer – a cancer and leukemia group B study. J Clin Oncol 1: 138–145

9. Tormey DC, Gelman R, Band PR, Sears M, Rosenthal SN, DeWys W, Perlia C, Rice MA (1982) Comparison of induction chemotherapies for metastatic breast cancer: an Eastern Cooperative Oncology Group Trial. Cancer 50: 1235–1244

10. Tormey DC, Falkson G, Crowley J, Falkson HC, Voelkel J, Davis TE (1982) Dibromodulcitol and adriamycin ± tamoxifen in advanced breast cancer. Cancer Clin Trials 5: 33–39

11. Tormey DC, Kalish L, Cummings FJ, Carbone PP (1983) Premenopausal breast cancer adjuvant chemotherapy – the Eastern Cooperative Oncology Group Trial (Abstr). Am Soc Clin Oncol 2: 102

12. Tormey DC, Taylor SG IV, Gray R, Olson JE (1984) Postmenopausal node positive comparison of observation to CMFP and CMFP + tamoxifen adjuvant therapy: An Eastern Cooperative Oncology Group Trial (this volume)

13. Tormey D, Fisher B, Bonadonna G, Carter S, Davis H, Glidewell O, Hahn RG, Payne S, Zelen M, Sears ME (1977) Proposed guidelines – report from the Combined Modality Trials Working Group. In: Carbone PP, Sears ME (eds) Breast cancer: Suggested protocol guidelines for combination chemotherapy trials and for combined modality trials. DHEW, Washington (DHEW publication no. NIH) 77-1192, pp 20–35

14. Kaplan EL, Meier P (1958) Nonparametric estimation from incomplete observations. J Am Stat Assoc 53: 457–481

15. Peto R, Peto J (1972) Asymptotically efficient rank invariant test procedures. J R Stat Soc [A] 135: 185–198

16. Cox DR (1972) Regression models and life tables (with discussion). J R Stat Soc [B] 34: 187–220

17. Lehman EL (1975) Nonparametrics: Statistical methods based on ranks. Holden Day, San Francisco

18. Fisher RA (1934) Statistical methods for research workers. Edinburgh

19. Bonadonna G, Valagussa P, Rossi A, Tancini G, Brambilla C, Marchini S, Veronesi U (1982) Multimodal therapy with CMF in resectable breast cancer with positive axillary nodes: The Milan Institute experience. Recent Results Cancer Res 80: 149–156

20. Bonadonna G, Rossi A, Tancini G, Bajetta E, Marchini S, Brambilla C, Tess JDT, Valagussa P, Banfi A, Veronesi U (1981) Adjuvant combination chemotherapy for operable breast cancer. Trials in progress at the Istituto Nazionale Tumori of Milan. Cancer Treat Rep 65: 61–65

21. Glucksberg H, Rivkin SE, Rasmussen S, Tranum B, Gad-El-Mawla N, Costanzi J, Hoogstraten B, Athens J, Maloney T, McCracken J, Vaugn C (1982) Combination chemotherapy (CMFVP) versus L-phenylalanine mustard (L-PAM) for operable breast cancer with positive axillary nodes. Cancer 50: 423–434

Adjuvant Therapy of Breast Cancer: A Southwest Oncology Group Experience

S. E. Rivkin, H. Glucksberg, and M. Foulkes

Southwest Oncology Group, 1221 Madison Street, Seattle, WA 98104, USA

Introduction

The disease-free interval and overall survival of women with operable breast cancer with positive axillary nodes has not improved over the past several decades despite a variety of local-regional approaches. The prognosis has not been significantly affected by the extent of surgery [9, 11] or the administration of postoperative radiation therapy [15]. Although the size of the primary tumor [3, 13] and the estrogen receptor status [12] are also significant, the status of the axillary lymph nodes [2] remains the most important prognostic factor. Approximately 50% of women with 1−3 and 75% of those with ≥ 4 involved axillary nodes have tumor recurrence by 5 years after initial treatment [2, 17]. Clearly, local-regional therapy is not adequate or curative for most women with axillary nodal metastases.

The majority of women with involved axillary nodes are not cured with local measures because microscopic deposits of tumor remain present at sites distant from the primary at the time of initial treatment. Therefore, only treatment (such as hormonal manipulation or chemotherapy) which reaches these distant sites, theoretically can affect disease-free survival in these women. The results of early trials with adjuvant chemotherapy (thiotepa, etc.), though conflicting, have been generally disappointing [4, 16]. However, these early trials involved short courses of chemotherapy aimed at eradicating malignant cells dislodged at the time of surgery. The currently accepted hypothesis, i.e., that micrometastases have already formed at the time of initial treatment, calls for a prolonged course of systemic treatment to eradicate these deposits [14].

In 1975 and 1976, the preliminary results of two controlled trials involving long-term adjuvant chemotherapy were reported. The National Surgical Adjuvant Breast Project (NSABP) reported on the efficacy of L-PAM [5] and Bonadonna et al. [1] reported on the efficacy of cyclic cylophosphamide, methotrexate, and 5-fluorouracil (CMF) vs surgery alone in women with operable breast cancer with histologically involved axillary nodes. The promising preliminary results of these two controlled studies prompted the Southwest Oncology Group (SWOG) to compare combination with single-agent adjuvant chemotherapy in women at high risk for relapse after local-regional therapy. Continuous, rather than intermittent combination chemotherapy, was used because the former was more effective in an earlier SWOG study of women with metastatic breast cancer [8].

This study evaluates the relative efficacy of continuous CMFVP (cyclophosphamide, methotrexate, 5-fluorouracil, vincristine, and prednisone) and melphalan (L-PAM) in terms of disease-free and total survival, and short- and long-term toxicity, in women with operable breast cancer with histologically involved axillary nodes. This report is an update of data previously reported with a mean follow-up of 5 years [7].

Patients and Methods

Selection of Patients

All women who had had a modified or radical mastectomy and who had one or more nodes positive on histologic examination with no evidence of metastatic disease were eligible for this study, provided they fulfilled specific criteria described in the protocol. These included: primary and axillary neoplasm completely removed as confirmed by the pathology report, tumors confined to the breast and axilla, tumors movable in relation to the underlying muscle and chest wall, axillary nodes movable in relation to the chest wall and neurovascular bundle, no preoperative arm edema, a leukocyte count $\geq$ 4,000, a platelet count $\geq$ 100,000, and a blood urea nitrogen (BUN) $\leq$ 25 mg/100 ml. Patients with inflammatory carcinoma or skin ulceration of more than 2 cm were excluded from the study. T_3 lesions were included if there was no fixation. Chemotherapy was initiated within 42 days of mastectomy.

This study was carried out on patients from 32 institutions affiliated with the SWOG. Patients were informed and signed consents stating they would receive either single-agent or combination chemotherapy after mastectomy.

Pretherapy Studies

All patients underwent the following studies: Bone scan, a complete blood count, transaminases, alkaline phosphatase, bilirubin, BUN, serum creatinine, serum calcium and phosphorus, and a chest X-ray. Liver and brain scans were obtained if symptoms, signs, or laboratory tests suggested possible metastases at these sites. Most patients also had mammography or xerography of the opposite breast.

Experimental Design

Stratification was done according to menopausal status, number of involved axillary nodes (1−3 and $\geq$ 4), and whether postoperative radiation was going to be administered. Patients were randomized to receive either 2 years of melphalan or 1 year of CMFVP. Treatment was begun 1−6 weeks after mastectomy.

Treatment

Adjuvant melphalan treatment consisted of 5 mg/m^2 daily by mouth for 5 days every 6 weeks for 2 years. CMFVP treatment consisted of cyclophosphamide 60 mg/m^2 daily by mouth, methotrexate 15 mg/m^2 i.v. weekly, and 5-fluorouracil (5-FU) 300 mg/m^2 i.v. weekly, all for 1 year. Vincristine 0.625 mg/m^2 was administered i.v. weekly for 10 weeks, and prednisone 30 mg/m^2 by mouth daily for days 1−14, 20 mg/m^2 daily for days 15−28, and 10 mg/m^2 for days 29−42, and discontinued thereafter. Drug doses were modified according to the presence and degree of toxicity.

Postoperative Irradiation

Irradiation was an option available to the primary physician and his patient in order to facilitate accrual on this study. The dose schedule and radiation fields were not standardized. Most patients received radiation to the supraclavicular and internal mammary nodal areas, some also to the anterior chest wall. When postoperative radiotherapy was used, it was started 10 weeks after combination chemotherapy or after three courses of melphalan had been administered. Twenty-six fully evaluable (18%) patients on the CMFVP arm and 39 (23%) patients on the melphalan arm received radiation.

Follow-up Studies

While receiving chemotherapy, patients had a monthly physical examination and a complete blood count was taken at each clinic visit; transaminases, alkaline phosphatase, serum calcium and phosphorus, serum creatinine, BUN data and a chest X-ray were obtained every 3 months; a bone scan was made every 12 months. After treatment was completed, the above blood tests were obtained every 3 months, a chest X-ray every 3−6 months, a bone scan and a mammogram every year.

Statistical Analysis

Statistical analysis of this study was based on time to first evidence of treatment failure, represented by local, regional, or distant recurrence, and on survival time. All patients with treatment failures were followed until death and the survival curves include both fully and partially evaluable patients. Disease-free interval (DFI) and survival curves were plotted using the life-table method of Kaplan and Meier [10]. A two-tailed generalized Wilcoxon test [6] was used to test for the differences between DFI and survival curves. In this trial, 356 fully and partially evaluable patients were analyzed, 184 in the L-PAM arm and 172 on the CMFVP arm. Randomization generated treatment groups with respect to age, race, tumor location, tumor size, and menopausal status.

Results

Table 1 shows recurrence patterns for both fully and partially evaluable patients in the two treatment arms, both overall and within patient subgroups. The median followup time for these patients is approximately 60 months and the minimum is 46 months. The difference in the overall rate of recurrence between CMFVP and melphalan (22% vs 41%) is highly significant ($P = 0.0001$). The difference in the observed proportion of treatment failures is also highly significant in favor of CMFVP compared with melphalan for the following subgroups: premenopausal women, 19% vs 44% ($P = 0.002$); postmenopausal women, 25% vs 39% ($P = 0.003$); women with 1−3 involved axillary nodes, 10% vs 25% ($P =$

Table 1. Characteristics of women treated with CMFVP and melphalam treatment with observed treatment failures

	Recurrences				
	Melphalan		CMFVP		
	No.	(%)	No.	(%)	Two-tailed P-value
Total	78/188	41	39/173	22	0.002
Nodal status					
1−3	18/72	25	8/77	10	0.017
≥ 4	60/116	52	31/96	32	0.002
Menopausal status					
Premenopausal	35/79	44	13/68	19	0.002
Postmenopausal	43/109	39	26/105	25	0.003

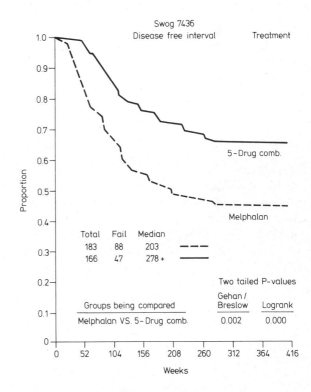

Fig. 1. Treatment failure time distribution for all fully and partially evaluable patients

0.017); and women with ≥ 4 involved axillary nodes, 32% vs 52% ($P = 0.002$). In the analysis of recurrence by menopausal status and number of involved nodes (1−3 and ≥ 4), there are differences favoring CMFVP in all subgroups.

Figure 1 shows Kaplan-Meier estimates of the time to treatment failure (DFI) of both fully (FE) and partially (PE) evaluable patients on the two treatment arms. The 5-year disease-free interval is 70% for CMFVP compared with 53% for melphalan ($P = 0.002$).

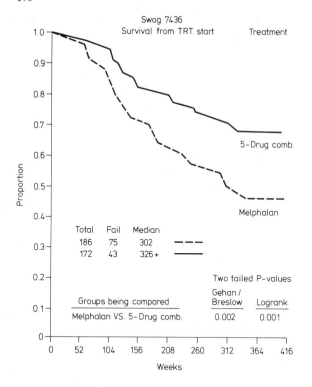

Fig. 2. Overall survival in fully and partially evaluable patients with CMFVP and melphalan

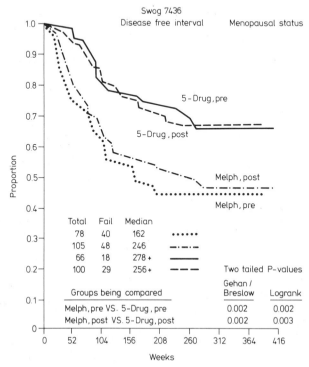

Fig. 3. Treatment failure time distribution in fully and partially evaluable pre- and postmenopausal patients

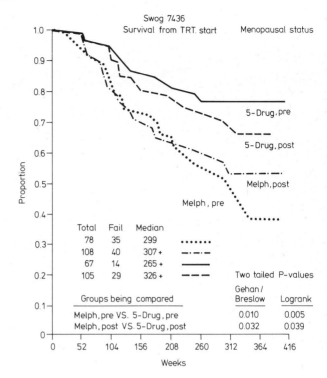

Fig. 4. Survival in fully and partially evaluable pre- and postmenopausal patients

Length of survival from onset of chemotherapy for all patients is shown in Fig. 2. The life-table estimate of survival at 5 years is 73% for CMFVP and 56% for melphalan; there is a significant difference in survival in favor of CMFVP over melphalan ($P = 0.002$).

Figure 3 compares DFI by menopausal status. The 5-year DIF is equal in both pre- and postmenopausal CMFVP patients (70% vs 68%). The 5-year DFI of premenopausal patients treated with melphalan is 50% and for postmenopausal patients 55%. Both pre- and postmenopausal patients treated with CMFVP have a significantly longer DFI compared with those treated with melphalan ($P = 0.002$ for premenopausal and $P = 0.003$ for postmenopausal patients).

Figure 4 compares the length of total survival by menopausal status. The 5-year survival for both pre- and postmenopausal patients treated with CMFVP is identical at 73%. The 5-year survival for premenopausal patients treated with melphalan is 51% and 58% for postmenopausal patients. Both pre- and postmenopausal patients treated with CMFVP have a significantly longer survival than those treated with melphalan ($P = 0.021$ for premenopausal; $P = 0.037$ for postmenopausal).

Figure 5 shows DFI by nodal status. The CMFVP-treated group has a 5-year DFI of 88% compared with 73% for patients treated with melphalan ($P = 0.017$). The lower two curves represent patients with a larger tumor burden, with four or more involved axillary nodes, and again CMFVP is highly significant. The 5-year DFI is 60% for CMFVP and 40% for melphalan ($P = 0.002$).

The length of survival by number of involved axillary nodes is shown in Fig. 6. The 5-year survival of patients treated with CMFVP is 81% compared with 67% for melphalan. This is not a significant difference in survival. The reason for this is twofold: (1) In the CMFVP group four patients died of unrelated causes. (2) In the melphalan group those patients

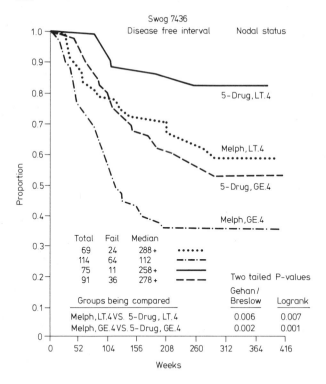

Fig. 5. Treatment failure time distribution in fully and partially evaluable patients with 1−3 and ≥ 4 involved axillary nodes

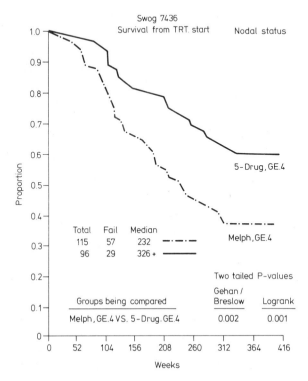

Fig. 6. Survival in fully and partially evaluable patients with ≥ 4 involved axillary nodes

Table 2. Side effects

Manifestation	CMFVP (%)	Melphalan (%)
Leukopenia[a]		
3,999−2,500	69	62
≤ 2500	12	6
Thrombocytopenia[b]		
99,000−50,000	15	21
≤ 50,000	1	3
Alopecia	40	0
Cystitis	5	0
Mucositis	16	0
Nausea	21	16

[a] Leukocyte per/mm^3
[b] Platelets per/mm^3

relapsing with local recurrence were effectively salvaged with CMFVP and local radiation.

Patients with four or more involved axillary nodes have a 67% survival at 5 years when treated with CMFVP compared with 41% when treated with melphalan ($P = 0.002$).

Toxicity

The side effects with both treatment arms are shown in Table 2. Nausea, vomiting, and malaise were more prominent with CMFVP than with melphalan. Cystitis, mucositis, and alopecia only occurred in patients treated with CMFVP. The eight patients who developed haemorrhagic cystitis secondary to cyclophosphamide were treated with chlorambucil. Approximately 40% of women treated with CMFVP developed significant alopecia. Leukopenia was a frequent complication in both treatment arms but was usually mild to moderate in degree. Less than 12% of patients on either treatment arm developed a leukocyte count ≤ 2,500 and/or platelet counts ≤ 50,000.

Subjective and objective toxicity, while more prominent in the CMFVP group, was acceptable with both treatment arms.

Three patients developed acute leukemia, one patient while on CMFVP therapy for 10 months. After completion of 2 years of therapy, two patients on the melphalan arm developed leukemia at about 3 and 5 years from the start of treatment.

Discussion

With a median follow-up of 5 years, our data show that women with operable breast cancer with histologically involved axillary nodes treated with continuous CMFVP show significantly longer disease-free and total survival than those treated with intermittent melphalan. This decrease in recurrence is demonstrated in both pre- and postmenopausal women resulting in prolonged total survival. Women with four or more axillary nodes have decreased recurrences and longer total survival than those treated with melphalan. Patients with one to three axillary nodes had a longer DFI but total survival was not significantly different because of deaths due to other causes and salvage therapy of local recurrences with surgery, radiotherapy, and chemotherapy.

Acknowledgements. This investigation was supported by the following grants awarded by the National Cancer Institute, U.S. Department of Health and Human Services: CA-03096, CA-03389, CA-04915, CA-04919, CA-04920, CA-12014, CA-12213, CA-12644, CA-13238, CA-13392, CA-14028, CA-16385, CA-16943, CA-16957, CA-20319, CA-21116, CA-22411, CA-22416, CA-22433, and CA-27057, and by Foreign Research Agreement 03-054-N.

References

1. Bonadonna G, Bursamolino E, Valagussa P et al. (1976) Combination chemotherapy as an adjuvant treatment in operable breast cancer. N Engl J Med 294: 405–410
2. Fisher B (1972) Surgical adjuvant therapy for breast cancer. Cancer 30: 1556–1564
3. Fisher B, Slack MH, Bross IDJ (1969) Cancer of the breast: Size of neoplasm and prognosis. Cancer 24: 1071–1080
4. Fisher B, Slack N, Katrych D, Wolmark N (1975). Ten-year follow-up results of patients with carcinoma of the breast in a cooperative clinical trial evaluating surgical adjuvant chemotherapy. Surg Gynecol Obstet 140: 528–534
5. Fisher B, Carbone P, Economou SG et al. (1975) L-Phenylalanine mustard (L-PAM) in the management of primary breast cancer: A report of early findings. N Engl J Med 292: 117–122
6. Gehan EA (1965) A generalized Wilcoxon test for comparing arbitrarily single-censored samples. Biometrika 52: 203–223
7. Glucksberg H, Rivkin SE, Rasmussen S et al. (1982) Combination chemotherapy (CMFVP) vs L-Phenylalanine mustard (L-PAM) for operable breast cancer with positive axillary nodes. A Southwest Oncology Group study. Cancer 50: 423–434
8. Hoogstraten B, George SL, Samal B et al. (1976) Combination chemotherapy and adriamycin in patients with advanced breast cancer. A Southwest Oncology Group study. Cancer 38: 13–20
9. Kaee S, Johansen H (1967) Prognostic factors in breast cancer. In: Forrest APM, Kunkler PB (eds) Proceedings of first tenovus symposium, Cardiff. Livingston, Edinburgh, pp 93–102
10. Kaplan EL, Meier P (1958) Nonparametric estimation from incomplete observations. J Am Stat Assoc 53: 457–481
11. Lacour J, Bucalossi P, Caceres E (1976) Radical mastectomy vs radical mastectomy plus internal mammary dissection: Five-year results of an international cooperative study. Cancer 37: 206–214
12. McGuire WL (1975) Current status of estrogen receptors in human breast cancer. Cancer 36: 638–644
13. Say CC, Donegan WL (1974) Invasive carcinoma of the breast: Prognostic significance of tumor size and involved axillary lymph nodes. Cancer 34: 468–471
14. Schabel FM Jr (1977) Rationale for adjuvant chemotherapy. Cancer 39: 2875–2882
15. Stjernsward J (1977) Adjuvant radiotherapy trials in breast cancer. Cancer 39: 2846–2867
16. Tormey DC (1975) Combined chemotherapy and surgery in breast cancer: A review. Cancer 36: 881–892
17. Valagussa P, Bonadonna G, Veronesi U (1978) Patterns of relapse and survival following radical mastectomy: Analysis of 716 consecutive patients. Cancer 41: 1170–1178

Short- or Long-term Chemotherapy for Node-Positive Breast Cancer: LMF 6 Versus 18 Cycles. SAKK Study 27/76

W. F. Jungi, P. Alberto, K. W. Brunner, B. Mermillod, L. Barrelet, and F. Cavalli*

Medizinische Klinik C, Kantonsspital, 9007 St. Gallen, Switzerland

Introduction

Type, dosage, and duration of adjuvant chemotherapy in breast cancer are chosen more or less empirically. Only five groups have addressed the question of optimal *duration* of treatment in prospective randomized studies. Bonadonna and his group have demonstrated that 6 cycles of CMF are equivalent to 12 for premenopausal patients at 6 years [1]. Henderson and co-workers have shown that three courses of adriamycin and cyclophosphamide are as good as 6 [2]. The ongoing study of the Southeastern Cancer Study Group [4] has to date failed to show any difference between 6 and 12 months of CMF (combined partly with radiation). No results have been published so far by the Southwestern Oncology Group. The Swiss Group (SAKK) decided in 1976 to examine the well-tolerated oral St. Gallen Leukeran (chlorambucil), methotrexate, fluorouracil (LMF) regimen in a randomized comparison of a short- and a long-term treatment in node-*positive* breast cancer patients. We hope that the prolonged treatment with its anticipated heavier drug toxicity would be compensated for by improved tumor control.

Study Design and Patients

The study design is given in Fig. 1. Eligible for the SAKK study 27/76 were women below 70 years of age with breast cancer of stages T1-3a with positive axillary nodes. Surgery was done by modified radical mastectomy. There was stratification for menopausal age and postoperative radiotherapy (optional). The adjuvant chemotherapy was identical to that used by Seen et al. (this volume). In group A patients received 6 monthly 14-day cycles of oral LMF, in group B 12 monthly cycles followed by one course of LMF every other month for a total of 18 courses over a period of 24 months.

In total, 419 node-positive breast cancer patients were entered between January 1976 and September 1978; 401 patients were fully eligible. Of these, 351 are fully evaluable; 50 patients are not evaluable for various reasons not specified here (see [3]).

---

* For the Schweizerische Arbeitsgruppe für Klinische Krebsforschung

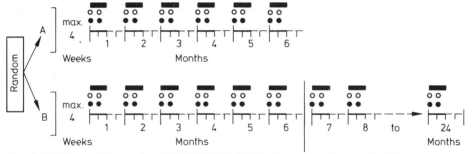

Fig. 1. LMF, 6 vs 24 months. (SAKK 27/76) (LMFq 2 months after cycle 12)

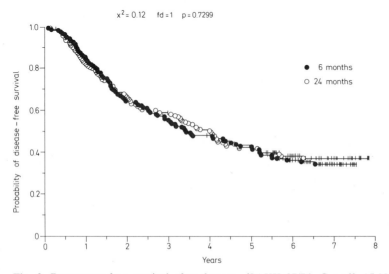

Fig. 2. Recurrence-free survival after 6 years. (SAKK 27/76. Cut-off: 15 Nov. 1983)

Results

After 6 years of mean observation time there are 218 recurrences among the 351 evaluable patients, giving a 62.1% overall recurrence rate. There is no difference if we consider all eligible or only the evaluable patients. As in our last analysis presented 3 years ago [3] there is no difference whatsoever between 6 and 18 cycles of oral LMF for the whole study population nor in any subgroup (neither in recurrence-free nor overall survival) (Figs. 2 and 3). Postmenopausal patients fared somewhat worse than pre- and perimenopausal. There is no detrimental effect of additional radiotherapy which, on the other hand, reduced local recurrences from 41% to 26%.

Conclusions

There is no change since our last analysis presented 3 years ago. The overall relapse rate of 62% at 6 years in node-positive breast cancer patients is again extremely high. It is higher

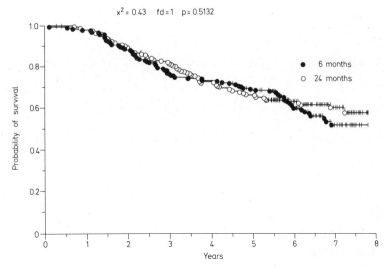

Fig. 3. Overall survival after 6 years mean observation time. (SAKK 27/76. Cut-off: 15 Nov. 1983)

than the corresponding number in the comparable node-positive patients treated with LMF + BCG (bacillus Calmette-Guérin) in the OSAKO study at 6 years (55% vs 72% in the controls). There is definitely no advantage in prolonging a well-tolerated, but still unpleasant oral LMF regimen up to 2 years. Does oral LMF have activity at all? This answer cannot be given from our study, as it lacks an untreated control group. It must be stressed that even with this low-dose LMF there were considerable dose reductions, more than in the previous OSAKO trial. LMF, as given in this trial, appears to be only marginally effective in treating node-positive breast cancer patients.

References

1. Bonadonna G, Rossi A et al. (1983) Adjuvant CMF in breast cancer. Lancet 1:1157
2. Henderson IC, Gelman R et al. (1982) 15 vs 30 weeks of adjuvant chemotherapy for breast cancer patients with a high risk of recurrence. Proc Am Soc Clin Oncol 1: C-290
3. Jungi WF, Alberto P et al. (1981) Short- or long-term adjuvant chemotherapy for breast cancer. In: Salmon SE, Jones SE (eds) Adjuvant treatment of cancer III. Grune and Stratton, New York London Toronto Sidney San Francisco, p 395
4. Velez-Garcia E, Moore M et al. (1983) Adjuvant chemotherapy with or without radiation therapy in patients with stage II breast cancer. A Southeastern Cancer Study Group study. Proc Am Soc Clin Oncol 2: C-432

Adjuvant Programs for Postmenopausal Women with Node-Positive Breast Cancer: Preliminary Analysis of 5-Year Results

A. Rossi, C. Brambilla, P. Valagussa, and G. Bonadonna

Istituto Nazionale per lo studio e la Cura dei Tumori, Via Venezian 1, 20133 Milano, Italy

Introduction

The results of the first CMF program (cyclophosphamide, methotrexate, and fluorouracil given for 12 monthly cycles) indicated only a slight benefit for the subgroup of postmenopausal patients with node-positive (N+) breast cancer [2, 9]. Although this finding was not consistently reported in all case series [3], several hypotheses were formulated to interpret the impact of adjuvant results on patients who are postmenopause [e.g., suboptimal drug-dose levels and proportion of estrogen receptor (ER) positive tumors].

In 1977, two prospective trials were simultaneously started by our group. We studied postmenopausal women with breast cancer N+ for the effect of (1) full-dose sequential drug regimens and, (2) a combined chemoendocrine therapy (Table 1). The purpose of this paper is to report the preliminary analysis of the results at 5 years with a median follow-up of about 50 months. For a definitive evaluation of the above-mentioned treatment protocols, a more prolonged observation will be necessary in this particular subset of women.

Sequential Non-Cross-Resistant Combinations (CMFP + AV)

Accrual into this study was limited to women aged ≤ 65 years, on the assumption that older patients would not be able to tolerate intensive chemotherapy. The adjuvant program included two sequential combinations, known through a previous study [5] to be

Table 1. Adjuvant programs in postmenopausal node-positive breast cancer. (Patient accrual: May 1977–September 1980)

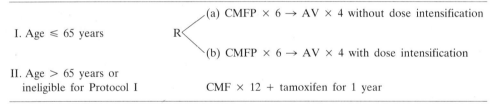

I. Age ≤ 65 years   R ⟨ (a) CMFP × 6 → AV × 4 without dose intensification
(b) CMFP × 6 → AV × 4 with dose intensification

II. Age > 65 years or ineligible for Protocol I   CMF × 12 + tamoxifen for 1 year

non-cross-resistant. CMF plus prednisolone (CMFP) given for six cycles was followed by adriamycin plus vincristine (AV) for four cycles. Taking into consideration some of the principles expressed by the Norton-Simon hypothesis [8], patients were randomly treated at 4-week intervals either (a) with conventional doses of CMFP (C 100 mg/m^2 p.o. day 1−14, M 40 mg/m^2 i.v. on day 1 and 8, F 600 mg/m^2 i.v. on day 1 and 8, P 40 mg/m^2 i.m. day 1−14) and AV (A 60 mg/m^2 i.v. on day 1, V 1.4 mg/m^2 i.v. on day 1 and 8) or (b) with dose intensification every two cycles of all drugs except P and V (C 50−100−150 mg/m^2, M 20−40−60 mg/m^2, F 400−600−800 mg/m^2, A 50−75 mg/m^2).

By the end of therapy, patients in both groups had received the same total dose of each drug. The cumulative dose of adriamycin did not exceed 250 mg/m^2. As one of the main goals of the trial, it was planned to administer chemotherapy without dose reduction. In the presence of myelosuppression (leukocytes < 3,800/mm^3, platelets < 100,000/mm^3) therapy was delayed on a weekly basis until complete bone marrow recovery occurred. After stratification according to the number of positive nodes (1−3, > 3), a total of 140 patients were randomized (no intensification 70, intensification 70). The main patient characteristics are shown in Table 2. In spite of an imbalance in subsets not considered for stratification, the two groups were comparable with respect to main prognostic factors. The majority of patients had N+ 1−3 and ER+ tumors. It is worthy of note that the incidence of extensive nodal involvement (N+ > 10) in this study was considerably higher (20%−26%) than in our previous CMF trials (8%−9%).

Table 2. Adjuvant programs in postmenopausal node-positive breast cancer. (Main patient characteristic in percent)

	CMFP − AV		CMF − T	
	No intensi-fication = 70	Intensi-fication = 70	≤ 65 years = 47	> 65 years = 74
Primary tumor ≤ 2 cm	61	40	49	53
> 2 cm	39	60	51	47
N+ 1−3	50	49	53	58
4−10	30	25	28	23
> 10	20	26	19	19
ER+	60	46	49	58
ER−	13	26	21	18
ER unknown	27	28	30	24
Median age (years)	57 (49−65)	57 (46−65)	62 (52−65)	68 (66−75)
Median follow-up (months)	52	50	48	49

Table 3. CMFP-AV: 5-year results related to the number of positive nodes (N+)

N+	No. of patients	RFS (%)	Survival (%)
1−3	69	76	87
4−10	39	41	68
> 10	32	11	35

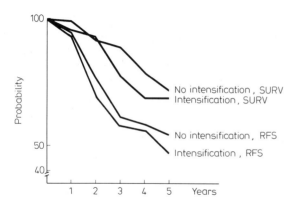

Fig. 1. CMFP-AV in postmenopausal breast cancer N+. RFS and total survival related to treatment arms (no intensification vs intensification)

Figure 1 shows relapse-free survival (RFS) and total survival in both treatment groups. No significant difference was evident in patients given sequential chemotherapy without dose itensification compared with those receiving progressive dose intensification. For this reason, all data will be further evaluated grouping patients of both treatment arms together. The impact of the sequential program on nodal subsets is detailed in Table 3. RFS and total survival rates confirmed the unfavorable prognosis for patients with a high number of involved nodes in spite of aggressive therapy. On the contrary, however, for women with N+ 1−3 our present results appear more favorable than those achieved in our previous studies of the same age population (RFS: control 50%, CMF 12 cycles 63%, CMF 6 cycles 63%; survival: control 73%, CMF 12 cycles 77%, CMF 6 cycles 69%). Treatment failure was documented most frequently in distant sites (33%) and in 13% of patients first recurrence was limited to the local-regional area. No contralateral breast cancer has been observed to date.

Immediate and early toxic manifestations from this adjuvant program did not differ from those commonly reported with CMFP and AV regimens [5]. Vomiting and loss of hair were common in both treatment arms. One or more episodes of leukopenia were slightly more frequent in patients receiving CMFP with dose intensification (76%) than in those treated without dose intensification (64%), while platelet fall was uncommon in both groups (10% vs 6%). Myelosuppression after AV, virtually represented by leukopenia, was reported in about one-third of women with no difference in relation to dose escalation. Prednisolone and vincristine markedly contributed to treatment toxicity in this age group. Edema and arterial hypertension were observed in about 60% and gastric disturbances in about 30% of women. These side effects forced discontinuance of prednisolone in 17% of women. Neurotoxicity was very frequent (80%), including prolonged adynamic ileus in 6% of women; vincristine was withheld because of toxicity in 18% of patients. Twenty-six patients (18%) refused to complete therapy although there was no marked objective toxicity, mainly for psychological reasons. In this group of women, adriamycin could be administered with no clinical evidence of cardiac toxicity. In particular, no episodes of congestive heart failure attributable to adriamycin were observed. Consideration of risk factors in pretreatment patient selection, as well as the planned total dose of the drug (≤ 250 mg/m^2), enabled this severe aspect of drug toxicity to be avoided. Data derived from monitoring cardiac function, during and after adjuvant chemotherapy, are detailed in a separate paper [4]. In short, no relevant modifications of some cardiac function parameters (i.e., PEP/LVET ratio, echocardiography, multigated scintiscan) were detected. Second neoplasms have been detected to date in three patients (2.1%). Bladder and colon cancers were documented in two women 50−59 months from start of adjuvant therapy. A third patient developed overt chronic lymphocytic leukemia 34 months after entering the study. (It is worthy to note that in this patient a relative lymphocytosis was present at the time of treatment start but was not further evaluated in the absence of any suspicious clinical signs or symptoms.)

Although in some patients dose attenuation had to be employed for prolonged myelosuppression, a dose level $\leq 85\%$ of all drugs was administered to about 80% of patients (no intensification 78%, intensification 84%). The treatment program could be completed within the scheduled period of time (about 10 months) for 50% of women receiving therapy at conventional doses but only for 34% of those treated with escalated doses. However, the majority of women completed the adjuvant treatment within 12 months (no intensification 76%, intensification 74%).

Combined Chemoendocrine Therapy

This prospective nonrandomized trial included patients older than 65 years as well as younger postmenopausal patients in whom the presence of other concomitant systemic diseases (e.g., cardiac or renal disease, diabetes) prevented the administration of some of the drugs (methotrexate, prednisolone, adriamycin) as planned in the above-mentioned sequential protocol. In this trial CMF was administered at the conventional dose schedule, as previously reported, in patients younger than 65 years. A lower dose schedule was applied to patients older than 65 years (M 30 mg/m^2, F 400 mg/m^2). Tamoxifen (T) was given orally at the dose of 20 mg daily for 1 year. Drug-dose reduction, as applied in previous CMF protocols [1, 2, 9], was planned in the presence of myelosuppression. For moderate toxicity (leukocytes 3,700−2,500/mm^3, platelets 99,000−75,000/mm^3), 50% of the calculated dose was given. For lower values treatment was delayed until at least 50% of the dose could be administered. The main characteristics of patient population in the two age subsets are reported in Table 2. Known prognostic factors appeared to be equally distributed between the two groups. The majority of patients had 1−3 positive nodes and ER+ tumors. Nearly 50% of women had a primary tumor of < 2 cm. A comparable percent had > 10 involved nodes.

RFS and total survival rates in the entire group are reported in Fig. 2. At 5 years, RFS was 63% and total survival 78%. No difference could be demonstrated in relation to age lesser or greater than 65 years (RFS: 65% vs 62%; survival: 83% vs 77%). RFS related to the number of positive nodes is shown in Fig. 3. Treatment appeared to be equally effective in the subsets with N+ 1−3 and N+ 4−10 (71% and 68%, respectively), while in the group with N+ > 10, RFS was significantly lower ($P = 0.001$). In this study no difference was observed relative to the presence or absence of ER (RFS: 59% vs 63%, survival: 80% vs 82%). New disease manifestations were observed more frequently in distant sites (29%) and only a small fraction of patients showed local-regional recurrence alone (2.5%). Contralateral breast cancer has occurred to date in only one patient.

Drug-induced side effects were those commonly observed with CMF. T produced mild toxicity in about 15% of patients (hot flashes and vaginal symptoms). Myelosuppression, in particular leukopenia, was frequently observed in both age groups (≤ 65 yrs: 93%; > 65 yrs: 96%). In about 25% of patients peripheral leukocytes fell below 2,500/mm^3. Bone marrow toxicity was the main cause of drug reduction. Only a minority of patients (about 20%) in both groups could receive $\leq 85\%$ of planned doses.

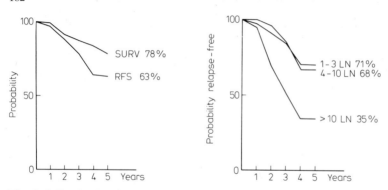

Fig. 2 (*left*). CMF-T in postmenopausal breast cancer N+. RFS and total survival in the total population

Fig. 3 (*right*). CMF-T. RFS related to the number of N+

Second malignancies were observed in seven patients: rectal cancer (two), skin cancer (two), colon cancer (one), anal cancer (one), endometrial cancer (one). These tumors were detected 14−54 months from start of therapy.

Comment

Adjuvant therapy for breast cancer patients who are postmenopausal and have positive axillary nodes has so far been an area of controversy. The experience of our group indicated only a marginal benefit with 12 cycles of CMF as given in the first study [2, 9]. However, recent data for the second CMF program showed a favorable effect from 6 cycles of CMF, irrespective of menopause [1, 10].

Two different treatment approaches were tested prospectively in postmenopausal patients. Preliminary analyses of 5-year results for patients with 1−3 positive nodes show a favorable trend for both of these treatment protocols compared with our previous results. In fact, while mindful of the limits of a retrospective comparison with a patient population of different size and followed for a longer period of time, we can say that RFS after CMFP-AV and CMF-T appeared superior to RFS with surgery + CMF or surgery alone in the same age subset. However, these results need to be confirmed by longer follow-up observation.

Treatment morbidity with intensive chemotherapy given at full doses was acceptable in postmenopausal women with no serious side effects; in this group vincristine and prednisone markedly contributed to toxicity. Adriamycin could be administered without evidence (at 5 years) of drug-induced late effects. In addition, in the older patient group CMF-T could be safely administered by applying dose attenuation. In both studies no increased incidence of second neoplasms was evident.

Interpretation of present results is not definitive for either study. Whether the effect of sequential combinations was a consequence of full-dose administration during the first 6 cycles of CMFP, or was secondary to the cell kill of resistant cell sublines induced by AV combination, remains to be established. Although results with 6 cycles of CMF seem to stress the importance of short-term effective chemotherapy, the problem of optimal treatment duration utilizing non-cross-resistant regimens is still open to discussion. On the other hand, CMF-T was effective irrespective of ER status and in spite of low drug dose.

These troublesome findings can in part be explained by the absence of information in this case series on progesterone receptors, which have been repeatedly reported to be stronger predictors for response to endocrine therapy than is ER, also in the adjuvant setting [6, 7]. Furthermore, benefit of CMF-T in spite of low-dose regimen can be in part interpreted as a consequence of the additive effect of cytotoxic and hormonal compounds as well as of the rather indolent course of breast cancer in elderly women.

Optimal adjuvant chemotherapy for postmenopausal high-risk breast cancer is still to be defined. Current trials should take into account all known prognostic variables, in particular the proportion of extensive nodal involvement (> 10 positive nodes) as well as ER and progesterone receptor tumor content.

Acknowledgement. This study was supported in part by contract N01-CM-33714, Department of Cancer Treatment, National Cancer Institute, National Institutes of Health.

References

1. Bonadonna G, Rossi A, Tancini G, Valagussa P, Veronesi U (1984) CMF adjuvant programs at the Milan Cancer Institute. (this volume)
2. Bonadonna G, Rossi A, Valagussa P, Banfi A, Veronesi U (1977) The CMF program for operable breast cancer with positive axillary nodes. Updated analysis on the disease-free interval, site of relapse, and drug tolerance. Cancer 39: 2904–2915
3. Bonadonna G, Valagussa P (1983) Chemotherapy of breast cancer: current views and results. Int J Radiat Oncol Biol Phys 9: 279–297
4. Brambilla C Manuscript in preparation
5. Brambilla C, De Lena M, Rossi A, Valagussa P, Bonadonna G (1976) Response and survival in advanced breast cancer after two non-cross-resistant combinations. Br Med J 1: 801–804
6. Clark GM, McGuire WL (1983) Prognostic factors in primary breast cancer. Breast Cancer Res Treat 3: 69–72
7. Fisher B, Redmond C, Brown A, Wickerham DL, Wolmark N, Allegra J, Escher G, Lippman M, Savlov E, Wittlipp J, Fisher ER, with the contribution of Plotkin D, Bowman D, Wolter J, Bornstein R, Desser R, Frelick R, and other NSABP Investigators (1983) Influence of tumor estrogen and progesterone receptor levels on the response to tamoxifen and chemotherapy in primary breast cancer. J Clin Oncol 1: 227–241
8. Norton L, Simon R (1977) Tumor size, sensitivity to therapy, and the design of treatment schedule. Cancer Treat Rep 61: 1307–1317
9. Rossi A, Bonadonna G, Valagussa P, Veronesi U (1981) Multimodal treatment in operable breast cancer: five-year results of the CMF program. Br Med J 282: 1427–1431
10. Tancini G, Bonadonna G, Valagussa P, Marchini S, Veronesi U (1983) Adjuvant CMF in breast cancer: comparative five-year results of 12 vs 6 cycles. J Clin Oncol 1: 2–10

Review: Experience of Randomized Trials Without Surgical Controls

D. C. Tormey

Department of Human Oncology, K4/666, Clinical Science Center,
600 Highland Avenue, Madison, WI 53792, USA

The trials presented in this section deal with four major issues in the adjuvant treatment of breast cancer: the optimal duration of therapy, treatment intensity, implications regarding drug schedule, and the role of combining tamoxifen with chemotherapy.

Duration of Therapy

It was noted that an earlier analysis of 24 months of CMF as delivered by CALGB appeared to be equivalent to the 12 months regimen used in Milan [1]. The SAKK trial demonstrated that 18 cycles of LMF over 24 months did not differ from 6 cycles over 6 months and the Milan study continues to show no significant difference between 12 and 6 months of CMF. These results all suggest that treatment beyond 6 months with a single regimen may not confer any therapeutic advantage. Indeed, there is a suggestion in the Milan trial that 12 months of CMF may be slightly inferior to 6 months. This observation could be very important, especially in view of animal data from Southern Research Institute indicating that treatment over prolonged time-frames may be detrimental. The hypothesis that therapy can be shortened should soon be settled as survival data from these trials will shortly extend to 10 years.

The suggestion that the treatment period with these regimens can be shortened would enable a greater treatment-free period (Fig. 1). It can be argued that providing patients with a treatment-free period that is in excess of that achieved without systemic therapy may increase the overall quality of survival. More formal analyses of this endpoint might, therefore, usefully be included in future reports from these trials.

Treatment Intensity

There are many approaches to increasing treatment intensity aside from changes in the drug schedule. Three major approaches were presented in this section: (1) the addition of more drugs, (2) a fixed cross-over, and (3) an escalation of drug dosages. Such considerations as very high dose regimens, rotating therapy, and combining systemic therapy with radiotherapy have only recently been studied in various centers.

The addition of more drugs to CMF has its basis in advanced-disease trials wherein either response rate, time to treatment failure, or survival appeared to be improved with the

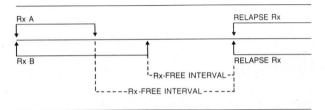

Fig. 1. The impact of systemic treatment interval if the treatment regimens are equally effective. It is assumed that relapse will be delayed due to treatment but that the duration of treatment beyond, e.g., 6 months, does not further delay relapse. In that case the shorter treatment *(Rx A)* will yield a longer treatment-free interval than will the longer treatment *(Rx B)*. *Rx,* systemic treatment

addition of vincristine and prednisone (VP) to CMF [2], prednisone to CMF [3, 4], and tamoxifen to CMF [5], or to dibromodulcitol and adriamycin [6]. These trials in advanced disease provided advantages in only one or two of these major treatment endpoints. The corresponding CALGB and ECOG adjuvant trials presented at these meetings have not found an advantage of these additions to CMF except within selected patient cohorts. However, the use of CMFVP was distinctly superior to L-PAM across the entire population and most patient cohorts examined. Assuming CMFVP is at least equivalent to CMF, this result is in keeping with the superiority of CMF over L-PAM demonstrated for all major treatment endpoints in the ECOG advanced-disease trial [7]. Thus, it would appear that a major treatment intensity advantage needs to be observed in advanced disease before that difference can be appreciated in at least the first 5–6 years of adjuvant therapy.

The Milan experience comparing standard-dose CMFP → AV with the same regimen, starting at "low dose" and escalating through "standard dose" to "high dose", provided no statistical differences. Perhaps in retrospect the "escalating arm" should have started at "standard dose." Thus, it is not clear that this disproves the underlying hypothesis. The cross-over design in this trial from CMFP to AV appears to be doing better than historical CMF data, but the lack of an appropriate CMF or CMFP control group makes its true impact difficult to assess. There is a suggestion in advanced disease that time to treatment failure using a cross-over from AV to CMF may be slightly superior to CMF alone [3, 8] but, again, this is a minor difference which may not translate to the adjuvant setting at 5 or 6 years.

Treatment Schedule Modifications

There were no direct tests of treatment schedule modifications presented but data from three of the trials bear on this issue. The CALGB's 6 weeks of continuous induction with CMF prior to initiating intermittent therapy did not appear to confer an advantage over the Milan intermittent CMF. The SWOG continuous CMFVP was distinctly superior to L-PAM. Since advanced-disease trials suggest that continuous CMFVP is only borderline superior to intermittent CMFVP [9, 10], and that CMFVP is only borderline superior to CMF [2], the marked advantage of continuous CMFVP in the SWOG study may be the first clue to a necessity to use continuous therapy in postoperative patients.

The other modification in these trials involved lengthening the treatment cycles in year 2 in the CALGB and SAKK trials in an attempt to kill slow-growing cells. The apparent failure of this approach does not refute the tactic, only the means by which it was executed. Taken in concert with the SWOG trial a more appropriate tactic might be to provide a true continuous therapy reinduction at one or more specified times after an initial 6 months of therapy.

Role of Tamoxifen with Combination Chemotherapy

It was of interest that the only early trends favoring the addition of tamoxifen to CMF-based chemotherapy occurred in ER− patients. The use of CMFT in patients > 65 years by the Milan group is difficult to assess due to the lack of a concurrent control group. Certainly the advanced-disease trials suggest a greater initial cell kill by using tamoxifen in combination with cytotoxic drugs [5, 6]. The present maturing adjuvant trials all stop tamoxifen concurrently with termination of chemotherapy. Both in vitro and in vivo data suggest that the antiestrogen provides a G_1 block of sensitive cells [11, 12]. It is therefore reasonable to consider continuing the drug indefinitely beyond chemotherapy in order to continue to control the sensitive cells in this apparently heterogeneous disease. This has been done in a pilot trial at Wisconsin with promising results [13] and has led to recently activated randomized trials in ECOG to test this concept. Blood levels of tamoxifen and its major two metabolites have been found to be stable over at least the first 5 years of therapy [13].

Thus, the trials in this section suggest that initial induction therapy can be reduced to 6 months or less, that only major advanced-disease differences will translate to adjuvant results at 5−6 years, that the treatment schedules should perhaps be based on continuous rather than intermittent therapy schedules, and that the addition of tamoxifen to cytotoxic drugs may provide benefit in ER− cohorts and perhaps should be continued indefinitely beyond the chemotherapy in all cohorts.

References

1. Holland JF (1983) Breaking the cure barrier. J Clin Oncol 1: 75−90
2. Muss HB, White DR, Cooper R, Richards II F, Spurr CL (1977) Combination chemotherapy in advanced breast cancer. Arch Intern Med 137: 1711−1714
3. Tormey DC, Gelman R, Band PR, Sears M, Rosenthal SN, DeWys W, Perlia C, Rice MA (1982) Comparison of induction chemotherapies for metastatic breast cancer: an Eastern Cooperative Oncology Group trial. Cancer 50: 1235−1244
4. Tormey DC, Gelman R, Falkson G (1983) Prospective evaluation of rotating chemotherapy in advanced breast cancer: An Eastern Cooperative Oncology Group trial. Am J Clin Oncol 6: 1−8
5. Engelsman E, Mouridsen HT, Palshof T, Sylvester R (1981) CMF vs CMF plus tamoxifen in advanced breast cancer in postmenopausal women. An EORTC study. Rev Endocrine Related Cancer [Suppl] 9: 427−438
6. Tormey DC, Falkson G, Crowley J, Falkson HC, Voelkel J, Davis TE (1982) Dibromodulcitol and adriamycin ± tamoxifen in advanced breast cancer. Cancer Clin Trials 5: 33−39
7. Canellos GP, Pocock SJ, Taylor SG III, Sears ME, Klaasen DJ, Band PR (1976) Combination chemotherapy for metastatic breast carcinoma. Prospective comparison of multiple drug therapy with L-phenylalanine mustard. Cancer 38: 1882−1886
8. DeLena M, Brambilla C, Morbito A, Bonadonna G (1975) Adriamycin plus vincristine compared to and combined with cyclophosphamide, methotrexate, and 5-fluorouracil for advanced breast cancer. Cancer 35: 1108−1115

9. Tormey DC, Weinberg VE, Leone LA, Glidewell OJ, Perloff M, Kennedy BJ, Cortes E, Silver
    RT, Weiss RB, Aisner J, Holland JF (to be published) A comparison of intermittent vs
    continuous and of adriamycin vs methotrexate 5-drug chemotherapy for advanced breast cancer
    − a cancer and leukemia group B study. Am J Clin Oncol
10. Hoogstraten B, George SL, Samal B, Rivkin SE, Costanzi JJ, Bonnet JD, Thigpen T, Braine H
    (1976) Combination chemotherapy and adriamycin in patients with advanced breast cancer.
    Cancer 38: 13−20
11. Osborne CK, Blodt DH, Clark GM, Trent JM (1983) Effects of tamoxifen on human breast
    cancer cell cycle kinetics: accumulation of cells in early G_1 phase. Cancer Res
    43: 3583−3585
12. Jordan VC, Dix CJ, Allen KE (1979) The effectiveness of long-term tamoxifen treatment in a
    laboratory model for adjuvant hormone therapy of breast cancer. In: Jones SE, Salmon SE (eds)
    Adjuvant therapy of cancer II. Grune and Stratton, New York, pp 19−26
13. Tormey DC, Jordan VC (to be published) Adjuvant chemotherapy and chemohormonal therapy
    in postoperative N+ patients. In: Breast cancer − Therapeutic modalities, current and
    future

Remaining Problems of Adjuvant Chemotherapy in Breast Cancer

Second Malignant Neoplasms in Operable Carcinoma of the Breast

E. E. Holdener, R. Nissen-Meyer, G. Bonadonna, S. E. Jones, A. Howell, R. Rubens, and H. J. Senn

Division für Onkologie und Hämatologie, Abteilung für Medizin C, Kantonsspital, 9007 St. Gallen, Switzerland

Introduction

Development of a second malignant neoplasm (SMN) following prolonged cytotoxic therapy is a potential delayed consequence of tumor treatment [1, 5, 6, 20, 26, 27, 31, 34, 46, 48, 49, 51]. In addition, specified primary neoplasms are associated with the development of other primary malignancies through either a common etiology or an impaired patient's defense mechanism [44]. The oncogenic potential of adjuvant chemotherapy in early breast cancer may, therefore, best be analyzed by looking at the occurrence of SMNs in prospective randomized trials using a similar, nontreated patient population (surgical control). This report summarizes the frequency of SMNs in five controlled adjuvant chemotherapy trials and two studies with no surgical control group.

Materials and Method

Scandinavian Adjuvant Chemotherapy Study Group (SACSG)

A cooperative, randomized clinical trial with single-agent short course chemotherapy (Table 1) was started in January 1965 and terminated in Spetember 75. Overall, 1,136 eligible patients with operable breast cancer (T_1-T_3, N$-$/N+) were randomized in this trial. A detailed review of the study case material has been published previously [42].

Milan Trials

Between June 1973 and September 1975 a total of 386 patients with operable breast cancer (T_1-T_{3a}, N+) were randomly allocated to receive either adjuvant chemotherapy or no further treatment (Table 1). A more detailed study design has previously been reported [3]. In a second consecutive trial, which lasted from September 1975 to May 1978, a prospective randomized study compared 12 cycles of CMF to 6 cycles of CMF as adjuvant chemotherapy in 459 patients with operable breast cancer [55].

Recent Results in Cancer Research. Vol. 96
© Springer-Verlag Berlin · Heidelberg 1984

Table 1. Treatment schedules used as adjuvant chemotherapy in breast cancer patients

Institution	Treatment	Schedule	
SACSG	RM vs RM + CTX:	5 mg/kg/d × 6 days	
Milan	RM vs RM + CTX:	100 mg/m² p.o. d_1-d_{14}	
	+ MTX:	40 mg/m² i.v. $d_1 + d_8$	q4w × 12
	+ 5-FU:	600 mg/m² i.v. $d_1 + d_8$	
OSAKO (St. Gallen)	RM vs RM + CLB:	6–8 mg p.o. d_1-d_{14}	
	+ MTX:	5–7.5 mg p.o. $d_1-d_3 + d_8-d_{10}$	q4w × 6
	+ 5-FU:	500–750 mg p.o. $d_1 + d_8$	
	+ BCG:	× 1/month × 18 after LMF	
Manchester/Guy's	RM vs RM + CTX:	80 mg/m² p.o. d_1-d_{14}	
	+ MTX:	32 mg/m² i.v. $d_1 + d_8$	q4w × 12
	+ 5-FU:	480 mg/m² i.v. $d_1 + d_8$	
	RM vs RM + L-PAM:	0.15 mg/kg/d × 5	q6w for 2 years
Milan	12 cycles CMF vs 6 cycles CMF		
Arizona	ADM:	30 mg/m² i.v. d_1	q3w × 8
	CTX:	150 mg/m² p.o. d_3-d_6	

Abbreviations: *d*, day; *w*, week; *RM*, radical mastectomy; *CTX*, cyclophosphamide; *MTX*, methotrexate; *5-FU*, 5-fluorouracil; *CLB*, chlorambucil; *BCG*, bacillus Calmette-Guèrin; *L-PAM*, melphalan; *CMF*, CTX + MTX + 5-FU; *ADM*, adriamycin; *LMF*, leukeran (= CLB) + MTX + 5-FU

OSAKO Trial

Between April 1974 and December 1977, 240 evaluable patients with operable breast cancer (T_1-T_{3a}, N_{0-1}) were randomized to adjuvant chemo(immuno)therapy (Table 1) or no further treatment after radical mastectomy [50].

Manchester/Guy's Trials

The two studies were set up in a similar manner in order to combine their results, using the same melphalan (L-PAM) regime, as shown in Table 1. The Guy's Hospital study randomized patients with operable breast cancer (T_1-T_3, N+) for melphalan or no further therapy. The Manchester trial was designed as a three-arm study comparing CMF vs melphalan vs no further treatment following radical mastectomy. Patients with operable breast cancer (T_1-T_3, N+ and T_3N_0) were eligible for this study [7].

Arizona Trial

Since 1973 a total of 232 patients with operable breast cancer (stage II, N+) have recieved two-drug adjuvant chemotherapy as outlined in Table 1 [25].

Table 2. SMNs after radical mastectomy with or without adjuvant chemotherapy

Center or group	Regimen	Number of patients	Median follow-up (years)	SMNs Excluding contra- lateral breast cancer (%)	Contra- lateral breast cancer only (%)
SACSG	Surgical controls	577	14	22 (3.8)	15 (2.6)
	CTX × 6 days	559		17 (3.0)	13 (2.3)
Milan	Surgical controls	179	8	4 (2.2)	6 (3.4)
	CMF × 12 months	207		5 (2.4)	8 (3.7)
Milan	CMF × 6 months	216	7	2 (0.9)	6 (2.8)
	CMF × 12 months	243		4 (1.7)	8 (3.3)
OSAKO (St. Gallen)	Surgical controls	123	8	7 (5.7)	2 (1.6)
	LMF × 6 months + BCG	117		6 (5.1)	1 (0.9)
Tucson	ADM + CTX × 6 months	232	> 4	6 (2.6)	4 (1.7)
Manchester/Guy's	Surgical controls	161	3	2 (1.2)	–
	CMF × 12 months	165		3 (1.8)	–
	Surgical controls	183	4	3 (1.6)	–
	Melphalan	187		2 (1.0)	–
Overall (five studies)	Surgical controls	1,223	–	38 (3.1)	
	Adjuvant chemotherapy	1,235	–	33 (2.7)	

See Table 1 for definition of abbreviations

Results

The numbers of extramammary SMNs and contralateral, metachronous breast cancers are shown in Table 2. A total of 2,458 patients (five studies) were randomly allocated to receive either adjuvant chemotherapy or no further treatment after radical mastectomy. Thirty-eight (3.1%) SMNs were found in the surgical controls and 33 (2.7%) in patients with adjuvant chemotherapy. Two trials using no surgical controls (Arizona, Milan second trial) found a total of 12 (1.7%) SMNs in 691 patients. Contralateral breast cancer occurred in 23 of 879 (2.6%) patients with no further treatment after radical mastectomy and in 22 of 883 (2.5%) patients with adjuvant chemotherapy. The SMNs are listed by site in Table 3. Although there is a slightly higher number of lung cancers, colorectal cancers, and ovarian cancers and a lower number of lymphomas, leukemias, and melanomas in patients with adjuvant chemotherapy, neither difference is statistically significant compared to surgical controls. In the SACSG trial, with a median observation time of 14 years, six of 22 SMNs in the surgical control group were tumors from the gastrointestinal tract (four stomach, one colon, one pancreas) and six were endometrial carcinomas. Among the remaining 48% of SMNs were two bladder cancers and two non-Hodgkins lymphomas. Seventeen patients with adjuvant chemotherapy developed SMNs, 47% of which originated in the gastrointestinal tract, predominantly in the colon and rectum. Gynecological tumors and lung cancer were the next most frequent tumor types. The median interval from

Table 3. Number of SMNs (excluding contralateral breast cancer) in patients with operable breast cancer

Site/type	Surgical controls ($n = 1,223$)	Adjuvant chemotherapy ($n = 1,235$)
Lung	3	5
Esophagus	0	2
Stomach	4	2
Pancreas	2	2
Colon/rectum	3	7
Gallbladder	0	1
Ovary	2	5
Uterus	4	2
Cervix	3	1
Fallopian tube	0	1
Oropharynx	1	1
Parathyroid	1	0
Thyroid	1	0
Kidney	1	0
Urinary bladder	2	1
CNS	1	1
Lymphoma	2	1
Leukemia	3	1
Sarcoma	2	1
Melanoma	3	0

Pooled data from 5 randomized studies (SACSG, Milano, OSAKO, Manchester/Guy's)

mastectomy to the diagnosis of SMN was 5 years (range 3−160 months) for patients in the surgical control group and 9.5 years (range 14−190 months) for patients with adjuvant chemotherapy. Both at 5 and at 10 years there is no statistically significant difference ($P = 0.1$) in the number of SMNs between the control group and the adjuvant chemotherapy group. The median survival of patients with SMNs was 13.3 years in the surgical control group and 11.7 years in the adjuvant chemotherapy group. Seventy-five percent and 78% died from SMNs respectively.

In the first Milan trial, four SMNs were found in the surgical control group, two of them gynecological tumors. Gastrointestinal tumors and gynecological tumors were the most frequent SMNs in the adjuvant chemotherapy group. The median interval from mastectomy to the SMN was 30.5 months (range 3−59) in the surgical control group and 71 months (range 38−101) in the adjuvant chemotherapy group. In the second Milan trial, all patients with SMNs were alive at the time of this analysis, with median survival times of 90 months (control) and 86 months (adjuvant chemotherapy) since mastectomy.

In the OSAKO trial (St. Gallen) two patients in the surgical control arm developed acute leukemia (ALL, AML) as SMNs. Third malignant tumors, which developed in one patient in each group, were included in this analysis and are responsible for the somewhat higher rate of SMNs than in the other trials. The median time from mastectomy to the diagnosis of SMN was 40.5 months (range 11−65) in surgical controls and 26 months (range 9−71) in the adjuvant chemotherapy group. Eight of nine patients have died from the SMNs.

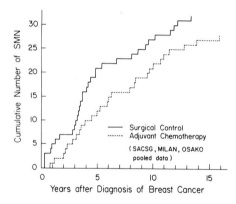

Fig. 1. Occurrence of SMNs (contralateral breast cancer excluded) over a median follow-up of 8–14 years in three prospective, randomized trials. SMNs in surgical controls, $n = 33$; SMNs in adjuvant chemotherapy groups, $n = 28$

The three above-cited prospective trials, with a median follow-up of 8–14 years, showed a median interval to SMN of 3.7 years for surgical controls and 5.8 years for the adjuvant chemotherapy group (Fig. 1).

In the Manchester/Guy's trials, one patient in the CMF arm developed acute leukemia.

In the Arizona trial, two melanomas, one colon cancer, one esophageal carcinoma, one lung cancer, and one endometrial carcinoma were found after a median interval of 30 months (range 20–61) after radical mastectomy and adjuvant chemotherapy. Four (66%) of these patients were alive at the time of this analysis.

Discussion

The overall rate of SMNs other than breast cancer was 2.6%. In a retrospective study of 1985 breast cancer patients [23], the rate of SMNs was 2.1%.

Iatrogenic leukemia has been linked to the chemotherapeutic agents used to treat breast cancer [9, 13, 30, 34, 43, 46–48]. AML was found to be the most frequent SMN after cytotoxic chemotherapy with cyclophosphamide for a variety of primary tumors, predominantly Hodgkin's disease, and occured with an average dose of 45,000 mg after an average interval of 49 months [49]. In another series of 335 patients with SMNs, 51% developed leukemia (ANLL 79%) after an average duration of chemotherapy of 4 years and 3 months [45]. Foucar et al. [16] reported on 15 patients with various malignancies who developed AML after a median interval of 60 months (range 31–182). All patients but one had received an alkylating agent as single drug or in combination with other cytostatic drugs. Curtis et al. [8] reported that patients with breast cancer have greater risk for AML in the 3–7 year period. Portugal et al. [46] found four patients with breast cancer who developed ANLL after a median interval of 66.5 months from the start of chemotherapy for metastatic disease. All four had been treated with cyclophosphamide, with a median total dose of 54,150 mg and a median exposure time of 37.5 months. Rosner et al. [48] found 24 patients with breast cancer who developed acute leukemia. However, only five had received chemotherapy alone, and ANNL was diagnosed after a median interval of 4 years (range 2.5–8). In the same series, six patients without treatment after mastectomy also developed acute leukemia (five ANLL, one ALL), after a median interval of 4.5 years (range 0.25–14). The same authors reviewed the literature, where only three of 54 patients with breast cancer developed acute leukemia after being treated with chemotherapy alone;

Fig. 2. Frequency of contralateral breast cancers. Each *circle* represents the data of one study reported in the literature. The *regression line* (r^2 = 0.723; slope 0.025 ± 0.003) is drawn as the number of contralateral breast cancers *(ordinate)* as a function of the number of patients with breast cancer *(abscissa)*. The *dashed lines* encompass the 95% confidence range [4, 10, 11, 15, 17–19, 21–24, 28, 29, 32, 33, 35, 36, 38, 39, 41, 52, 53, 56]

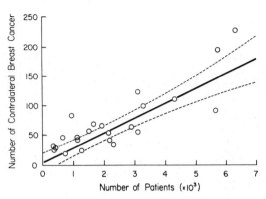

leukemia was diagnosed 4, 18, and 48 months after diagnosis of breast cancer. In the present studies only four leukemias could be observed; three of them (one AML, one ALL, one CLL) developed in patients in the surgical control groups after intervals of 44, 65, and 97 months. Assuming a high body surface area of 2 m² and an application of full doses over 12 cycles of CMF treatment, a patient could theoretically receive cyclophosphamide in a maximum dose of 33,600 mg. As only 17% of the patients could tolerate a full or nearly full (≥ 85%) dose of CMF [2], most have received a total dose far below 30,000 mg. In addition, the exposure time to the drug was shorter than in most other studies. These two important factors may be responsible for the lack of increased rate of leukemias observed in the combined studies presented here.

The most frequent SMNs after cyclophosphamide therapy other than leukemia were bladder cancer and squamous cell carcinoma of the skin in a review of 303 cases of reported SMNs [49]. We did not observe an excess of bladder carcinoma in patients treated with adjuvant chemotherapy. Bladder cancers associated with cyclophosphamide therapy were reported after total doses of more than 150,000 mg [12, 14].

The overall rate of contralateral breast cancer in the present studies was 2.55%–2.6% in the surgical control groups and 2.5% in the adjuvant chemotherapy groups. In a retrospective study the frequency of contralateral breast cancer was 2.1% [23]. A review of the literature on contralateral breast cancer revealed an average rate of 2.5 ± 0.3% in 49,449 patients reported (Fig. 2).

Enough data have accumulated to demonstrate that the tumor incidence is directly dependent on the dose of chemical carcinogen in experimental animals and in man [20]. There are various in vitro short-term tests which predict in vivo tumorgenicity reasonably well [37, 40, 57, 58]. More in vitro/in vivo correlation studies are required, however, in order to optimize the test systems and verify their predictive value.

This will finally improve our understanding as to which agents potentially lead to late toxicity and endanger the patient's future despite immediate therapeutic usefulness [54].

In conclusion, we did not observe an increase of SMNs in patients receiving adjuvant chemotherapy for early breast cancer after median follow-up of 8–14 years in three prospective, randomized trials. Further follow-up will show whether this holds true for much longer observation periods.

Acknowledgements. We would like to thank U. Gessner for helping with the statistical analysis and E. Mettler and I. Schuster for preparing the manuscript.

References

1. Boice JD Jr, Grenne MH, Killen JY Jr, Ellenberg SS, Keehn RJ, McFadden E, Chen TT, Fraumeni JF Jr (1983) Leukemia and preleukemia after adjuvant treatment of gastrointestinal cancer with semustine (methyl-CCNU). N Engl J Med 309: 1079–1084
2. Bonadonna G, Valagussa P (1981) Dose-reponse effect of adjuvant chemotherapy in breast cancer. N Engl J Med 304: 10–15
3. Bonadonna G, Brusamolino E, Valagussa P, Rossi A, Brugnatelli L, Brambilla C, De Lena M, Tancini G, Bajetta E, Musumeci R, Veronesi U (1976) Combination chemotherapy as an adjuvant treatment in operable breast cancer. N Engl J Med 297: 405–410
4. Busk T, Clemmensen J (1947) The frequency of left- and right-sided breast carcinoma. Br J Cancer 1: 345–351
5. Carey RW, Holland JF, Sheehe PR, Graham S (1967) Association of cancer of the breast and acute myelocytic leukemia. Cancer 20: 1080–1088
6. Chan PYM, Sadoff L, Winkley JH (1977) Second malignancies following first breast cancer in prolonged thiotepa adjuvant chemotherapy. In: Salmon SE, Jones SE (eds) Adjuvant therapy of cancer. Elsevier/North-Holland Biomedical, Amsterdam, pp 597–607
7. Crowther D (1979) Controlled adjuvant chemotherapy trials for breast cancer in the United Kingdom. In: Jones SE, Salmon SE (eds) Adjuvant therapy of cancer, vol II. Grune and Stratton, New York, pp 237–244
8. Curtis RE, Hankey BF, Myers MH, Young JL (1984) Risk of leukemia associated with the first course of cancer treatment: an analysis of the surveillance, epidemiology and end results program experience. JNCI 72: 531–544
9. Davis HL Jr, Prout MN, McKenna PJ, Cole DR, Korbitz BC (1973) Acute leukemia complicating metastatic breast cancer. Cancer 31: 543–546
10. Desaive P (1949) Le cancer mammaire bilatéral. J Radiol [D] 30: 335–338
11. Devitt EF (1971) Bilateral mammary cancer. Ann Surg 174: 774–778
12. Durkee C, Benson R (1980) Bladder cancer following administration of cyclophosphamide. Urology 16: 145–148
13. Ershler WB, Robins HI, Davis HL (1982) Emergence of acute non-lymphocytic leukemia in breast cancer patients. Am J Med Sci 284: 23–31
14. Fairchild WV, Spence CR, Solomon HD, Gangai MP (1979) The incidence of bladder cancer after cyclophosphamide therapy. J Urol 122: n 163–164
15. Farrow DH (1969) Bilateral mammary cancer. Cancer 9: 1182–1188
16. Foucar K, McKenna RW, Bloomfield CD, Bowers TK, Brunning RD (1979) Therapy-related leukemia: A panmyelosis. Cancer 43: 1285–1296
17. Haagensen CD, Lance N, Lattes R, Bodian C (1978) Lobular neoplasia (so-called lobular carcinoma in situ) of the breast. Cancer 42: 737–769
18. Harnett W (1948) A statistical report on 2,529 cases of cancer of the breast. Br J Cancer 2: 212–238
19. Harrington SW (1946) Survival rates of radical mastectomy for unilateral and bilateral carcinoma of the breast. Surgery 19: 154–166
20. Harris CC (1976) The carcinogenicity of anticancer drugs: a hazard in man. Cancer 37: 1014–1024
21. Hawkins JW (1944) Evaluation of breast cancer therapy as a guide to control programs. J Natl Cancer Inst 4: 445–460
22. Herrman JB (1955) Bilateral mammary carcinoma. Acta UICC II: 433–439
23. Holdener EE, Osterwalder J, Senn HJ, Enderlin F, Gloor F (1982) Zweitmalignome bei operiertem Mammakarzinom. Schweiz Med Wochenschr 112: 1800–1804
24. Hubbard TB, Montgomery MD (1953) Nonsimultenaous bilateral carcinoma of the breast. Surgery 34: 706–723
25. Jones SE, Salmon SE, Allen H, Giordano GF, Davis S, Chase E, Moon TE, Hensinkveld RS (1982) Adjuvant treatment of node-positive breast cancer with adriamycin-cyclophosphamide with or without radiation therapy: interim results of an ongoing clinical trial. Recent Results Cancer Res 80: 162–169

26. Karchmer RK, Amare M, Larsen WE, Mallouk AG, Caldwell GG (1974) Alkylating agents as leukomogens in multiple myeloma. Cancer 33: 1103–1107
27. Kardinal CG, Donegan WL (1980) Second cancers after prolonged adjuvant thiotepa for operable carcinoma of the breast. Cancer 45: 2042–2046
28. Kesseler HJ, Grier RN, Seidmann I, McIlveen SJ (1970) Bilateral primary breast cancer. JAMA 236: 278–280
29. Kilgore AR, Bell HG, Ahlquist RE (1956) Cancer in the second breast. Am J Surg 92: 156–161
30. Koyama H, Wada T, Takahashi Y, Nishizawa Y, Iwanaga T, Aoki Y, Terasawa T, Kosaki G, Kajita A, Wada A (1980) Surgical adjuvant chemotherapy with mitomycin C and cyclophosphamide in Japanese patients with breast cancer. Cancer 46: 2373–2379
31. Kyle RA, Pierre RV, Bayrd ED (1975) Multiple myeloma and acute leukemia associated with alkalyting agents. Arch Intern Med 135: 185–192
32. Lapis K, Kis A (1956) Über beiderseitige Brustkrebse. Zentralbl Chir 81: 680–689
33. Leis HP Jr, Mersheimer WL, Black MM, Chabon A (1965) The second breast. NY State J Med 65: 2460–2468
34. Lerner HJ (1978) Acute myelogenous leukemia in patients receiving chlorambucil as long-term adjuvant chemotherapy for stage II breast cancer. Cancer Treat Rep 62: 1135–1138
35. Lewis D, Rienhoff WF Jr (1932) A study of the results of operations for the cure of cancer of the breast. Ann Surg 95: 336–409
36. Lewison EF, Neto AS (1971) Bilateral breast cancer at the Johns Hopkins Hospital. A discussion of the dilemma of contralateral breast cancer. Cancer 28: 1297–1301
37. Marquardt H (1977) Induction of malignant transformation and mutagenesis in cell cultures by cancer chemotherapeutic agents. Cancer 40: 1930–1934
38. Martynjuk UU, Kalinikna VI (1968) Cancer of the second breast. Vopr Onkol 14: 92–95
39. McWilliams CA (1925) Bilateral mammary cancer operations. Ann Surg 82: 63–80
40. Medina D (1977) Enhancement of mammary tumor formation in mice by a cytostatic drug, melphalan. Cancer Res 37: 317–319
41. Moertel CG, Soule EH (1957) The problem of the second breast: A study of 118 patients with bilateral carcinoma of the breast. Ann Surg 146: 764–771
42. Nissen-Meyer R, Kjellgren K, Malmio K, Mansson B, Norin T (1978) Surgical adjuvant chemotherapy. Results with one short course with cyclophosphamide after mastectomy for breast cancer. Cancer 41: 2088–2098
43. Nowell P, Glick JH, Bucolo A, Finan J, Creech R (1981) Cytogenic studies of bone marrow in breast cancer patients after adjuvant chemotherapy. Cancer 48: 667–673
44. Penn I (1981) Depressed immunity and the development of cancer. Clin Exp Immunol 46: 459–474
45. Penn I (1982) Second neoplasms following radiotherapy of chemotherapy for cancer. Am J Clin Oncol 5: 83–96
46. Portugal MA, Falkson HC, Stevens K, Falkson G (1979) Acute leukemia as a complication of long-term treatment of advanced breast cancer. Cancer Treat Rep 63: 177–181
47. Robins HI, Ershler WB, Hafez GR, Dohlberg S, Arndt C (1980) Acute nonlymphocytic leukemia in breast cancer: Therapy related or de novo? Lancet I: 91–92
48. Rosner F, Carey RW, Zarrabi MH (1978) Breast cancer and acute leukemia: report of 24 cases and review of the literature. Am J Hematol 4: 151–172
49. Schmähl D, Habs M, Lorenz M, Wagner I (1982) Occurrence of second tumors in man after anticancer drug treatment. Cancer Treat Rev 9: 167–194
50. Senn HJ, Jungi WF, Amgwerd R (1979) Divergent effect of chemoimmunotherapy with LMF/BCG in node-negative and node-positive breast cancer. In: Jones SE, Salmon SE (eds) Adjuvant therapy of cancer, vol II. Grune and Stratton, New York, pp 245–252
51. Sieber SM (1975) Cancer chemotherapeutic agents and carcinogenesis. Cancer Chemother Rep 59: 915–918
52. Slack NH, Bross IDJ, Nemoto T, Fisher B (1973) Experiences with bilateral primary carcinoma of the breast. Surg Gynecol Obstet 136: 433–440

53. Smithers DW, Rigby-Jones P, Gatton DAG, Payne PM (1952) Cancer of the breast. A review. Br J Radiol [Suppl 4]
54. Strauss BS (1977) Molecular biology of the response of cells to radiation and to radiomimetic chemicals. Cancer 40: 471–480
55. Tancini G, Bonadonna G, Valagussa P, Marchini S, Veronesi U (1983) Adjuvant CMF in breast cancer: comparative 5-year results of 12 versus 6 cycles. J Clin Oncol 1: 2–10
56. Webber BL, Heise H, Neifeld JP, Costa J (1981) Risk of subsequent contralateral breast carcinoma in a population of patients with in-situ breast carcinoma. Cancer 47: 2928–2932
57. Weisburger EK (1977) Bioassay program for carcinogenic hazards of cancer chemotherapeutic agents. Cancer 40: 1935–1949
58. Weisburger JH, Griswold DP Jr, Prejean JD, Casey AE, Wood HB, Weisburger EK (1975) The carcinogenic properties of some of the principal drugs used in clinical cancer chemotherapy. Recent Results Cancer Res 52: 1–17

Tamoxifen and Combination Chemotherapy as Adjuvant Treatment in Postmenopausal Women with Breast Cancer

A. Wallgren, E. Baral, U. Beling, J. Carstensen, S. Friberg, U. Glas, M. Kaigas, and L. Skoog

Stockholm-Gotland Oncologic Centre, Radiumhemmet, Karolinska Hospital, 107 01 Stockholm, Sweden

Introduction

The general acceptance of breast cancer as a systemic disorder with lymph node metastases as an indicator of poor prognosis has stimulated the search for effective means to control micrometastases. While the early trials on prolonged adjuvant chemotherapy significantly delayed the onset of relapse in premenopausal women, breast cancer in the postmeno-pausal group of patients was apparently less affected [1, 2]. In postmenopausal women tamoxifen has proved to be of value in the palliative treatment of advanced breast cancer and has usually few and mild side effects. Several groups of investigators have therefore included tamoxifen in the adjuvant treatment of breast cancer, either alone or in combination with cytotoxic chemotherapy; for a review consult Mouridsen and Palshof [3].

In 1976, studies were initiated in the Stockholm-Gotland health care region in Sweden, aimed at exploring the efficacy of adjuvant systemic treatment of operable breast cancer. These studies included tamoxifen in postmenopausal women (irrespective of stage) and cytotoxic combination chemotherapy in premenopausal and postmenopausal women with large tumors or axillary node involvement. Postmenopausal women then, with this stage of disease were included in both studies; this is an interim report of the results of their treatment.

Material and Methods

Patients

Postmenopausal women who had been treated with a modified radical mastectomy for breast carcinoma were eligible for the present study if they were less than 71 years of age and the tumor was greater than 30 mm in the surgical specimen or there were lymph node metastases.

Between November 1976 and December 1982, 331 patients entered this trial. In a two-by-two fashion these patients were randomly allocated to adjuvant cytotoxic chemotherapy or to postoperative radiotherapy, and to tamoxifen or to no further endocrine treatment. The distribution of patients by treatment combinations is given in Table 1. During a period of the study more patients were randomized to chemotherapy

Recent Results in Cancer Research. Vol. 96
© Springer-Verlag Berlin · Heidelberg 1984

Table 1. Number of patients and number of patients with treatment failure in the treatment groups

Treatment group	No. of patients	No. of patients with failure			
		Local	Distant	Death	Any
Adjuvant chemotherapy	173	42	62	50	83
Tamoxifen	86	17	27	23	35
Controls	87	25	35	27	48
Radiotherapy	158	14	44	38	51
Tamoxifen	82	7	22	17	25
Controls	76	7	22	21	26
Total	331	56	106	88	134

than to radiotherapy because of a temporary shortage of radiation treatment machine capacity. There were no lymph node metastases in 11% of the cases. In 54% there were 1−3 metastatic nodes, and in 34% more than three nodes were involved. The distribution of cases with different numbers of lymph node metastases was similar in all treatment combinations.

Estrogen Receptors

These were determined in one laboratory using isoelectric focusing on slabs of polyacrylamide gel [4]. Quantitative receptor data were obtained for 82% of the tumors. A level of 0.10 fmol/µg DNA constitutes the arbitrary distinction between receptorpoor and receptorrich tumors. In 28% of the cases, the tumors were poor in receptor protein.

Tamoxifen

This treatment was given for 2 years and the daily dose prescribed was 40 mg.

Cytotoxic Chemotherapy

The regimen consisted of 12 courses of 5-fluorouracil at 600 mg/m^2, and of methotrexate at 40 mg/m^2, i.v. on days 1 and 8 of each course. Initially, chlorambucil was given orally in a dose of 10−15 mg on days 1 through 8 and the next course was given on day 42. After a year and a half, chlorambucil was replaced by cyclophosphamide, 100 mg/m^2, orally on days 1 through 14 and the next course was started on day 28. The treatment policy was changed because chlorambucil caused progressive depression of the thrombocytes. The doses were reduced in women 65 years of age or older, and according to hematologic toxicity as outlined by Bonadonna et al. [2].

The doses of chemotherapy have been calculated as described by Bonadonna and Valagussa [5]. They were expressed as percentages of the total dose which would have been given in 12 courses with no reduction. No reduction was calculated for those over 64 years of age. If a woman experienced a recurrence before 12 courses had been given, the total "ideal" dose was calculated only up to and including the last course before the relapse.

Postoperative radiotherapy

This was given by high voltage machines. The target area included the chest wall and the lymph node regions of the axilla, the supra- and infraclavicular fossae and the ipsilateral internal mammary region. The treatment was delivered with a daily dose of 2.0 Gy, 5 days a week to a total dose of 46.0 Gy.

Follow-up

The follow-up includes all eligible patients, irrespective of whether treatment was given or not. The mean follow-up period was 49 months with a range of 12−87 months.

Statistical Analysis

Time to any failure (local or distant recurrence or death) and to death from any cause were analysed using the log-rank test [6]. The Cox regression model was used to study the simultaneous influence of several factors including interaction between the variables [7]. Significance levels are represented by P-values for two-sided tests.

Results

Complicance

Tamoxifen was generally well tolerated. Side effects, including gastrointestinal disturbance and hot flashes, were usually mild, but were the reason for a premature interruption of the treatment in 14% of the patients.

Cytotoxic chemotherapy caused the commonly encountered side effects, such as nausea, mucositis, and lethargy. The patients were prerandomized and 4% of them refused to accept the treatment. They were, however, included in the analyses. The doses were reduced in many patients, mainly due to hematologic toxicity as prescribed in the protocol. Only 27% of the patients received more than 84% of the dose according to the protocol. Furthermore, since the protocol prescribed a dose reduction in women 65 years of age or older only 18% of the patients received more than 84% of the unreduced dose. In 51%, including 4% who refused any treatment, the dose was less than 65% of the "ideal" dose.

Prognostic importance of lymph node metastases and estrogen receptors

Both number of lymph node metastases (0, 1−3, 4+) and estrogen receptor status were significant predictors of relapse and death. The predictive information in both variables were independent of each other and of the treatment modalities.

Table 2. Relative recurrence rates (95% confidence limits) in the different treatment comparisons. The rates were obtained from a Cox regression analysis including an interaction term between chemotherapy/radiotherapy and tamoxifen

Treatment comparisons	Relative recurrence rates
Chemotherapy vs radiotherapy	
Total material	1.52 (1.07−2.16)
Tamoxifen group	1.33 (0.80−2.23)
No tamoxifen group	1.70 (1.05−2.75)
Tamoxifen vs no tamoxifen	
Total material	0.64 (0.46−0.90)
Chemotherapy group	0.58 (0.38−0.91)
Radiotherapy group	0.75 (0.43−1.30)

Effect of Treatment on Relapse Rate and Death Rate

The number and type of failures are given in each of the treatment groups in Table 1.

Adjuvant Cytotoxic Chemotherapy/Radiotherapy

There were significantly more recurrences in the chemotherapy group than in the radiotherapy group (Table 2, relative recurrence rate 1.52/1, $P = 0.01$). As is seen in Table 1, the main reason for the difference is the much higher frequency of local-regional recurrences after chemotherapy than after radiotherapy.

In patients for whom the dose of chemotherapy exceeded 84% of the "ideal" dose, the rate of recurrence was approximately 70% of that for patients who received lower doses, but this difference was not statistically significant ($P = 0.26$).

There was no significant difference in mortality rates in the chemotherapy group and the radiotherapy group (relative mortality rates 1.2/1, $P = 0.36$).

Adjuvant Tamoxifen

Tamoxifen significantly decreased the rate of recurrence compared to the controls (Table 2, relative recurrence rate 0.66/1, $P = 0.02$).

In the Cox regression model both cytostatic chemotherapy/radiotherapy and tamoxifen independently influenced the rate of recurrence (Table 2). No interaction was found between any of the treatments and the lymph node status. Though there was no significant interaction between tamoxifen and chemotherapy/radiotherapy ($P = 0.49$), the interaction factor indicated that tamoxifen may have been slightly more effective in the chemotherapy group than in the radiotherapy group (Table 2).

In Table 3 the relative recurrence rates of the tamoxifen patients compared to those of their controls are given by dose of chemotherapy for the chemotherapy groups of patients. Tamoxifen reduced the rate of recurrence at all dose levels and no consistent relation is visible between the effect of tamoxifen and the dose of chemotherapy.

Table 3. Relative recurrence-rates of tamoxifen-treated patients in comparison to their controls according to dose levels of chemotherapy among patients randomized to receive adjuvant chemotherapy

Dose level of chemotherapy (%)	Relative recurrence rates (95% confidence limitis)
< 65	0.73 (0.41−1.31)
65−84	0.37 (0.16−0.83)
> 84	0.79 (0.23−2.76)
Total	0.60 (0.39−0.94)

In the present material there was little interaction between the effect of tamoxifen and estrogen receptor status on the recurrence rate. The relative recurrence rate of the tamoxifen patients compared to that of the controls was $0.61/1$ ($P = 0.16$) for patients with receptor-poor tumors and $0.63/1$ ($P = 0.04$) if the tumor was receptor rich.

The mortality rate was not significantly influenced by tamoxifen treatment (relative mortality rate $0.76/1$, $P = 0.20$).

Discussion

Despite the fact that several randomized trials have been conducted, the merit of adjuvant cytotoxic chemotherapy in postmenopausal women remains controversial. The subject of adjuvant treatment has recently been reviewed by Mouridsen and Palshof [3]. Bonadonna and Valagussa [5] concluded from a retrospective analysis of their trials that the generally low doses delivered to postmenopausal women were the reason for the discrepant effectiveness in premenopausal and postmenopausal women. However, attractive this hypothesis may seem, it has not yet been supported by a properly designed prospective trial. A recent report from the Southwest Oncology Group on CMFVP vs melphalan indicated that CMFVP for 1 year improved the freedom from relapse and survival in both premenopausal and postmenopausal women [8]. Since CMFVP probably is more effective than melphalan in the treatment of advanced disease, this study might give some support for the hypothesis of a dose-related response. Unfortunately, it is difficult to know whether such conclusions can be derived from that trial. For instance, approximately 33% of the patients were entirely or partially excluded from analysis for various reasons, including refusal to continue treatment and early death. Such exclusions were slightly more common in one of the treatment groups and may well have biased the results.

The dose levels achieved in our trial were similar to those in the Milan trials [5]. Whether the doses were insufficient or there is a general resistance to the drugs, the treatment was less effective than postoperative radiotherapy in preventing local-regional relapses. In fact, the results of chemotherapy treatment resembled those of no further treatment in our previous study on preoperative and postoperative treatment in operable breast cancer [9]. So far, we have not seen any difference in survival between the treatment groups. Because of the side-effects of adjuvant cytotoxic chemotherapy, a major impact on survival is necessary before this type of treatment should be routinely recommended.

The efficacy of tamoxifen in the treatment of advanced breast cancer and the few and mild side effects made this drug an attractive alternative or complement to cytotoxic chemotherapy in the adjuvant treatment of breast cancer. Several groups have included tamoxifen in their adjuvant armory. Most of the reported results indicate a prolongation of the relapse-free interval [3, 10−14]. The British group also recently reported a significantly prolonged survival in the tamoxifen-treated patients [16].

Results of treatment with a combination of tamoxifen and cytotoxic chemotherapy have also been reported [13, 14]. As in our trial, the addition of tamoxifen to cytotoxic chemotherapy improved the relapse-free survival in these studies.

At the present time, no definite conclusions can be drawn concerning the place of adjuvant therapy of breast cancer in postmenopausal women. It is obvious, that the impact on survival of any of the reported combinations has been less than what may have been anticipated on the receipt of the initial optimistic reports [1, 2]. Such treatment, therefore, should still be considered as experimental. Future trials should be designed to improve treatment results as well as to find the least toxic treatment combinations able to prolong the most critical part of the woman's life after treatment for breast cancer, i.e., the time to the first recurrence if it was not cured [15, 16]. Therefore, locally effective treatment, using surgery and radiotherapy, should be included in trials. Because of the low toxicity of tamoxifen, this drug might be useful for the adjuvant treatment even if the ultimate cure rate is little influenced.

Acknowledgement. This study was supported with grants from the King Gustav V Jubilee Fund.

References

1. Fisher B, Carbone P, Economou SG, et al. (1975) L-Phenylalanine mustard (L-PAM) in the management of primary breast cancer. A report of early findings. N Engl J Med 292: 117−122
2. Bonadonna G, Brusamolino E, Valagussa P, et al. (1976) Combination chemotherapy as an adjuvant treatment in operable breast cancer. N Engl J Med 294: 405−410
3. Mouridsen HT, Palshof T (1983) Adjuvant systemic therapy in breast cancer; a review. Eur J Cancer Clin Oncol 19: 1753−1770
4. Wrange Ö, Nordenskjöld B, Gustafsson J-Å (1978) Cytosol estradiol receptor in human mammary carcinoma: An assay based on isoelectric focusing in polyacrylamide gel. Anal Biochem 85: 461−475
5. Bonadonna G, Valagussa P (1981) Dose-response effect of adjuvant chemotherapy in breast cancer. N Engl J Med 304: 10−15
6. Peto R, Pike MC, Armitage P, et al. (1977) Design and analysis of randomized clinical trials requiring prolonged observation of each patient. II. Analysis and examples. Br J Cancer 35: 1−39
7. Cox DR (1972) Regression models and life tables. JR Stat Soc [B] 34: 187−220
8. Knight WA, Rivkin SE, Glucksberg H, et al. (1983) Adjuvant therapy of breast cancer: the Southwest Oncology Group experience. Breast Cancer Res Treat [Suppl 1] 3: 27−33
9. Strender L-E, Wallgren A, Arndt J, et al. (1981) Adjuvant radiotherapy in operable breast cancer: correlation between dose in internal mammary nodes and prognosis. Int J Radiat Oncol Biol Phys 7: 1319−1325
10. Nolvadex Adjuvant Trial Organisation (1983) Controlled trial of tamoxifen as adjuvant agent in management of early breast cancer. Lancet 1: 257−261
11. Wallgren A, Baral E, Glas U, et al. (1981) Adjuvant treatment of breast cancer with tamoxifen and combination chemotherapy in postmenopausal women. In: Salmon SE, Jones SE (eds) Adjuvant therapy of cancer III. Grune and Stratton, New York, pp 345−350
12. Palshof T, Mouridsen HT, Daehnfeldt JL (1980) Adjuvant endocrine therapy of primary operable breast cancer. Report on the Copenhagen breast cancer trials. Eur J Cancer 16: 183−187

13. Pearson OH, Hubay CA, Marshall JS, et al. (1983) Adjuvant endocrine therapy, cytotoxic chemotherapy, and immunotherapy in stage-II breast cancer: five-year results. Breast Cancer Res Treat [Suppl 1] 3:61–68
14. Fisher B (1983) Treatment of primary breast cancer with L-PAM/5-FU and tamoxifen: an interim report. Breast Cancer Res Treat [Suppl 1] 3:7–17
15. Baum M, Brinkley DM, Dossett JA, et al. (1983) Improved survival amongst patients treated with adjuvant tamoxifen after mastectomy for early breast cancer. Lancet 1:450
16. Baum M (1982) Scientific empirism and clinical medicine. In: Baum M, Kay R, Scheurlen H (eds) Clinical trials in early breast cancer. Birkhäuser, Basel, pp 35–46

Ludwig Breast Cancer Trials LBCS III and IV: Adjuvant Endocrine Treatment in Postmenopausal Patients

A. Goldhirsch*

Ludwig Institut für Krebsforschung. Inselspital, 3010 Bern, Switzerland

Introduction

In July 1978, the Ludwig Breast Cancer Study (LBCS) Group (see Appendix A) initiated four complementary randomized controlled clinical trials to evaluate adjuvant therapy in both pre- and postmenopausal patients with operable breast cancer and axillary lymph-node involvement. The postmenopausal patients who were randomly allocated to receive either endocrine therapy alone or mastectomy alone are the subject of this report (Fig. 1). The studies terminated accrual of patients on August 31, 1981.

Materials and Methods

Postmenopausal women, defined by menstrual history or by endocrine testing (Table 1) who were 80 years of age or less and who had histologically confirmed, noninflammatory, unilateral breast carcinoma with axillary lymph node metastasis, were considered for eligibility in the two studies. Treatment of the primary was by total mastectomy and axillary clearance for disease staged according to the International TNM Classification as $T_{1A \text{ or } B}$, $T_{2A \text{ or } B}$, T_{3A}, $N_{0 \text{ or } 1}$ (but with histologically proven axillary node metastasis); M_0 was a requirement. A chest radiograph and bone scan (with X-rays of "hot spots", if applicable) were required for exclusion of detectable metastatic disease. A peripheral white blood cell count of $\geq 4,000/mm^3$, a platelet count of $\geq 100,000/mm^3$, creatinine of $< 130 \, \mu mol/l$, bilirubin $< 20 \, \mu mol/l$ and SGOT of < 60 IU were also required.

Treatment with endocrine therapy was started within 6 weeks of surgery and continued for 12 months. Standardized follow-up assessment were required every 3 months for 2 years and every 6 months thereafter. All study records (eligibility, treatment, toxicity, and recurrence) were reviewed centrally by the study coordinator.

Estrogen and progesterone receptor results of ≥ 10 fmol/mg cytosol protein were considered positive and values below this as negative. Estrogen receptor (ER) results were available for 49% of the patients and progesterone receptor (PR) results for 44%. Histological type and grade based on a central pathology review were available for 96% of the patients. A total of 629 patients were available for the comparison of adjuvant endocrine therapy with observation (Fig. 1). The distribution of relevant patient

---

* Ludwig Breast Cancer Study Group, see pp. 208, 209

Recent Results in Cancer Research. Vol. 96
© Springer-Verlag Berlin · Heidelberg 1984

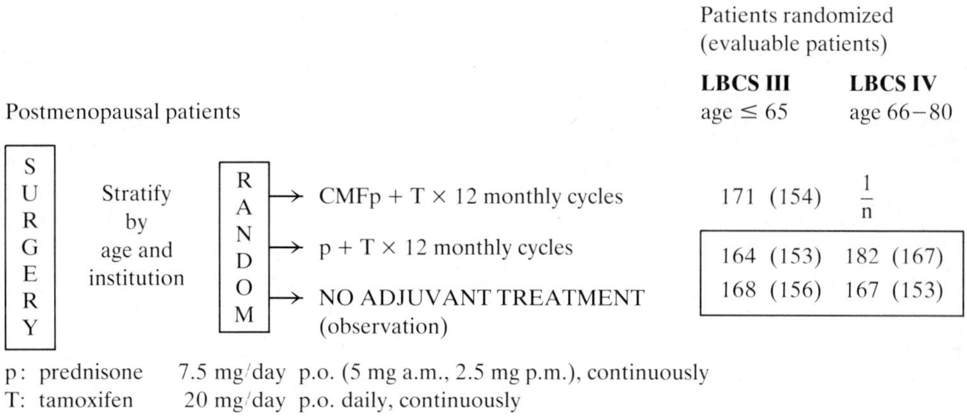

Patients randomized
(evaluable patients)

| | LBCS III
age ≤ 65 | LBCS IV
age 66−80 |

Postmenopausal patients

					LBCS III age ≤ 65	LBCS IV age 66−80

S
U   Stratify   R
R   by   A   → CMFp + T × 12 monthly cycles   171 (154) $\frac{1}{n}$
G   age and   N
E   institution   D   → p + T × 12 monthly cycles   164 (153)   182 (167)
R   O
Y   M   → NO ADJUVANT TREATMENT   168 (156)   167 (153)
                                        (observation)

p: prednisone   7.5 mg/day p.o. (5 mg a.m., 2.5 mg p.m.), continuously
T: tamoxifen   20 mg/day p.o. daily, continuously

Fig. 1. Protocol in LBCS III and IV. The abbreviation p (rather than P) stress the fact that low-dose prednisone was given

Table 1. Definition of postmenopausal patients

Condition	Age
A) At least 1 year amenorrhea, no hysterectomy	> 52 years
B) At least 3 years amenorrhea, no hysterectomy	≤ 52 years
C) Biochemical evidence of cessation of ovarian function for doubtful patients with regard to A and B	Any age
D) Hysterectomy without bilateral oophorectomy	≥ 56 years
E) More than 1 year after bilateral oophorectomy	Any age

characteristics (extent of nodal involvement, tumor size, ER and PR status, histological type and grade, extent of surgical procedure) were balanced between the two treatment regimens.

This analysis was performed on data available on all eligible patients as of October 1, 1983, with a median follow-up of 36 months. The treatment comparison was performed using a stratified analysis combining LBCS III and IV. For analysis of disease-free survival (DFS), *failure* was defined as any recurrence, appearance of a second primary malignancy, or death, whichever occurred first.

The Kaplan-Meier method [1] was used to estimate survival distributions for DFS and overall survival. The log-rank procedure [2] was utilized to assess the statistical significance of treatment differences between these survival distributions. Times were measured from the data of randomization. Tests of significance for treatment effects were carried out adjusting for prognostic factors (nodal status and ER status), using the Cox proportional hazard regression model [3].

Results

Disease-free survival was significantly increased for women who received prednisone + tamoxifen (p + T) as compared with those who had no adjuvant therapy (observation),

Table 2. LBCS III and IV: Endocrine therapy vs observation − DFS and overall survival by treatment (36 months median follow-up)

	p + T	Observation	P^a
Total no. patients	(320)	(309)	
A) 3-year DFS			
1. Overall	58 ± 3[a]	44 ± 3	0.001
2. Nodal status			
N+ 1−3	70 ± 4	53 ± 4	0.003
N+ ≥ 4	42 ± 5	31 ± 4	0.07
B) 3-year overall			
survival	75 ± 3	80 ± 3	0.032

For DFS, failure is defined as recurrence, second primary, or death, whichever occurred first
Results expressed as Kaplan-Meier percent ± SE
[a] Stratified by study (LBCS III or IV)

Table 3. Endocrine treatment in LBCS III and IV: DFS by treatment and ER and PR content in the tumor

3-year DFS	p + T	Observation	P^a
ER+	67 ± 5[a] (104)	49 ± 5 (100)	0.02
ER−	30 ± 7 (51)	40 ± 8 (50)	0.86
PR+	73 ± 6 (65)	59 ± 7 (60)	0.2
PR−	42 ± 6 (74)	38 ± 6 (77)	0.64
ER+/PR+	77 ± 6 (56)	57 ± 7 (54)	0.035
ER−/PR−	27 ± 8 (39)	35 ± 8 (42)	0.49
ER unknown	61 ± 4 (165)	43 ± 4 (159)	0.002

Results expressed as Kaplan-Meier percent (%) ± SE with no. of patients in parentheses
[a] Stratified by study

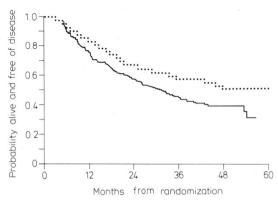

Treatment	Failed / total	3-year DFS (±s.e.)
..... p+T	131 / 320	58% (± 3%)
—— OBS	169 / 309	44% (± 3%)

Fig. 2. DFS in LBCS III and IV

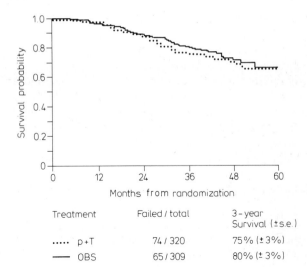

Treatment	Failed / total	3-year Survival (±s.e.)
····· p+T	74 / 320	75% (±3%)
—— OBS	65 / 309	80% (±3%)

Fig. 3. Survival in LBCS III and IV

both in patients ≤ 65 years (LBCS III; $P = 0.008$) and in patients 66–80 years old (LBCS IV; $P = 0.05$). The effect of treatment, using the combined data (stratified by study), is shown in Table 2 and Fig. 2. No survival advantage has been observed ($P = 0.32$) (Fig. 3). Treatment results according to ER and PR content are summarized in Table 3. Comparison of sites of first failure showed that p + T decreased only the number of local and regional disease relapses: There were 42 local and/or regional first failures for p + T-treated patients as compared with 85 for the control group. First failures in distant sites were the same for the two populations (72 patients failed in each).

Toxic Effects

The frequency of severe hematologic and nonhematologic toxic effects of p + T was 3.5%, of which thrombosis and/or embolism occurred in 1% of the treated patients. Although no fatalities were definitely attributable to treatment, seven of the 16 patients who expired without evidence of recurrent cancer died within the first year.

Discussion

In these trials endocrine therapy consisted of a combination of tamoxifen and low-dose prednisone given continuously for 1 year. At a median follow-up of 36 months, the endocrine therapy was shown to significantly increase the DFS of treated patients with operable breast cancer and lymph node metastases in the axilla ($0 = 0.001$) (Fig. 2). This advantage was noted in patients with ER+ tumors while those with ER− tumors did not benefit from the treatment. In our randomized controlled trial, patients with unknown hormone receptor content had treatment results similar to those of patients whose tumors were ER+. This is probably due to the fact that more than two-thirds of the postmenopausal patient population will have ER+ tumors. In our study the proportion increased with age (61% ER+ in LBCS III, 74% in LBCS IV). Information about progesterone receptor content might add prognostic significance to the data available concerning ER content (Table 3, ER+ vs ER+/PR+). Analysis of sites of first failure high-lighted the fact that DFS anvantage for the endocrine-treated population was due to control of local and/or regional disease. No difference between the frequency of first failure in distant sites has been observed. No survival differences were observed, in contrast to another trial using tamoxifen [4] in which an overall survival advantage appeared at an average follow-up time of 35 months. Further follow-up is necessary for an evaluation of the place of adjuvant endocrine therapy in the treatment of postmenopausal women with breast cancer. At the present time it seems clear that this form of endocrine therapy is useful for control of local and regional disease.

Ludwig Breast Cancer Study Group: LBCS (Toxicity Report. Pilot and First Series)

Institution	
Ludwig Institute for Cancer Research, Inselspital, Bern, Switzerland	A. Goldhirsch (*Study Coordinator*), W. Hartmann, B. Davis, D. Zava, M. de Marval
Frontier Science and Technology Research Foundation, Boston, USA	R. Gelber (*Study Statistician*), M. Isley, L. Szymoniak, M. Zelen
Auckland Breast Cancer Study Group, Auckland, New Zealand	R. G. Kay, J. Probert, B. Mason, H. Wood, E. G. Gifford, J. F. Carter, J. C. Gillmann, J, Anderson, L. Yee, I. M. Holdaway, G. C. Hitchcock, M. Jagusch
Groote Schuur Hospital, Cape Town, Rep. of South Africa	A. Hacking, D. M. Dent, J. Terblanche, A. Tiltman, A. Gudgeon, E. Dowdle, R. Sealy, P. Palmer
University of Essen, West German Tumor Center, Essen, Germany	C. G. Schmidt, F. Schüning, K. Höffken, L. D. Leder, H. Ludwig, R. Callies, P. Faber, H. Bender, H. Bojar
Swedish Western Breast Cancer Study Group, Göteborg, Sweden	C.-M. Rudenstam, E. Cahlin, H. Salander, I. Branehög, G. Jäderström, R. Hultborn, U. Wannholt, S. Nilsson, J. Fornander, J. Säve-Söderbergh, Ch. Johnsén, O. Ruusvik, G. Ostberg, L. Mattsson, C. G. Bäckström, S. Bergegardh, U. Ljungqvist, I. Dahl, Y. Hessman, S. Holmberg, S. Dahlin, G. Wallin
The Institute of Oncology, Ljubljana, Yugoslavia	J. Lindtner, J. Novak, J. Cervek, O. Cerar, P. Mavec, R. Golouh, J. Lamovec, J. Jancar, S. Sebek
Madrid Breast Cancer Group, Madrid, Spain	H. Cortés-Funes, F. Martinez-Tello, F. Cruz Caro, M. L. Marcos, M. A. Figueras, F. Calero, A. Suarez, F. Pastrana, R. Huertas
Anti-Cancer Council of Victoria, Melbourne, Australia	J. Collins, I. Russell, M. A. Schwarz, J. F. Forbes, P. R. B. Kitchen, L. Sisely, R. Reed, E. Guli, R. C. Bennett, J. W. Funder, L. Harrison, G. Brodie, W. I. Burns, R. D. Snyder, P. Jeal, J. H. Colebatch

Institution	
Sir Charles Gairdner Hospital Nedlands, Western Australia	M. Byrne, P. M. Reynolds, H. J. Sheiner, S. Levitt, D. Kermode, K. B. Shilkin, R. Hähnel
SAKK (Swiss Group for Clin. Cancer Res.) − Basel, Kantonsspital	J. P. Obrecht, F. Harder, A. C. Almendral, U. Eppenberger, J. Torhorst
− Bern, Inselspital	K. Brunner, P. Aeberhard, H. Cottier, K. Bürki, A. Zimermann, E. Dreher, G. Locher, M. Berger, M. Walther, R. Joss, A. Gervasi, P. Herrmann
− Geneva, Hopital Cantonal Universitaire	P. Alberto, F. Krauer, R. Egeli, R. Mégevand, M. Forni, P. Schäfer, E. Jacot des Combes, A. M. Schindler, F. Leski
− Neuchatel, Hôpital des Cadolles	P. Siegenthaler, V. Barrelet, R. P. Baumann
− St. Gallen, Kantonsspital	W. F. Jungi, H. J. Senn, A. Mutzner, U. Schmid, Th. Hardmeier, E. Hochuli, O. Schildknecht
− Bellinzona, Ospedale San Giovanni	F. Cavalli, M. Varini, P. Luscieti, E. S. Passega, G. Losa
− Zurich, Universitätsspital	G. Martz, T. Muller, R. Maurer, E. S. Siebenmann, W. E. Schreiner, V. Engeler, C. Genton, H. J. Schmid
Ludwig Institute for Cancer Research, and Royal Prince Alfred Hospital, Sydney, Australia	M. H. N. Tattersall, R. Fox, A. Coates, D. Raghavan, F. Niesche, R. West, S. Renwick, D. Green, J. Donovan, P. Duval, A. Ng, T. Foo, D. Glenn, T. J. Nash, R. A. North, J. Beith, G. O'Connor
Wellington Hospital, Wellington, New Zealand	J. S. Simpson, L. Hollaway, C. Unsworth

References

1. Kaplan EL, Meier P (1958) Nonparametric estimation from incomplete observation. J Am Statist Assoc 53: 457−481
2. Peto R, Pike MC, Armitage P, Breslow NE et al. (1977) Design and analysis of randomized clinical trials requiring prolonged observation of each patient Br J Cancer 35: 1−39
3. Cox DR (1972) Regression models and life tables (with discussion). J R Statist Soc B (Methodol) 34: 187−220
4. Baum M, Brinkley DM, Dossett JA, McPherson K, Patterson GS, Rubens RD, Smiddy FG, Stoll BA, Wilson A, Lea JC, Richards D, Ellis SM Improved survival amongst patients treated with adjuvant tamoxifen after mastectomy for early breast cancer

Problems of Combined Adjuvant Radiochemotherapy

P. C. Veraguth

Klinik für Radiotherapie, Universitätsklinik, Inselspital, 3010 Bern, Switzerland

Adjuvant chemotherapy has been found to improve recurrence-free survival time for stage II breast cancer after mastectomy, at least for premenopausal patients [3, 9]. On the other hand, we are aware of the fact that a routinely applied postoperative radiotherapy for all operated mammary carcinoma, stage I and II does not influence the survival time. Nevertheless, the Scandinavien randomized study with 960 patients, reported by Wallgren [18] has to be mentioned. Compared with a group of patients treated only by surgery the post- or preoperative radiotherapy improves the relapse-free survival time after 6 years by about 15% (Fig. 1). This difference appears even more distinct for tumors localized in the inner quadrants (Fig. 2). This same study showed that local and lymph node recurrences diminished about three times as much in the radiotherapy group (pre- and postoperative) as in the surgically treated patients, but the distant metastases were equally frequent in all three groups (between 22% and 25% at 6 years) (Table 1).

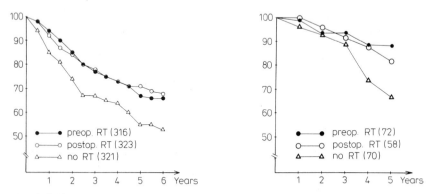

Fig. 1 (*left*). Actuarial survival at 6 years of operable breast carcinoma, stage II, treated by surgery alone or by surgery with preoperative or postoperative radiotherapy. Randomized study. The figures in *parentheses* are numbers of patients. The figures on the *ordinate* signify the percentage of relapse-free survivors (Wallgren [18])

Fig. 2 (*right*). Same study as shown in Fig. 1, but concerning only the tumors in the *inner* quadrants. The difference between patients treated by surgery alone and those treated by surgery and adjuvant radiotherapy (preoperative or postoperative) is significant (Wallgren [18])

Recent Results in Cancer Research. Vol. 96
© Springer-Verlag Berlin · Heidelberg 1984

Table 1. Number of patients with recurrences (Wallgren [18])

Treatment group	Locoregional recurrence	Distant metastases	All recurrences
Preoperative irradiation	23	73	81
Postoperative irradiation	21	76	79
No irradiation	69	84	115
Total	113	233	275

Relying on these facts, in order to improve results, it seems reasonable to try a combination of radio- and chemotherapy as an adjuvant method for stage II breast cancer with positive axillary lymph nodes.

In connection with this the following questions arise and will be discussed briefly:

1. Will the long-term results be improved by adding irradiation to chemotherapy or do the combined methods have an adverse effect?
2. Is there an enhancement of early toxicity or of late tissue alterations, and to what extend should the adjuvant treatment possibly be adapted?
3. Is it possible to combine a definitive irradiation for primary breast cancer (tumorectomy) with adjuvant chemotherapy?

There are not a great number of randomized studies dealing with question 1. The first study, reported in 1978 by Ahmann [1] compared the effect of L-phenylalanine mustard (L-PAM) to cyclophosphamide, 5-FU and prednisone (CFP) with and without irradiation for operated breast cancer, stage II. Based on 3 years-survival time, the recurrence rate for the L-PAM group was 42%. The adjuvant treatment group with CFP yielded better results, with (15%) or without (13%) radiotherapy; therefore, no further improvement was accomplished by the addition of irradiation. Acute myelotoxicity in the CFP group was about the same with or without radiotherapy, but after irradiation an edema of the arm was observed twice as frequently.

L-PAM and cyclophosphamide, methotrexate (MTX), and 5-FU (CMF) − combined or not with radiotherapy − were submitted to a comparative study by Cooper from the Bowman Gray and the Piedmont Oncology Association [7]. For the CMF group, with and without postoperative irradiation, the MTX dose was lowered to half ($20 \, mg/m^2$), compared with the original Bonadonna scheme [3]. CMF given alone had a better effect than did L-PAM, but the recurrence rate for the CMF + radiotherapy series was higher than for CMF given alone.

A comparative study, not entirely randomized, was undertaken by Allen [2] and completed by Jones [11], using adriamycin and cyclophosphamide (AC), with or without radiotherapy. The chemotherapy alone was administered in 3-week cycles, with a total of 8 cycles. For the combined group 2 cycles of AC were given followed by radiotherapy 1 week after the second adriamycin application in order to avoid a too strong skin toxicity. In this way the combined radio- and chemotherapy was well supported, and a decrease of the dose was needed in a few cases only. On the whole, the relapse-free survival time after 5 years reached about 65% for all node-positive cases (Fig. 3). For the group of patients with 1−3 positive lymph nodes the results were far better for the combined treatment AC + radiotherapy (Fig. 4), but in presence of more than four positive lymph nodes this difference disappeared and the subset of combined treatment patients had even a worse result (Fig. 5).

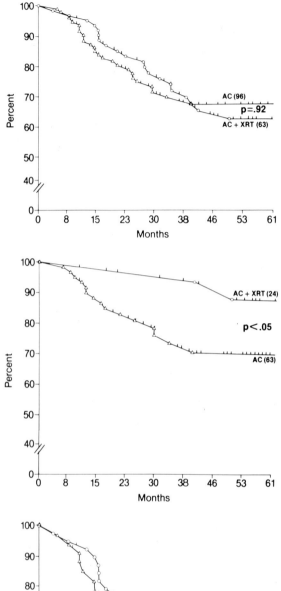

Fig. 3. Relapse-free survival rate over 5 years of stage II operable breast cancer treated by adriamycin + cyclophosphamide *(AC)* alone or by *AC* + radiotherapy *(XRT)*. The irradiation of the chest wall and of the regional lymph nodes (44 Gy) was started after the second cycle of *AC*. Number of patients are shown in parentheses (Allen [2])

Fig. 4. Same treatment schedules for cases with 1−3 axillary positive lymph nodes. The difference in favor of the combined treatment modality including radiotherapy approaches statistical relevance (Allen [2])

Fig. 5. For patients with more than 3 positive axillary lymph nodes additional radiotherapy offers no advantages. The group *AC* + *XRT* has an even lower survival rate (by about 15%) than the *AC* group (Allen [2])

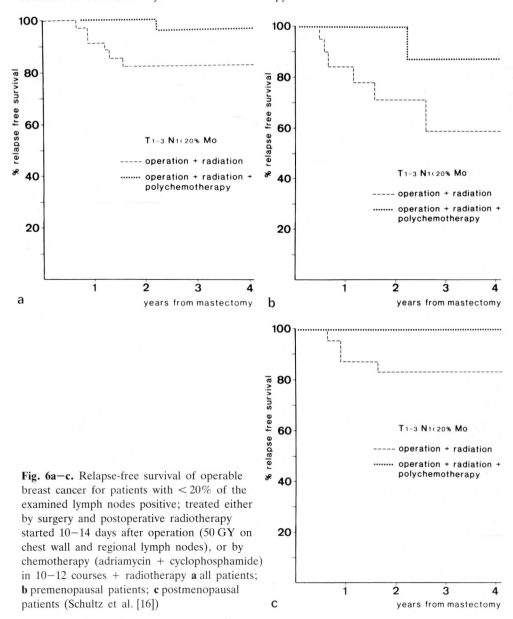

Fig. 6a–c. Relapse-free survival of operable breast cancer for patients with < 20% of the examined lymph nodes positive; treated either by surgery and postoperative radiotherapy started 10–14 days after operation (50 GY on chest wall and regional lymph nodes), or by chemotherapy (adriamycin + cyclophosphamide) in 10–12 courses + radiotherapy **a** all patients; **b** premenopausal patients; **c** postmenopausal patients (Schultz et al. [16])

A similar study was undertaken by Schulz [16] for stage II premenopausal breast cancer patients: at least 10 axillary lymph nodes were examined. According to the number of positive lymph nodes (more or less than 20%) two subsets were formed, group II and group III; group I, without lymph node metastases (pN0), will not be considered here. An immediate postoperative radiotherapy was applied (50 Gy) to the patients of group II followed by 12 cycles of AC every 3 to 4 weeks (Fig. 6a) − that means that the chemotherapy regime started only 6 to 7 weeks after mastectomy. The difference is apparent in premenopausal (Fig. 6b) as well as in postmenopausal patients (Fig. 6c). For group III, with more than 20% positive lymph nodes, a subset was treated by adjuvant

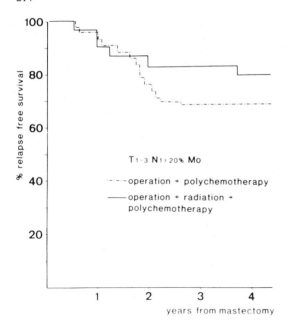

Fig. 7. Relapse-free survival of operable breast cancer for patients with > 20% of the examined lymph nodes positive (Schulz et al. [16])

chemotherapy AC within 10−14 days of operating, whereas the others received radiotherapy first and the entire chemotherapeutic treatment later on (Fig. 7). Relapse-free survival is enhanced by 11% in cases with more than 20% positive axillary lymph nodes, if a combined treatment including radiotherapy is applied [16]. On the whole, a trend favoring patients treated *with* additional radiotherapy is noted, especially in the case of premenopausal women, but the limited time of observation leaves this inconclusive.

Astonishingly, in cases with more than four positive lymph nodes the gain of additional radiotherapy does not seem to meliorate the relapse-free survival time. Further randomized series should be made to determine whether a chemotherapeutic regimen with AC + radiotherapy yields better results than a regime containing MTX.

Preliminary conclusions

Consideration of these data suggests reintroduction for well-determined groups of patients, of a limited postoperative radiotherapy in additon to the adjuvant chemotherapy. This combined regime would be suitable for: (a) patients (pre- and postmenopausal) with 1−3 positive axillary lymph nodes to whom radiotherapy would be applied on the thoracic wall and the supraclavicular region; and (b) patients with primary tumors located in the inner quadrants, in which case the retrosternal region would be irradiated.

As was to be expected, acute toxicity of combined radio- and chemotherapy is more intense; MTX- and CYT-containing therapy schedules show an increased myelotoxicity and patients treated with ADM and MTX had strong skin reactions.

Based upon the findings of Nissen-Meyer [13], it seems important that adjuvant chemotherapy take place immediately after the mastectomy and not only 2−4 weeks later (Fig. 8). Otherwise, the effect of the complementary therapy will fail. Therefore, planned complementary chemo/radiotherapy has to be started as an early postoperative treatment,

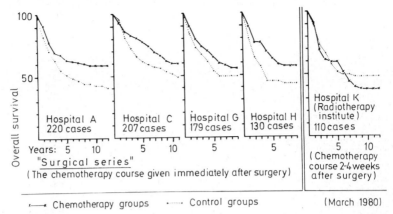

Fig. 8. Long-lasting effect of adjuvant chemotherapy for operable breast cancer, stage II, applied immediately after surgery (the four graphs on the *left*) compared with the same chemotherapeutic treatment not instituted until 2–4 weeks postoperation (graph on the *right*) (Nissen-Meyer [13])

in any case, with chemotherapy followed by radiotherapy only after the first 2 or 3 cycles. This also seems to be the appropriate method for more advanced inoperable stages III and IV.

Concerning the CMF therapy Bonadonna et al. [3] pointed out that an incomplete chemotherapy dose impairs the success of adjuvant therapy; therefore, care should be taken to ensure that a large decrease of leuco- and thrombocytes does not lead to reducing the dose to below 65% of that planned. If it is intended to combine the two modalities of adjuvant treatment, the best way should be to administer only ADM and CYT (AC) or CYT and 5-FU (CF) instead of CMF before the radiotherapy. Furthermore, the volume of the irradiation fields has to be reduced and adapted to the tumor situation; a lower single dose of 170–180 rad should be chosen instead of the usual 200 rad.

These considerations form the guidelines for a combined radio- and chemotherapy after the *breast-preserving operation* for initial primary tumors (T1/T2 up to a diameter of 3 cm), for patients with 1–3 lymph nodes, or even for micrometastases in the axilla (stage II). As the relapse-free survival time decreases in the presence of positive lymph nodes, even when few in number (four), it seems mandatory to add a supplementary treatment to the radiotherapy after tumorectomy.

According to recent studies [2, 5, 10, 12] combined irradiation and chemotherapy can be carried out after local excision of the primary tumor and axillary clearing. The chemotherapy may consist of CMF, but this treatment carries the risk of a heavy thrombocytopenia when more than 6 cycles are administered [5]. A better tolerance is expected if CMF + prednisone or CF alone (without MTX) is used before irradiation. There is an ongoing study [10] with two randomized schemes: the first group (A) receives irradiation (on the preserved breast and the lymph node regions) immediately after tumorectomy and after 12 cycles of chemotherapy with CMF or CMFP. In a second group (B) the tumorectomy is followed first by 2 cycles of CF, then the radiation treatment is installed and thereafter it is completed by 10 cycles of CMFP.

In a first synopsis [8] it is shown that the complications after combined radio/chemotherapy were not significantly higher, except regarding the arm edema, and that a more pronounced contraction of the breast was to be expected (Table 2).

Table 2. Complications following primary radiotherapy and adjuvant chemotherapy, Stage I and II breast cancer (Danoff [8])

Complication	Control group	Adjuvant chemotherapy		
		CMF	CF → CMFP	All patients
Arm edema	0	2	4	6
Rib fracture	0	1	0	1
Symptomatic pneumonitis	1	0	0	0
Necrosis (axilla)	0	0	1	1
Brachial plexis injury	0	0	0	0

At a combined radio/chemotherapy the inclusion of the whole axilla in the treatment fields is not even mandatory in cases of operatively cleared positive axillary lymph nodes [8, 15]. By avoiding irradiation of the operated axilla, the frequency of arm edema can be reduced. Also the ongoing study by the Milan group stops irradiation of the axilla when chemotherapy is effected [17].

Through a corresponding adjustment of the volume of irradiation − not of the total dose − combined adjuvant radiochemotherapy following a reduced operation of the mammary carcinoma, stage II, is practicable without grave myelotoxicity and with an only moderate increase of the retarded alterations in the irradiated region. It seems advisable to choose a chemotherapeutic scheme without MTX or an association of A + C, instead of CMF, when irradiation is planned together with a chemotherapy regime. The appraisal of eventual late tissue damage may require more than 2−3 years, as would irradiation only with curative intention after tumorectomy of the breast.

As in the combined surgical-radiotherapeutic treatment of the mammary carcinoma, the two methods of combined radio/chemotherapy have to be coordinated. Through adjustment of the volume of irradiation and maintenance of the required total dose [14], the total amount of chemotherapy first planned should be retained in order to guarantee the success of this multidisciplinary treatment method.

References

1. Ahmann DL, Scanlon PW, Bisel HF, Edmonson JH, Frytak S, Payne WS, O'Fallon JR, Hahn RG, Ingle JN, O'Connell MJ, Rubin J (1978) Repeated adjuvant chemotherapy with phenylalanine mustard or 5-fluorouracil, cyclophosphamide, and prednisone with or without radiation, after mastectomy for breast cancer. Lancet 1: 893−896
2. Allen H, Brooks R, Jones SE, Chase E, Heusinkveld RS, Giordano GF, Ketchel SJ, Jackson RA, Moon TE, Salmon SE (1981) Adjuvant treatment for stage II (node positive) breast cancer with adriamycin − cyclophosphamide (AC) +/−radiotherapy (XRT). In: Salmon SE, Jones SE (eds) Adjuvant therapy of cancer III. Grune and Stratton, New York, pp 453−463
3. Bonadonna G, Brusamolino E, Valagussa P, et al. (1976) Combination chemotherapy as an adjuvant treatment in operable breast cancer. N Engl J Med 294: 405−410
4. Bonadonna G, Valagussa P, Rossi A, Tancini G, Brambilla C, Marchini S, Veronesi U (1982) Multimodal therapy with CMF in resectable breast cancer with positive axillary nodes: the Milan Institute experience. Recent Results Cancer Res 80: 149−156
5. Bonadonna G, Valagussa P, Zucali R, Del Vecchio M, Veronesi U (1983) Feasibility of adjuvant chemotherapy plus radiotherapy in operable breast cancer. In: Harris JR, Hellman S, Silen W (eds) Conservative management in breast cancer. Lippincott, Philadelphia, pp 329−336

6. Botnick LE, Come S, Rose CM, Goldstein M, Lange R, Tishler S, Schnipper L (1983) Primary breast irradiation and concomitant adjuvant chemotherapy. In: Harris JR, Hellman S, Silen W (eds) Conservative management in breast cancer. Lippincott, pp 321−328
7. Cooper MR, Rhyne AL, Muss HB, et al. (1981) A randomized comparative trial of chemotherapy and irradiation therapy for stage II breast cancer. Cancer 47: 2833−2839
8. Danoff BF, Goodman RL, Glick JH, Haller DG, Pajak TF (1983) The effect of adjuvant chemotherapy on cosmesis and complications in patients with breast cancer treated by definitive irradiation. Int J Radiat Oncol Biol Phys 9: 1625−1630
9. Fisher B, Redmond C, Wolmark N (1981) Breast cancer studies of the NSABP: An editorialized overview. In: Salmon SE, Jones SE (eds) Adjuvant therapy of cancer III. Grune and Stratton, New York, pp 359−369
10. Glick JH, Danoff BF, Haller DG, Weiler C, Goodman RL (1983) Adjuvant chemotherapy in patients undergoing definitive irradiation for primary breast cancer − the University of Pennsylvania experience. In: Harris JR, Hellman S, Silen W (eds) Conservative management of breast cancer. Lippincott, Philadelphia, pp 311−320
11. Jones SE, Salmon SE, Allen H, Giordano GF, Davis S, Chase E, Moon TE, Heusinkveld RS (1982) Adjuvant treatment of node-positive breast cancer with adriamycin-cyclophosphamide with or without radiation therapy: interim-results of an ongoing clinical trial. Recent Results Cancer Res 80: 162−169
12. Lichter AS, Lippman ME, Gorell CR, D'Angelo TM, Edwards BK, deMoss EV (1983) Adjuvant chemotherapy in patients treated primarily with irradiation for localized breast cancer. In: Harris JR, Hellman S, Silen W (eds) Conservative management of breast cancer. Lippincott, Philadelphia, pp 299−310
13. Nissen-Meyer R, Kjellgren K, Mansson B (1982) Adjuvant chemotherapy in breast cancer. Recent Results Cancer Res 80: 142−148
14. Notter G, Turesson I (1983) Zur prä- und postoperativen Bestrahlung beim Mammakarzinom. Strahlentherapie 159: 259−266
15. Sarrazin D, Le M, Fontaine F, Arriagada R (1983) Conservative treatment vs mastectomy in T1 or small T2 breast cancer: the experience of the Institute Gustave-Roussy. In: Harris JR, Hellman S, Silen W (eds) Conservative management of breast cancer. Lippincott, Philadelphia, pp 101−111
16. Schulz K-D, Schmidt-Rhode P, Weyman P, Herrmann F, Wuerz H, Kaiser R (1981) Consecutive radiation and chemotherapy in the adjuvant treatment of operable breast cancer. In: Salmon SE, Jones SE (eds) Adjuvant therapy of cancer III. Grune and Stratton, New York, pp 411−418
17. Veronesi U, Sacozzi R, Del Vecchio M, Bafi A, Clemente C, et al. (1981) Comparing radical mastectomy with quadrantectomy, axillary dissection and radiotherapy in patients with small cancers of the breast. N Engl J Med 305: 6−11
18. Wallgren A, Arner O, Bergstroem J, Blomstedt B, Granberg P, Karnstroem L, Silfverswaerd C (1980) The value of preoperative radiotherapy in operable mammary carcinoma. Int J Radiat Oncol Biol Phys 6: 287−290

The Present Dilemma of Adjuvant Chemotherapy: Acceptance and Risks Versus Benefits

P. P. Carbone

Wisconsin Clinical Cancer Center, K4/662, Clinical Science Center, 600 Highland Avenue, Madison, WI 53792, USA

Introduction

Currently the role of adjuvant chemotherapy (ACT) is clearly experimental, the effectiveness is not definitively established for most subsets of patients and is still subject to verification. The role of ACT is probably most proven in premenopausal node-positive women, particularly in the 1−3 node group. In this population the survival differences are consistently significant in the largest and best-controlled studies [1, 2]. In the other patients the study results presented are either premature, inconsistent, or still showing improvement only in disease-free interval (DFI). Table 1 shows the summary of the trials done by the Eastern Cooperative Oncology Group (ECOG) and the impact on DFI and survival. What is the acceptance of ACT and what are the benefits and risks?

Table 1. ECOG-NSABP adjuvant studies

Study	Subset (by age)	Nodes	P-value	5-Year survival	
EST 0771-B05	< 50	1−3+	0.02	L-PAM 0.88	Placebo 0.74
EST 1175-B07	> 50	4+	0.04	L-PAM + FU 0.40	L-PAM 0.29
EST 3176-B08	−	−	−	L-PAM + FU	L-PAM + FU + MTX

ECOG studies 1977−1984[a]

Study	Subset (by age)	Nodes	Treatment
EST 5177	< 50	+	CMF*CMFP*CMFPT
EST 6177	> 50	+	Surgery*CMFP*CMFPT
EST 1178	> 65	+	Surgery*tamoxifen
EST 1180		−	Surgery*CMFP(6)
EST 5181	< 50	+	CMFPT −/+ tamoxifen (60 months) CMFPTH/TsAVbTH −/+ tamoxifen
EST 4181	> 50	+	CMFPT(12)*CMFPT(4)* CMFPT(12) + tamoxifen (60 months)

[a] No significant impacts on survival or too early to analyze

Acceptance

At the present time the practising oncologist undoubtedly assumes that there is an advantage for ACT in all women with positive nodes. Most of the patients referred to our center for second opinions or after primary failure have been on some form of cyclophosphamide, 5-fluorouracil, methotrexate (CMF) treatment. In general, these women have not been treated with added prednisone and/or tamoxifen. At least in the Midwest, few nonstudy patients have been treated with adriamycin combinations. In addition, few patients are given tamoxifen only as adjuvant treatment. For the node-negative patients ACT is probably not given routinely. In the ECOG we showed that breast cancer patients make up about 30% of the patients [3]. We also showed that the proportion of patients who go on study as a fraction of the patients eligible is about 24%. Thus, in the 200 hospitals participating in ECOG, one would predict that 2,000 patients are treated with ACT since we access about 500 patients per year on our adjuvant protocols. The data on the protocol status of the ECOG population are shown in Table 2.

In the academic institutions where protocol studies are more likely to be used, ACT has achieved acceptance in the research studies for all node-positive patients. This is particularly true for the ECOG institutions since none of our trials contain a surgery-only arm for these patients. In fact, the treatment options are rather aggressive for some subsets of patients (Table 1). As can be seen, the possibilities range from a 4-month CMFPT option to the possibility of 12 months of alternating CMFPT and DAVTH followed by 4 more years of tamoxifen. The calculated expense for this regimen must be several thousand dollars, at least for the first year. Fortunately, the prolonged tamoxifen cost is underwritten in part by the pharmaceutical industry, but the laboratory and clinic costs are not.

For women who are node negative in the ECOG there are several options, depending on the size of the tumor and the ER status. At least two of the three options include a surgery-only arm. This possibility exists for all patients who have small tumors (< 3 cm) that are ER positive. For patients who are ER negative with any tumor size and for those who have tumors larger than 3 cm whatever their ER status, a randomization occurs between 6 months of CMFPT or surgery alone. Thus, we are beginning to see an acceptance of ACT for these node-negative patients as well.

Table 2. Breast cancer patients in oncology centers (expressed in percent). From Begg et al. [3]

Cancer patients with breast cancer	30
Incidence of new cases	14
Stage of disease	
Localized	15
Regional	25
Metastatic	59
On protocol	24
Treatment influenced by protocol	61
Reasons for not being on protocol	
Physicians preference for specific Rx	52
Patient refusal	19
Other medical problem	9
Difficulty with follow-up	8
Other reasons	12

Another group of patients who are highly likely to receive ACT are those women with stage III disease. In addition to ACT they will undoubtedly be subjected to surgery and radiation therapy. It appears that this is being done not only in the university hospitals but also in the community centers. There is at least one other subset that will receive ACT or at least combined modality treatment and that is patients with inflammatory carcinoma. At the University of Wisconsin, we have recently shown a rather good 5-year survival overall, but unfortunately we did not have a controlled study [4] and apparently no one else does either.

Thus, ACT seems to have become widely accepted both in private practice and in the university setting. The current trends lean towards aggressive combinations that undoubtedly will produce toxicities. When such therapies are administered in a protocol that is well designed, the patient will be well served. Not only will we learn by the randomized clinical trial, but we will clearly determine whether we will have done any harm. Unfortunately, the tendency of most oncologists is to assume therapeutic value and not to put the bulk of patients on trials. The temptation to offer therapy as proven satisfies the need of the patient to have something done and allows the physician to appear as if he is doing good. The difficulties of explaining all the options and the need for randomization often imply lack of knowledge on the part of the specialist. A great deal of time on the doctor's part is needed to explain the concepts of randomization to the patient.

Risks

The risks of ACT are in part due to the toxicities of the drugs used in the combinations. The major ones relate to the bone marrow, and the gastrointestinal, central nervous, endocrine, and cardiovascular systems. The most distressing to the patient are alopecia, weight gain, fatigue, anxiety, and nausea and vomiting. Tables 3 and 4 summarize the moderate-to-severe side effects reported in two current ECOG studies. Fatal side effects occurred in only one patient. As can be seen, the major toxicities seen in our trials have been life-threatening leukopenia, stroke, and pulmonary emboli.

The distressing side effects such as nausea and vomiting are often associated with the development of anticipatory vomiting and anxiety. Recent studies by Nerenz have indicated that these distressing symptoms are most likely to occur in the younger patient and increase with duration of treatment [5]. In a recent paper by Meyerwitz and colleagues, the distress associated with ACT lasted for many months [6]. These authors reported that almost half of the 35 patients who received adjuvant therapy had long-term disruption in their lives up to 2 years after chemotherapy. In another study, McArdle reported psychiatric morbidity in 13 of 34 patients 1 year after chemotherapy [7].

In my own patients one of the most distressing side effects has been weight gain. Patients who have a tendency to weight excess will gain 10–15 kilos and despite self-enforced measures the excess weight will persist for months. Very few seem to have the willpower to restrict their calories beforehand, but his is not a problem restricted to women receiving adjuvant therapy.

Endocrine problems such as amenorrhea, menopausal symptoms, ovarian cysts, etc. can occur following ACT administration. These symptoms have been well-characterized by Rose and Davis [8]. Tamoxifen undoubtedly plays a role in the incidence of these problems.

There are some possible effects on the germ cells beyond cessation of ovulation. In the child-bearing ages there is a finite risk of inducing fetal abnormalities. In my own

Table 3. Toxicity of ACT (CMFP) EST 1180 (expressed in percent)

	Mild to moderate	Severe	Life-threatening
Leukopenia	48	27	9
Thrombocytopenia	9	9	3
Nausea and vomiting	52	6	0
Stomatitis	15	0	0
Alopecia	61	0	0
Clotting problems	6	3	12

Pulmonary embolism occurred in 4/85 patients

Table 4. Toxicity ACT EST 5181 (expressed in percent)

	CMFPT			CMFPTH/TsAVbTH		
	Mild to moderate	Severe	Life-threatening	Mild to moderate	Severe	Life-threatening
Leukopenia	64	20	2	46	24	2
Thrombocytopenia	14	0	20	8	0	0
Nausea and vomiting	54	0	0	66	4	0
Infection	36	0	0	24	0	0
Alopecia	56	0	0	64	0	0
Clotting problems	6	2	2	6	0	2
Weight gain	30	4	0	22	2	0

Three of 152 patients developed clotting problems (CVA, arterial clot in leg)

experience this has not been a clinical problem, since most of these women seem to avoid pregnancies while on the drugs or seem to have their breast cancers detected after term. There is no data on the long-term effects of these combinations that are very likely to contain alkylating agents.

One of the most distressing aspects of ACT is the long-range impact on the incidence of second tumors particularly acute leukemias [9]. In 1978 Rosner and colleagues reported 24 patients with breast cancer who developed acute leukemia. They estimated a sevenfold risk increase. The comparable experience, when looked at at the University of Wisconsin by Ershler, indicated that since breast cancer is a relatively common disease, this supposed increased association may in fact be an independent occurence of two diseases [10]. They suggested that the induced leukemias may be differentiated from those spontaneously occurring by analysis of the cytogenetics of the acute leukemia cells. Still most studies utilizing relatively short-term chemotherapy have not reported a marked increase in the incidence of acute leukemia.

Benefits

The benefits of adjuvant therapy have been analyzed in a variety of ways with relative general agreement that more trials need to be done. At a 1980 National Cancer Institute –

sponsored consensus meeting the panel agreed that an increase in DFI and survival has been seen in premenopausal patients with positive nodes [11]. No figures of the actual benefit were given but looking at the data from the Milan group, 15% and 12% improvements for the two parameters were reported [2]. In the National Surgical Adjuvant Breast Project (NSABP) the major benefit was seen in the 1−3 node positive group treated with L-PAM [1]. However, the interstudy comparisons and the use of historical control groups leave much to be desired and should not be accepted as proven; there are some studies that are contradictory [12−14]. The data in postmenopausal patients are less convincing; definitive studies have not been reported.

The ultimate benefits of the successful treatment of micrometastases will undoubtedly be an improvement in survival with decreased morbidity. A 10% increase in survival could result in saving several thousand lives per year. My feeling is that the biological information derived from the current trials suggests that this goal is possible. The use of minimal treatment with chemotherapy is not likely to be succesful. Neither is the use of low-dose combinations [13]. The use of hormonal therapy combined with chemotherapy, particularly the long-term use of tamoxifen, looks promising [15].

Overall, the benefits of minimal surgery and the use of shorter durations of adjunctive treatment with long-term use of relatively nontoxic treatments such as tamoxifen may encourage physicians and patients to seek earlier treatment with smaller tumors and negative lymph nodes. The major reason for this change in attitude will be the opportunity to utilize the less radical procedures and the less toxic short-term treatment. Biologically one would expect less likelihood of distant metastases and the possibility that the long-term use of tamoxifen would suppress the development of second cancers. Only time and clinical trials will tell.

Summary

The acceptance of ACT has been very rapid since 1974 although earlier studies by Nissen-Meyer and the NSABP in the 1960's originally suggested the effectiveness of modest short-term chemotherapy [16, 17]. The current practice is to administer combination chemotherapy for at least 6 months in all node-positive women. The survival benefits are clearly established only for women who are premenopausal and who have fewer than three positive nodes. Trials in other groups of patients are highly suggestive but have lacked some or all of the rigorous standards of the randomized clinical trial. The reasons for this widespread acceptance of ACT are not clear, but both patients and physicians are able to appreciate the concepts and bear the costs in terms of money as well as toxicity. The risks of ACT are mainly short term and reversible. Long-term consequences are not so readily apparent as yet. The benefits of improved survival will only be appreciated as more time passes, either through the long-term analyses of the current trials or the overwhelming success of a new strategy. Then all the past arguments about one therapy or another will become irrelevant. At that point this new miracle treatment will be so good that none will ask whether CMF is better than surgery alone. In essence, the old standard has become the control.

Acknowledgement. This study was supported in part by ECOG Operations Office Grant CA-21115.

References

1. Fisher B, Carbone P, Economou SG, Frelick R, Glass A, Lerner H, Redmond C, Zelen M, Band P, Katrych DL, Wolmark N, Fisher ER (1975) L-Phenylalanine mustard (L-PAM) in the management of primary breast cancer. A report of early findings. N Engl J Med 292: 117–122
2. Bonadonna G (1981) Recent progress in multimodal therapy for resectable breast cancer. Isr J Med Sci 17: 916–921
3. Begg CB, Zelen M, Carbone PP, McFadden ET, Brodovsky H, Engstrom P, Hatfield A, Ingle J, Schwartz B, Stolbach L (1983) Cooperative groups and community hospitals. Measurement of impact in the community hospitals. Cancer 5: 1760–1767
4. Loprinzi CL, Carbone PP, Tormey DC, Rosenbaum PR, Caldwell W, Kline JC, Steeves RA, Ramirez G (to be published) Aggressive combined modality therapy for advanced local-regional breast carcinoma. J Clin Oncol
5. Nerenz DR, Leventhal H, Love RR (1982) Factors contributing to emotional distress during cancer chemotherapy. Cancer 50: 1020–1027
6. Meyerowitz BE, Watkins IK, Sparks FC (1983) Psychosocial implications of adjuvant chemotherapy. A two-year follow-up. Cancer 52: 1541–1545
7. McArdle CS, Calman KC, Cooper AF, Hughson AVM, Russell AR, Smith DC (1981) The social, emotional and financial implications of adjuvant chemotherapy in breast cancer. Br J Surg 68: 261–264
8. Rose DP, Davis TE (1980) Effects of adjuvant chemohormonal therapy on the ovarian and adrenal function of breast cancer patients. Cancer Res 40: 4043–4047
9. Rosner F, Carey RW, Zarrabi MH (1978) Breast cancer and acute leukemia: report of 24 cases and review of the literature. Am J Hematol 4: 151–172
10. Ershler WB, Robins HI, Davis HL, Hafez GR, Meisner LF, Dahlberg S, Arndt C (1982) Emergence of acute non-lymphocytic leukemia in breast cancer patients. Am J Med Sci 284: 23–31
11. NIH Consensus-Development Panel (1980) Adjuvant chemotherapy of breast cancer. N Engl J Med 303: 831–832
12. Senn HJ (1982) Current status and indications for adjuvant therapy in breast cancer. Cancer Chemother Pharmacol 8: 139–150
13. Hubay CA, Pearson OH, Marshall JS, Stellato TA, Rhodes RS, DeBanne SM, Rosenblatt J, Mansour EG, Hermann RE, Jones JC, Flynn WJ, Eckert C, McGuire WL (1981) Adjuvant therapy of stage II breast cancer. Br Cancer Res Treat 1: 77–82
14. Rubens RD, Knight RK, Fentiman IS, Howell A, Crowther D, George WD, Hayward JL, Bulbrook RD, Chaudary M, Bush H, Sellwood RA, Howat JMT (1983) Controlled trial of adjuvant chemotherapy with melphalan for breast cancer. Lancet 1: 839–843
15. Nissen-Meyer R, Kjellgren K, Malmio K, Mansson B, Norin T (1978) Surgical adjuvant chemotherapy. Results with one short course with cyclophosphamide after mastectomy for breast cancer. Cancer 41: 2088–2098
16. Nissen-Meyer R (1979) Comparison of effects obtained with various types of adjuvant treatments – a commentary. Cancer Treat Rep 6: 101–104
17. Fisher B, Slack N, Katrych D, Wolmark N (1975) Ten year follow-up results of patients with carcinoma of the breast in a co-operative clinical trial evaluating surgical adjuvant chemotherapy. Surg Gynecol Obstet 140: 528–534

Are Current Worldwide Studies Going to Answer the Important Questions Remaining in Adjuvant Chemotherapy of Breast Cancer?

K. W. Brunner

Institut für Medizinische Onkologie, Inselspital, 3010 Bern, Switzerland

Introduction

Despite nearly 20 years of experience with adjuvant chemotherapy of operable breast cancer with thousands of patients involved, many important questions for its routine use remain either unanswered or controversial. Therefore, it has to be said that adjuvant chemotherapy of breast cancer at present remains an experimental procedure of limited and possibly only temporary benefit for the majority of patients. Most would maintain that it should only be used in well-designed clinical trials.

It must be asked, whether present or future studies will ever be able to answer the important questions which past and current studies so far have not answered. Basically the question is whether adjuvant chemotherapy will ever become routine treatment in clearly defined patient populations with a predictable beneficial effect in an acceptable percentage of patients who undergo such a treatment. Or, will many important questions remain unanswered by prospective clinical trials? Is this instrument, which made so many valuable contributions for the improvement of cancer treatment in the past, facing its scientific and logistic limits in the difficult field of adjuvant therapy of breast cancer? Are other methods in sight to answer those questions?

Table 1. Unsolved problems in adjuvant chemotherapy of operable breast cancer

1. What is the definition of "optimal" adjuvant chemotherapy in various subgroups?

2. Is adjuvant combined hormono-chemotherapy superior to chemotherapy alone or hormonal treatment alone, overall or in subgroups?

3. What is the optimal duration of adjuvant therapy in breast cancer?

4. What is the optimal timing of adjuvant chemotherapy? (pre-, peri-, postoperative)?

5. Is there a need for better selection and/or exclusion criteria for adjuvant chemotherapy, especially in overall low-risk groups with small high-risk subpopulations (e.g., N-patients)?

6. What is the meaning of an increase in disease- or relapse-free survival in relation to final overall survival, or in terms of benefit to patient?

7. What are the long-term effects of adjuvant chemotherapy with regard to: long-term toxicity, second neoplasms, course of disease, and prospects of further systemic therapy in relapsing patients?

Table 2. Adjuvant chemotherapy trials with a mastectomy-alone control group in node-positive breast cancer

Group	Years follow-up	Treatment	Benefit[a]		Subgroup with greatest benefit
			Overall	Best groups	
NSABP: B-06 [9, 10]	5	L-PAM vs placebo	16	54	< 49 years, N+ 1–3
Milano [3]	8	CMF vs control	20	33	Premenopausal
OSAKO [30]	7	LMF vs control	28	51	Postmenopausal
Guy's/Manchester [29]	5	L-PAM vs control	16	26	N+ 1–3
Manchester [15]	3	CMF vs L-PAM vs control	60	72	Premenopausal
MBCCG [34]	3	CMF/CVM vs control	25	NA	NA
LBCS III [19]	3	CMFp + T vs p + T vs control (Postmenopausal, ≤ 65 years, N+)	47	–	–

[a] Benefit = % of decrease in relapses
Boxed figures = statistically significant difference in DFS/RFS
Boxed and underlined figures = statistically significant difference in DFS/RFS and OS; *NA*, not available

Table 3. Adjuvant chemotherapy trials with L-PAM treated control group in node-positive breast cancer

Group	Years follow-up	Treatment	Benefit[a]		Subgroup with greatest benefit
			Overall	Best groups	
NSABP: B-07 [10]	4	PF vs L-PAM	NA	35	> 50 years, N+ ≥ 4
SWOG [13]	5	CMFVP vs L-PAM	35	52	All N+ 1–3
Manchester [15]	3	CMF vs L-PAM	39	75	Postmenopausal
COG [7]	4	CMFV vs L-PAM	32	$P = 0.01$	Postmenopausal (≥ 50 years)
U of Alabama [5]	3	CMF vs L-PAM	33	–	in favour of L-PAM
Bowman-Gray [6]	2	CMF ± RT vs L-PAM ± RT	59	67	≥ 50 years
Northwest UV [4]	2	CFP ± BCG vs L-PAM	59	61	Postmenopausal
Mayo clinic [1]	2	CFP ± RT vs L-PAM	32	77	Premenopausal
Fox Chase [6a]	?	CMF vs L-PAM	9	20	Premenopausal

[a] Benefit = % of decrease in relapses
Boxed figures = statistically significant difference in DFS/RFS
Boxed and underlined figures = statistically significant difference in DFS/RFS and OS
Underlined figures = significant difference in mortality (overall survival); *NA*, not available

Table 4. Adjuvant hormone therapy trials in breast cancer

Group	Years follow-up	Treatment	Benefit[a]		Subgroup with greatest benefit
			Overall	Best groups	
Copenhagen [24] (Pre- and post-MP N+, N$_0$T$_3$)	3	Pre-Mp: tamoxifen vs placebo	40	–	–
	3	Post-Mp: tamoxifen vs DES vs placebo	38	–	–
Danish BC group [28] (Post-MP, N+, T$_3$N$_0$ + RT.)	3	Tamoxifen vs control	22.5	38	N+ ≥ 4
Christie + Holt [26]	5	Pre-Mp: tamoxifen vs radiation castration	21		
Pre- and post-Mp Stage I–III, RT to N+		Post-Mp: tamoxifen vs control		Survival advantage	Post-Mp, N+ ≥ 4
UK ("NATO") [23] Pre- and Post-Mp N– and N+	1.75	Tamoxifen vs control	31	41	ER ≥ 30 fmol
Toronto [25] Post-Mp ± RT	3	Tamoxifen vs control	25	53	No RT
LBCS III + IV [19] Post-Mp, N+	3	P + tamoxifen vs control	25	–	–

[a] Benefit = % decrease in relapses

Boxed figures, statistically significant difference in DFS/RFS

Boxed and underlined figures, statistically significant difference in DFS/RFS and OS; *Mp*, menopause; *RT*, radiation therapy; *P*, prednisone; *DES*, diethystilboestrol

Table 5. Adjuvant combined hormone chemotherapy trials in breast cancer

Group	Years follow-up	Treatment	Benefit[a] Overall	Benefit[a] Best groups	Subgroup with greatest benefit
NSABP: B-09 [11]	3	PFT vs PF	23	41	$\geq$ 50 years, N+ $\geq$ 4 (ER $\geq$ 10, PR $\geq$ 10)[b]
ECOG [32]	2–3	CMFPT vs CMFP vs CMF (Premenopausal)	20	32	N+ $\geq$ 4
Case Western [16]	4	CMFT $\pm$ BCG vs CMF	16	21	ER+
LBCS III [19]	3	CMFp + T vs p + T vs control (Postmenopausal)	47	47	–

[a] Benefit = % decrease in relapses

[b] (NSABP-study): adverse effect of PFT in patients < 50 years old with PR 0–9 (ER+) (77% more deaths!) or with ER < 10fmol (32% more deaths!) Boxed figures, statistically significant difference in DFS/RFS; boxed and underlined figures, statistically significant difference in DFS/RFS and OS; P, prednisone; F, 5-fluorouracil; T, tamoxifen; c, cyclophosphamide; M, methotrexate; p, low-dose prednisone; BCG, bacillus Calmette-Guérin

Table 1 summarizes the unsolved problems and existing questions in adjuvant chemotherapy of breast cancer. The majority of problems listed in this table are related to the basic question, of whether such a heterogenous disease with so many prognostic subgroups can be adequately studied and reliable results produced in randomized clinical trials of limited patient populations within a reasonable time.

Ongoing Clinical Trials

In order to judge which problems may be solved and which may not, we have to look at the presently available results of ongoing clinical trials. This is done in Tables 2–5, which summarize the relevant results of all important clinical trials with adjuvant chemotherapy, with adjuvant hormone therapy, and adjuvant combined hormone-chemotherapy in node-positive patients with operable breast cancer[1]. The "benefit" described in the tables is defined as percent decrease in relapses (or percent avoided relapses) as demonstrated in Fig. 1. This percentage is calculated from reported figures over certain periods of time in disease-free survival (DFS) or relapse-free survival (RFS). If this percentage is boxed, the difference is statistically significant. If in addition, the figure is underlined, it means, that there is also a statistically significant difference in overall survival (OS) (not identical with the figures). Underlined figures mean a decrease in deaths (or percent avoided deaths). The terms DFS, RFS, and OS are further explained in Fig. 2. Unfortunately, definitions are neither always the same in the various papers, nor always clear in an individual paper. This is one of the reasons that comparisons of different studies are so difficult. If we look at the summaries of the published results of ongoing trials on adjuvant chemotherapy of breast cancer, the picture is very confusing. Not surprisingly, the confusion is similar to that in the area of systemic treatment of metastatic breast cancer. In both areas, from the huge number of published results, no single treatment, or sequence of treatments, emerges which could be called optimal for all patients. Nor can subgroups be clearly defined, for which any one particular therapeutic regimen could be called optimal.

In trials where adjuvant chemotherapy is compared with untreated controls (mastectomy only, Table 2), the overall benefit in terms of avoided relapses observed between 3 and 8 years is 16% for L-PAM in two studies and varies 20%–60% in four studies with CMF, CMFpT (p = low-dose prednisone, T = tamoxifen), or LMF (L = Leukeran, chlorambucil). The subgroups (menopausal status and/or degree of nodal involvement (N+ 1–3 or N+ ≥ 4)) which benefited most from adjuvant chemotherapy vary from study to study. The percentage of avoided relapses in the best subgroup of each study varies 26%–72%. In two studies, only premenopausal patients (in one of them only those with 1–3 positive nodes) had a significant benefit from adjuvant chemotherapy; in both of these studies DFS and OS were improved. In two other studies, the group with the greates benfit were postmenopausal patients. One of the two studies with L-PAM vs controls was not significant for L-PAM. The percentages of avoided relapses were similar; but the patient population was smaller. The Ludwig trial III (LBCS III) for postmenopausal patients treated with CMFpT showed a significant benefit over the untreated control group in DFS, but to date not in OS. It has to be pointed out, that no study with an observation period of less than 5 years demonstrated a significant benefit in overall survival. There may be a trend for DFS or RFS to become smaller with increasing observation periods, but also for

---

1 The modified summaries are based on a review paper by Aron Goldhirsch [13a]

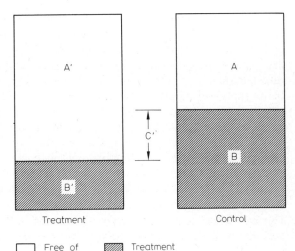

Fig. 1. The proportion of patients who benefitted from adjuvant treatment at a given point in time (*C'*). *A, A'*, free of disease; *B, B'*, treatment failures

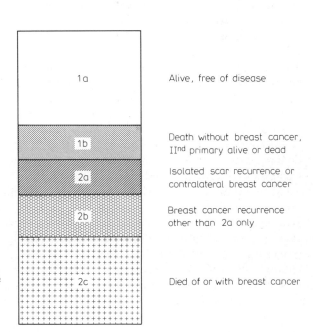

Fig. 2. The proportion of patients included in the definitions of the end points of clinical trials. *1a* = disease free (for DFS); *1a + b* = relapse free (for RFS); *1a + 2a* = free of systemic failure (for time to systemic failure, TSF); *1a +* alive *1b + 2a + 2b* = surviving (for OS)

OS to become significant; should this be confirmed in the future, it means that in some patients relapses are only postponed while in others they are avoided permanently.

The results are similarly confusing in the trials where different combination chemotherapies are compared with L-PAM alone (Table 3). In seven of nine studies, polychemotherapy is superior to L-PAM, with a decrease of relapses varying 9%−59% (30%−40% in five studies). One study showed better results for L-PAM than for CMF in terms of OS, which indicates an unexplained increase in mortality with CMF. In five of nine studies postmenopausal patients were the best subgroup (or patients > 50 years old); in two studies it was the premenopausal group; in one study it was the group with 1−3 positive nodes. The improvement in the best subgroups varies from 20%−77%. To date figures on OS are available in only two studies for the total study population; one of the two showed a benefit in OS after 5 years, the other showed no such benefit after 2 years. In another study (NSABP B-07), the best subgroup, consisting of patients older than 50 years with more than three positive nodes, has significantly better DFS and OS with polychemotherapy than with L-PAM.

In six trials with adjuvant hormone therapy (Table 4), mostly with tamoxifen (T), all studies show a decrease in relapses after 21–36 months of observation. This decrease is similar to the one observed with adjuvant chemotherapy and varies between 22% and 40% overall and between 38% and 53% for the best subgroup. The best subgroups are postmenopausal patients and/or patients with positive receptors and more than three positive nodes (in two studies). A detailed analysis of postmenopausal patients in the Ludwig trials III and IV (LBCS III + IV) suggests that the benefit of adjuvant tamoxifen is limited to local recurrences only, the rate of distant metastases remaining the same [19]. This is indirectly supported by the observation in the Toronto trial [25], which included patients with and without postoperative radiotherapy; only the patients without radiotherapy had a decrease in relapses after 3 years.

Four studies, which compared combined hormone- and chemotherapy with chemotherapy alone or hormone therapy alone, are summarized in Table 5. The largest is the NSABP [11] study, which compared L-PAM/5-fluorouracil/tamoxifen (PFT) with PF, demonstrating a significant disease-free and overall survival benefit after 3 years for the whole group with tamoxifen and especially for postmenopausal patients with more than three positive nodes. But in the same study, a highly significant adverse effect was observed in ER− and even more in PR− premenopausal patients, when tamoxifen was added to PF-therapy. This shows, that despite positive overall results, different subgroups may behave differently or may even be adversely affected. The same has been demonstrated in some studies with advanced breast cancer. The Ludwig trial III (LBCS III [19]) shows a similar benefit for CMFpT over controls as for PFT in the NSABP study in postmenopausal patients. Contrary to the NSABP study, no adverse effect (but also no significant positive effect) could be observed in the ECOG study [32] by adding tamoxifen to CMF or CMFP in premenopausal patients. The same is true for the Case Western study [16].

With regard to the optimal duration of adjuvant chemotherapy, there are five studies, which suggest that prolonged chemotherapy does not improve overall results. Two studies comparing 6 vs 12 months of CMF demonstrated no significant difference in overall results after 60 and 33 months respectively [31, 33]. The same was true for one study comparing 6 vs 24 months of oral chlorambucil/methotrexate/5-fluorouracil (LMF) [17]. In another study, 5 cycles of adriamycin/cyclophosphamide was compared with 10 cycles of treatment in high-risk patients (N+ ≥ 4 positive high axillary nodes). There was no difference after a median observation time of 2.5 years and a maximum of 6 years [14]. An ongoing study of the Southwest Oncology Group (SWOG) showed no difference between 12 and 24 months adjuvant therapy with CMFVP in ER− patients, but it is still in an early phase (18 months) [27].

Despite the evidence that overall results probably cannot be improved by treating patients longer than 6 months, it is not known whether this is true for all important subgroups of patients. Effect upon disease-free survival and overall survival for longer observation periods also remains unknown.

Based upon this analysis of present results we may return to the list of unsolved problems in adjuvant chemotherapy of operable breast cancer and try to arrive at some conclusions as to which questions may be answered in the future and which probably will remain unanswered.

Optimal Adjuvant Chemotherapy

It is unlikely, that current or future clinical trials will be able to define an "optimal" adjuvant chemotherapy in terms of number of drugs, schedule, or duration which is optimal for all important subgroups of patients. Maximum therapy with the most intensive regimens and schedules, which usually are also the most toxic, may produce the best overall results. Such treatment may, however, not be necessary. It may fail to improve results in important subgroups and may even have undectable adverse effects in certain subsets of patients. There are two main reasons for the difficulty in defining optimal adjuvant chemotherapy in breast cancer: First, there are simply too many subgroups of patients who should be studied, or at least analyzed, separately. Second, because of the heterogeneity of breast cancer, the time needed to answer a simple question is too long and the number of questions which can be answered in a reasonable time are too limited.

Subgroup Analysis

The first point is demonstrated in Table 6, which summarizes known risk factors determining the final outcome in operable breast cancer. The factors in brackets are not normally used in subgroup analysis of present studies, but have been found to have prognostic significance [11, 12]. Even if not all factors listed in the table are independant determinants of prognosis, the number of possibly relevant subsets (from 24 to more than 120) is so great, that meaningful subgroup analysis or stratification in present studies with total accruals of a few hundred patients is impossible. If, nevertheless, such analysis is performed, the possibility exists, that some differences will be found by chance and not be real. This may explain at least some of the variability of the results found in different studies. Presently used stratification criteria, e.g., N+ 1−3 and ≥ 4 for degree of nodal involvement, are insufficient to produce homogeneous groups and balanced treatment arms, as has recently been demonstrated [12].

Observation Time

The other point, necessary time of observation for meaningful results, is also a factor which seriously limits the potential of clinical trials in breast cancer. Observation periods up to 5

Table 6. Subgroups of operable breast cancer

Lymph nodes	Tumor size	Menopausal status	Hormone receptors	Histological grade
N_0		Premenopause	ER+, PR+	I
N+ 1−3	T < 3 cm		(ER+, PR−)[a]	
N+ $\geq$ 4		(Perimenopause)[a]		II
(N+ 4−6)	T > 3 cm		(ER+, PR+)	
(N+ 6−13)		Postmenopause		III
(N+ > 13)			ER−, PR−	
3−5	2	2−3	2−4	3

Number of subgroups: Min: 24 (without stage); Max: 120
Figures in last line of table give numbers of *potential* risk groups
[a] Not fully established as a risk factor

years are necessary to allow conclusions about disease- or relapse-free survival. A much longer observation time is probably required for reliable estimates on overall survival. This is well demonstrated by the observation that in operable breast cancer the overall survival curve approaches the curve of a normal population with a similar age distribution only after more than 20 years.

We have seen previously that most studies in adjuvant chemotherapy of breast cancer to date demonstrate a significant decrease in relapses. Only a few studies report on overall survival. Where such figures are available, a majority of studies to date show no difference in favor of adjuvant therapy, or only for subgroups (premenopause, N+ 1−3, etc.). This is cited as proof by some critics that adjuvant therapy has not lasting effect and only postpones relapses. This interpretation is certainly not the only possible one and therefore is not entirely correct. It has been demonstrated in some studies that significant differences in overall survival may appear only after an observation time of more than 5 years because of the natural history of operable breast cancer [8, 20, 21]. An early increase of DFS or RFS may have three possible meanings:

1. It may mean that relapses are merely postponed and that the final or overall outcome is not affected by adjuvant therapy.
2. It may be the first sign that the natural history of the breast cancer is changed and that after many more years of observation this will translate into a definite increase in the overall survival. Without here going into possible explanations why an increase in OS may lag behind the increase in DFS or RFS, suffice to say that many such explanations exist and some are beginning to be confirmed in some studies [19].
3. Most probably an early increase in DFS or RFS means both; in some subgroups of patients relapse is merely postponed and in others it is possibly prevented permanently.

Current and future clinical trials will certainly demonstrate whether and to what degree a decrease in relapses is finally reflected in an increase in overall survival. It is very doubtful that these studies will be able to define all or even only some of the subgroups in which relapse is only temporarily and those in which it is permanently avoided. This is probably another serious limitation of clinical trials in this area.

Combined Treatment

With regard to adjuvant hormone- and chemotherapy vs chemotherapy or endocrine treatment alone, current studies − at best − may show whether or not overall results are improved with the combined modality. But, as in advanced disease, it is doubtful that these studies are able to define subgroups which are or are not benefited by combined treatment, or where such therapy may even have an antagonistic or adverse effect.

Duration

The question of optimal duration and the problems involved with this question have already been dealt with. Here again, some gross approximations to the truth may be possible by present studies, but not precise answers for individual groups of patients can be expected. Only the development of methods to monitor minimal residual disease in each individual patient could solve this, as well as many other, important problems of adjuvant therapy.

Optimal Timing

Optimal timing (pre-, peri-, early postoperative or conventional postoperative therapy) is presently being studied in several trials [7, 18, 21]. It would seem that the simple hypothesis, derived from a biological rationale, that early adjuvant chemotherapy may produce superior results, should be confirmed or rejected by current studies without too much difficulty. Here no subgroup differences are likely to interfere with the interpretation of the results. But large numbers of patients and long observation periods are needed.

Criteria for Selection of Patients

At present, the criteria for the selection of patients for adjuvant chemotherapy are unsatisfactory for three reasons:
1. No subsets of patients can be defined in which more than half of the treated patients have a temporary or lasting benefit from presently available adjuvant therapies. This means that over 50% of all patients and probably as many as 80% have no benefit from adjuvant treatment, either because they fail despite treatment or because they are already cured by surgery alone. This unsatisfactory situation may be improved in the future by current studies to a certain, though limited, degree − but it is unlikely that it will change fundamentally.
2. No characterization of those patients who fail on adjuvant chemotherapy, and possibly should not receive it, is possible to date. In fact, such retrospective analyses of failing patients have not as yet been performed on a large scale. It is possible that a pooling of all data of relapsing patients from all large studies and the proper use of available statistical methods may help to define at least a subset of patients who have no reasonable chance of benefit with presently available adjuvant therapies.
3. The most obvious reason for the unsatisfactory situation in the selection of patients for adjuvant chemotherapy is our inability − despite an ever-increasing number or risk factors known to influence the probability of residual disease − to define those patients who in fact do have residual disease. It is possible that by improved analyses of pooled data of ongoing large clinical trials some further progress in the definition of risk patients, especially in the overall low-risk groups such as N− and N+ 1−3, may be made. But the problem will only be solved in a satisfactory manner by the development of methods to detect and monitor residual disease.

Relationship of DFS/RFS to Overall Survival

The meaning of an increase in disease- or relapse-free survival in relation to final overall survival has already been dealt with. Some general answers will certainly come from presently ongoing clinical trials. Should it be demonstrated that despite highly significant improvements in DFS/RFS the final benefit in overall survival is marginal, then adjuvant therapy of breast cancer will remain a disputed area employing subjective judgment. Despite all the efforts and the huge amount of data, subjective judgment then will determine whether or not the benfit a patient accrues by spending more time disease free, symptom free, and without palliative therapy − but with only a minimal chance of remaining disease free − outweighs the cost of treatment, in terms of side-effects, psychological burden, and money. This brings us to the last question.

Cost of Adjuvant Chemotherapy

The cost of adjuvant chemotherapy in terms of short-term and long-term toxicity, second neoplasms, possibly adverse effect on the course of the disease in relapsing patients, and on results of further systemic therapies in such patients is not yet fully known. Fortunately, at least in this area, past, present, and future clinical trials certainly do provide necessary answers which are urgently needed — because adjuvant chemotherapy of operable breast cancer most probably will continue to be an area where subjective judgment on cost-benefit relations will remain an important component of the decision to treat or not to treat. However, this decision in individual patients can possibly never be based solely on objective data.

References

1. Ahmann DL, Payne WS, Scanlon PW, O'Fallon JR, Bisel HF, Hahn RG, Edmonson JH, Ingle JN, Frytak S, O'Connell MJ, Rubin J (1978) Repeated adjuvant chemotherapy with L-phenylalanine mustard or 5-fluorouracil, cyclophosphamide, and prednisone with or without radiation, after mastectomy for breast cancer. Lancet 1: 893–896
2. Baum M, Berstock D (1982) Breast cancer — adjuvant therapy. Clin Oncol 1: 901–915
3. Bonadonna G, Rossi A, Tancini G, Valagussa P (1983) Adjuvant chemotherapy in breast cancer. Lancet 1: 1157
4. Caprini JA, Oviedo MA, Cunningham MP, Cohen E, Trueheart RS, Khandekar JD, Scanlon EF (1980) Adjuvant chemotherapy for stage II and III breast carcinoma. JAMA 244: 243–246
5. Carpenter JT, Maddox WA (1983) Melphalan adjuvant therapy in breast cancer. Lancet 2: 450–451
6. Cooper MR, Rhyne AL, Muss HB, Ferree C, Richards E, White DR, Stuart JJ, Jackson DV, Howard V, Shore A, Spurr CL (1981) A randomized comparative trial of chemotherapy and irradiation therapy for stage II breast cancer. Cancer 47: 2833–2839
6a.Creech RH, Dayal H, Alberts R, Catalano RB, Sha MK, Grotzinger PJ (1983) A comparison of L-PAM and low-dose CMF as adjuvant therapy for breast cancer patients with nodal metastases. Proc Am Assoc Cancer Res 24: 148
7. Davis HL, Metter GE, Ramirez G, Grage TB, Cornell G, Fletcher W, Moss S, Multhauf P (1979) An adjuvant trial of L-phenylalanine mustard (L-PAM) versus cyclophosphamide (C), methotrexate (M), 5-fluorouracil (F) and vincristine (V) — CMF-V following mastectomy for operable breast cancer. Proc Am Soc Clin Oncol 20: 358
8. Fisher B, Slack NH, Katrych D, Wolmark N (1975) Ten years of follow-up results of patients with carcinoma of the breast in a cooperative clinical trial evaluating surgical adjuvant chemotherapy. Surg Gynecol Obstet 140: 528–534
9. Fisher B, Carbone P, Economou SG et al. (1975) L-phenylalanine mustard (L-PAM) in the management of primary breast cancer. A report of early findings. N Engl J Med 292: 117–122
10. Fisher B, Redmond C, Fisher ER (1980) The contribution of recent NSABP clinical trials of primary breast cancer therapy to an understanding of tumor biology — an overview of findings. Cancer 46: 1009–1025
11. Fisher B, Redmond C, Brown A, Wickerham DL, Wolmark N, Allegra J, Escher G, Lippman M, Savlov E, Wittliff J, Fisher ER, with the contributions of Plotkin D, Bowman D, Wolter J, Bornstein R, Desser R, Frelick R, and other NSABP investigators (1983) Influence of tumor estrogen and progesterone receptor levels on the response to tamoxifen and chemotherapy in primary breast cancer. J Clin Oncol 4: 227–241
12. Fisher B, Wickerham DL, Brown A, Redmond CK (1983) Breast cancer estrogen and progesterone receptor values: their distribution, degree of concordance, and relation to number of positive axillary nodes. J Clin Oncol 6: 349–358

13. Glucksberg H, Rivkin SE, Rasmussen S, Tranum B, Gad el Maula N, Costanzi J, Hoogstraten B, Athens J, Maloney T, McCracken J, Vaughn C (1982) Combination chemotherapy (CMFVP) versus L-phenylalanine mustard (L-PAM) for operable breast cancer with positive axillary nodes. A Southwest Oncology Group study. Cancer 50: 423−434

13a. Goldhirsch A (Unpublished) Adjuvant therapy in early breast cancer, a critical review

14. Henderson IC, Gelman R, Parker LM, Skarin AT, Mayer RJ, Garnick MB, Canellos GP, Frei E III (1982) 15 vs 30 weeks of adjuvant chemotherapy for breast cancer patients with a high risk of recurrence: a randomized trial. Proc Am Soc Clin Oncol 1: 75

15. Howat JMT, Hughes R, Durning P, George WD, Sellwood RA, Bush H, Phadke K, Grafton C, Crowther D (1981) A controlled clinical tral of adjuvant chemotherapy in operable cancer of the breast. In: Salmon SE, Jones SE (eds) Adjuvant therapy of cancer III. Grune and Stratton, New York, pp 371−376

16. Hubay CA, Pearson OH, Marshall JS, Stellato TA, Rhodes RS, DeBanne SM, Rosenblatt J, Mansour EG, Herman RE, Jones JC, Flynn WJ, Eckert C, McGuire WL (1981) Adjuvant therapy of stage II breast cancer. Breast Cancer Res Treat 1: 77−82

17. Jungi WF, Alberto P, Brunner KW, Cavalli F, Barrelet L, Senn HJ (1981) Short- or long-term adjuvant chemotherapy for breast cancer. In: Salmon SE, Jones SE (eds) Adjuvant therapy of cancer III. Grune and Stratton, New York, pp 395−402

18. Ludwig Breast Cancer Study Group (1983) Toxic effect of early adjuvant chemotherapy for breast cancer. Lancet 2: 542−544

19. Ludwig Breast Cancer Study Group (Unpublished data)

20. Nissen-Meyer R, Kjellgren K, Malmio K, Mansson B, Norin T (1978) Surgical adjuvant chemotherapy. Results with one short course of cyclophosphamide after mastectomy for breast cancer. Cancer 41: 2088−2098

21. Nissen-Meyer R, Høst H, Kjellgren K, Mansson B, Norin T (1982) Perioperative adjuvant chemotherapy vs postoperative chemotherapy for one year. Breast Cancer Res Treat 2: 391−394

23. Nolvadex Adjuvant Trial Organisation (1983) Controlled trial of tamoxifen as adjuvant agent in management of early breast cancer. Lancet 1: 257−261

24. Palshof, T, Mouridsen H,T Daehnfeldt JL (1980) Report on the Copenhagen breast cancer trials. Adjuvant endocrine therapy of primary operable breast cancer. In: Mouridsen HT, Palshof T (eds) Breast cancer − experimental and clinical aspects. Pergamon, Oxford, p 183

25. Pritchard KI, Meakin JW, Boyd NF, Ambus U, Dembo AJ, Evans WK, Sutherland DJA, Wilkinson RH, Bassett A, Campbell J, DeBoer G (1983) A prospective randomized controlled trial of adjuvant tamoxifen in postmenopausal women with axillary node-positive breast cancer. Proc Am Soc Clin Oncol 2: 104

26. Ribeiro G, Palmer MK (1983) Adjuvant tamoxifen for operable carcinoma of the breast: report of clinical trial by the Christie Hospital and Holt Radium Institute. Br Med J 286: 827−830

27. Rivkin SE, Knight WS, Foulkes M (1983) Adjuvant chemotherapy and hormonal therapy for operable breast cancer with positive axillary nodes. J Steroid Biochem 19: 2065

28. Rose C, Thorpe SM, Mouridsen HT, Andersen JA, Brincker H, Andersen KW, Danish Breast Cancer Cooperative Group (1983) Antiestrogen treatment of postmenopausal women with primary high risk breast cancer. Breast Cancer Res Treat: 77−84

29. Rubens RD, Hayward JL, Knight RK, Bulbrook RD, Fentiman IS, Chandary M, Howell A, Bush H, Crowther D, Sellwood RA, George WD, Howat JMT (1983) Controlled trial of adjuvant chemotherapy with melphalan for breast cancer. Lancet 1: 839−843

30. Senn HJ Seven-years results of the OSAKO study. Personal communication

31. Tancini G, Bonadonna G, Valagussa P, Marchini S, Veronesi U (1983) Adjuvant CMF in breast cancer: comparative 5-year results of 12 vs 6 cycles. J Clin Oncol 1: 2−10

32. Tormey DC, Kalish L, Cummings FJ, Carbone PP (1983) Premenopausal breast cancer adjuvant chemotherapy − the Eastern Cooperative Oncology Group Trial. Proc Am Soc Clin Oncol 2: 102

33. Vélez Garcia E, Moore M, Marcid V, Vogel C, Barolucci A, Liu C, Ketcham A, Smalley R
    (1983) Postoperative adjuvant chemotherapy with or without radiation therapy in patients with
    stage II breast cancer − A Southeastern Cancer Study Group (SECSG) Study. Proc Am Soc Clin
    Oncol 2: 111
34. Wheeler TK (1979) Four-drug combination chemotherapy following surgery for breast cancer.
    In: Salmon SE, Jones SE (eds) Adjuvant therapy of cancer II. Grune and Stratton, New York,
    pp 269−276

Closing Remarks and Outlook

G. A. Nagel

Medizinische Universitätsklinik, Abteilung für Hämatologie/Onkologie,
Robert-Koch-Strasse 40, 3400 Göttingen, Federal Republic of Germany

Introduction

The second International Conference on Adjuvant Chemotherapy of Breast Cancer brought together experts who have actively been engaged in adjuvant chemotherapy trials and who have been able to contribute original firsthand information based upon personal experience in the field.

The major crucial issues, such as problems of late toxicity, patient subsets, and the preclinical and clinical basis of adjuvant chemotherapy, have been dealt with. More questions have been asked than answered, and even after 10 years of intensive clinical evaluation, the experimental background and clinical results of adjuvant chemotherapy are still a matter of open scientific discussion. Nevertheless, it seems safe to state, that for postoperative patients treated within the framework of controlled trials, adjuvant chemotherapy has altered the natural course of the disease in patients with metastatic breast cancer and small remaining tumor burdens. This is demonstrable by looking at postoperative disease-free intervals (DFI) which are prolonged in some patient groups by 1–2 years. Furthermore, some, not all trials, show a survival benefit for given patient subgroups. Looking optimistically at late results of some of the earlier trials, like the Nissen-Meyer study, or at relapse rates in treatment arms compared with controls in NSABP trials, one might even speculate about possible increases in cure rates.

Results in general, however, have not fulfilled earlier expectations. This symposium was on occasion to reevaluate hypotheses leading to adjuvant chemotherapy trials in the past and to generate new hypotheses to be tested in future trials.

Respective summaries have been given (see earlier chapters). One major lesson is reemphasized here: microscopic postoperative disease is different from advanced metastatic breast cancer; new models will be needed to study and understand the biology of cancer in this very early stage.

Differences between Early and Advanced Metastatic Breast Cancer

Principles applied to the treatment of metastatic breast cancer in the early stage, i.e., of postoperative adjuvant chemotherapy, have been adopted from the experience with chemotherapy of advanced metastatic disease.

The major principle is to apply in the treatment of early cancer only drugs, dosage, and schedules whose efficacy has been proven in advanced disease. After this symposium one is

Recent Results in Cancer Research. Vol. 96
© Springer-Verlag Berlin · Heidelberg 1984

Table 1. Differences in treatment results with chemotherapy of metastatic breast cancer: microscopic, early breast cancer (postoperative adjuvant chemotherapy) vs macroscopic, advanced breast cancer

Microscopic	Macroscopic

Significant differences between different treatment regimes related to
  % Patients responding
  Prolongation of disease-free intervals
  Survival benefit
  Menopausal status
	No significant differences between different adequately dosed combination chemotherapy regimes (CMF, CMFVP, AC, FAC, VAG) related to
	  Remission rates
	  Remission duration
	  Survival benefit
	  Menopausal status

Treatment results delicately dependent upon drug-dose modifications	Drug-dose modifications have some influence on response rates but there is never a complete loss of activity even if doses are reduced to less than 50% of standard
Low response rate of chemotherapy: in the best subgroups, i.e., premenopausal patients, 1−3 lymph nodes, full-dose combination chemotherapy prolongs disease-free interval in 15−30% of patients	High response rate of chemotherapy: in subgroups of favorable prognosis, i.e., local-regional disease, no previous chemotherapy, full-dose chemotherapy applied, remission rates are above 60% with 20−30% complete remission
Long-term adjuvant chemotherapy results, such as Nissen-Meyer data, indicate possible cure of microscopic disease with adjuvant chemotherapy	In advanced breast cancer no cure achievable
Number of involved lymph nodes are of significant prognostic importance for therapeutic results	There is no correlation between number of lymph nodes involved at operation and treatment results in advanced disease

Also other prognostic factors might influence results of adjuvant chemotherapy
  Size of lymph node metastases
  Group of axillary nodes involved
  Tumor penetration into blood and lymph node vessels or through lymph node capsule
  Histological grading
  Receptor status
	These factors are not of prognostic significance in advanced disease

tempted to ask whether this principle should be questioned. Looking at treatment results of microscopic vs macroscopic breast cancer several differences become apparent (Table 1).

The most obvious observation is that therapeutic efficacy of adjuvant chemotherapy is lost if already minor reductions in drug dosages are made. It is an open question whether or not this is true for all drug combinations and patient subsets. In fact from some of the data presented it appears that adriamycin-containing drug combinations tolerate dose modifications better than CMF. Furthermore, dose reductions become more critical the more lymph nodes involved or the older the patient. Senn et al. have shown efficacy in node-negative patients with oral LMF − a rather mild regimen − which failed in lymph node-positive patients. Nissen-Meyer with his short-term postoperative chemotherapy and Fisher with L-PAM significantly improved operative treatment results in some patient subgroups. In advanced disease one would anticipate only marginal success with these drug regimens.

For the treatment of advanced breast cancer the standard procedure is to give drug combinations in pulses at consistent intervals. Rivkin presented data which indicate that within his regimen low-dose daily cytoxan yielded results, at least equal to the best data obtained with intermittent pulse-dose chemotherapy.

All these data suggest that minimal postoperative breast cancer is a different disease calling for a different chemotherapy approach than advanced metastatic disease. This view is further supported by two other findings. First, colorectal carcinoma, stomach and lung cancer have successfully been treated with chemotherapy. Controlled clinical trials, however, have failed to improve postoperative treatment results if drug regimens developed for advanced disease were used in the adjuvant setting [1, 2, 3, 5, 6]. Second, a heterogeneity in terms of treatment response between primary tumor and metastases has been shown in experimental tumor systems [4].

A Lesson from Adjuvant Chemotherapy for the Management of Advanced Disease

This lesson concerns the problem of objectively evaluating response in early- and advanced-stage breast cancer. As presented in Table 1, results of chemotherapy are more impressive for advanced disease than for adjuvant chemotherapy.

The question remains, however, whether the results of adjuvant chemotherapy expressed in percentage of patients with prolonged disease-free intervals after therapy as compared with untreated controls, really reflects what has been achieved with this form of treatment.

It is reasonable to assume that in patients with primary breast cancer and lymph node metastases there are not only many microscopic metastatic foci but also micrometastases which are heterogenous with respect to drug sensitivity. Prolongation of the disease-free interval will be achieved only if all metastatic foci are drug sensitive to some extent. Only then the total cell number in each micrometastases will be reduced and residual cell mass will need more cell cycles for its regrowth to clinically detectable macrometastases.

If, however, among a large number of micrometastases sensitive to chemotherapy, there are only a few resistant ones, it will not be possible to prolong the disease-free interval. Despite the fact that the cell number of the residual disease has been reduced in total, foci not influenced by chemotherapy will regrow and lead to clinically detectable macro-metastases in the same time as in untreated controls.

There is no other way to measure the effect of chemotherapy on subclinical disease than by the assessment of the disease-free interval. Complete and partial remissions as well as no-change status are response criteria not applicable for early metastatic cancer. DFI, however, appears to describe what has been gained by chemotherapy much more accurately than remission rates in advanced disease which do not necessarily translate into prolongation of survival times.

As already mentioned about 15%−30% of given patient subsets will experience prolongation of DFI by adjuvant chemotherapy. This figure does not compare to overall, but to complete remission rates in advanced disease. Under these aspects it will be of interest to reassess the true value of the so-called objective remission criteria for advanced disease.

Adjuvant Chemotherapy Outside Clinical Trials

A final conclusion from the data on adjuvant chemotherapy is that this treatment modality should still be considered experimental and not be recommended for routine postoperative use. The major arguments here are summarized as follows:

1. Data analysis has shown that only a minority of patients will profit from adjuvant chemotherapy.
2. Patient subsets being prime candidates for adjuvant chemotherapy are still poorly defined. Within the subsets particularly sensitive to adjuvant chemotherapy, i.e., premenopausal women with less than four lymph nodes involved, there are still over 70% of patients not responding to adjuvant chemotherapy.
3. Other subgroups, like patients with 10 or more lymph nodes involved, will not respond to adjuvant chemotherapy and for the typical older woman with receptor-positive tumors and relatively good prognosis, a true benefit of adjuvant chemotherapy remains to be shown.
4. The optimal drug selection and dosage problems appear so delicate that even within clinical trials there are exorbitant dropout rates and too many patients who are not able to tolerate drugs at dosages necessary for therapeutic efficacy.
5. All results with adjuvant chemotherapy hitherto reported are derived from clinical trials. It is unknown, what treatment results look like in an unselected patient population.

Outlook

Variations in treatment results reported with any given drug combination, i.e., various modifications of the CMF-regimens, support the view that further improvements in cancer chemotherapy might be possible not only if new compounds become available but also if better use is made of known drugs.

The large data pool of many well-controlled trials should allow cross-study comparisons of data related to variables such as prognostic patient factors, relapse patterns of the disease, and modifications of treatment regimens, etc. between trials.

Such a cross-examination might, for example, determine whether there are drug combinations which might tolerate better than others dose modifications without losing therapeutic potential. The answer to this question might not only help to better understand the action mechanism of chemotherapy in minimal disease but also to develop recommendations for the use of adjuvant chemotherapy outside study protocols and groups.

To improve adjuvant chemotherapy, better models are required to analyze the microenvironment of metastases in the early stages of development. It might well be that such conditions are better simulated in an in vitro than an in vivo system, assuming that the intercellular integration is minimal in the early phase of metastatic seeding. In this regard in vitro tumor stem-cell assays might be of particular importance in studying pharmacological effects of chemotherapeutic agents on small cell numbers not yet dependent upon host supportive systems such as feeder tissues or vascular supply.

The future will teach us, perhaps, not to look at early cancer as some sort of minimal advanced disease and apply similar treatment principles accordingly, but to look at early disease as something entirely different in terms of cell kinetics, drug resistance, tumor heterogeneity, and host-tumor relationship. Perhaps it might be more appropriate to the biological situation to look for parallels between early cancer and advanced disease in complete remission and to take complete remission rather than measurable disease as a model situation for the development of new adjuvant-therapy strategies.

References

1. Brunner KW, Marthaler TH, Müller W (1971) Unfavorable effects of long-term adjuvant chemotherapy with endoxan in radically operated bronchogenic carcinoma. Eur J Cancer 7: 285
2. Higgins G (1972) The use of chemotherapy as an adjuvant to surgery for bronchogenic carcinoma. Cancer 30: 1383
3. Macdonald IS, Haller DG, Kisner DL (1982) Adjuvant chemotherapy in colon and gastric cancer. Recent Results Cancer Res 80: 284
4. Schabel FM (1977) Experimental basis for adjuvant chemotherapy. In: Salmon SE, Jones SE (eds) Adjuvant chemotherapy of cancer. North-Holland, Amsterdam, p 3
5. Schlag P, Schreml W, Gaus W, Herfarth C, Linder MM, Queißer W, Trede M (1982) Adjuvant 5-fluorouracil and BCNU chemotherapy in gastric cancer: 3-year results. Recent Results Cancer Res 80: 278
6. Shields TW, Humphrey EW, Keehn RJ (1977) Adjuvant chemotherapy after resection of carcinoma of the lung. Cancer 40: 2057

Subject Index

Recent Results in Cancer Research

Managing Editors:
C. Herfarth, H. J. Senn

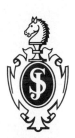

Springer-Verlag
Berlin
Heidelberg
New York
Tokyo

Volume 94
Predictive Drugs Testing on Human Tumor Cells
Editors: V. Hofmann, M. E. Berens, G. Martz
1984. 87 figures, 107 tables. XII, 287 pages. ISBN 3-540-13497-2

Volume 93
Leukemia
Recent Developments in Diagnosis and Therapy
Editors: E. Thiel, S. Thierfelder
1984. 36 figures, 63 tables. IX, 305 pages. ISBN 3-540-13289-9

Volume 92
Lung Cancer
Editor: W. Duncan
1984. 23 figures, 42 tables. IX, 132 pages. ISBN 3-540-13116-7

Volume 91
Clinical Interest of Steroid Hormone Receptors in Breast Cancer
Editors: G. Leclercq, S. Toma, R. Paridaens, J. C. Heuson
1984. 74 figures, 122 tables. XIV, 351 pages. ISBN 3-540-13042-X

Volume 90
Early Detection of Breast Cancer
Editors: S. Brünner, B. Langfeldt, P. E. Andersen
1984. 94 figures, 91 tables. XI, 214 pages. ISBN 3-540-12348-2

Volume 89
Pain in the Cancer Patient
Pathogenesis, Diagnosis and Therapy
Editors: M. Zimmermann, P. Drings, G. Wagner
1984. 67 figures, 57 tables. IX, 238 pages. ISBN 3-540-12347-4

Volume 88
Paediatric Oncology
Editor: W. Duncan
1983. 28 figures, 38 tables. X, 116 pages. ISBN 3-540-12349-0

Volume 87
F. F. Holmes
Aging and Cancer
1983. 58 figures. VII, 75 pages. ISBN 3-540-12656-2

Recent Results in Cancer Research

Managing Editors:
C. Herfarth, H. J. Senn

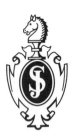

Springer-Verlag
Berlin
Heidelberg
New York
Tokyo

Volume 86
Vascular Perfusion in Cancer Therapy
Editors: **K. Schwemmle, K. Aigner**
1983. 136 figures, 79 tables. XII, 295 pages
ISBN 3-540-12346-6

Volume 85
Urologic Cancer: Chemotherapeutic Principles and Management
Editor: **F. M. Torti**
1983. IX, 151 pages
ISBN 3-540-12163-3

Volume 84
Modified Nucleosides and Cancer
Editor: **G. Nass**
1983. 217 figures, 89 tables. XII, 432 pages
ISBN 3-540-12024-6

Volume 82
Early Detection and Localization of Lung Tumors in High Risk Groups
Editor: **P. R. Band**
1982. 79 figures, 66 tables. XII, 190 pages
ISBN 3-540-11249-9

Volume 81
H.-P. Lohrmann, W. Schreml
Cytotoxic Drugs and the Granulopoietic System
1982. 6 figures, 87 tables. VIII, 222 pages
ISBN 3-540-10962-5

Volume 80
Adjuvant Therapies of Cancer
Editors: **G. Mathé, G. Bonadonna, S. Salmon**
1982. 108 figures, 146 tables. XVI, 356 pages
ISBN 3-540-10949-8

Volume 78
Prostate Cancer
Editor: **W. Duncan**
1981. 68 figures, 67 tables. X, 190 pages
ISBN 3-540-10676-6

Prices are subject to change without notice